S0-AEQ-062

OXFORD MEDICAL PUBLICATIONS

Cancer Risks and Prevention

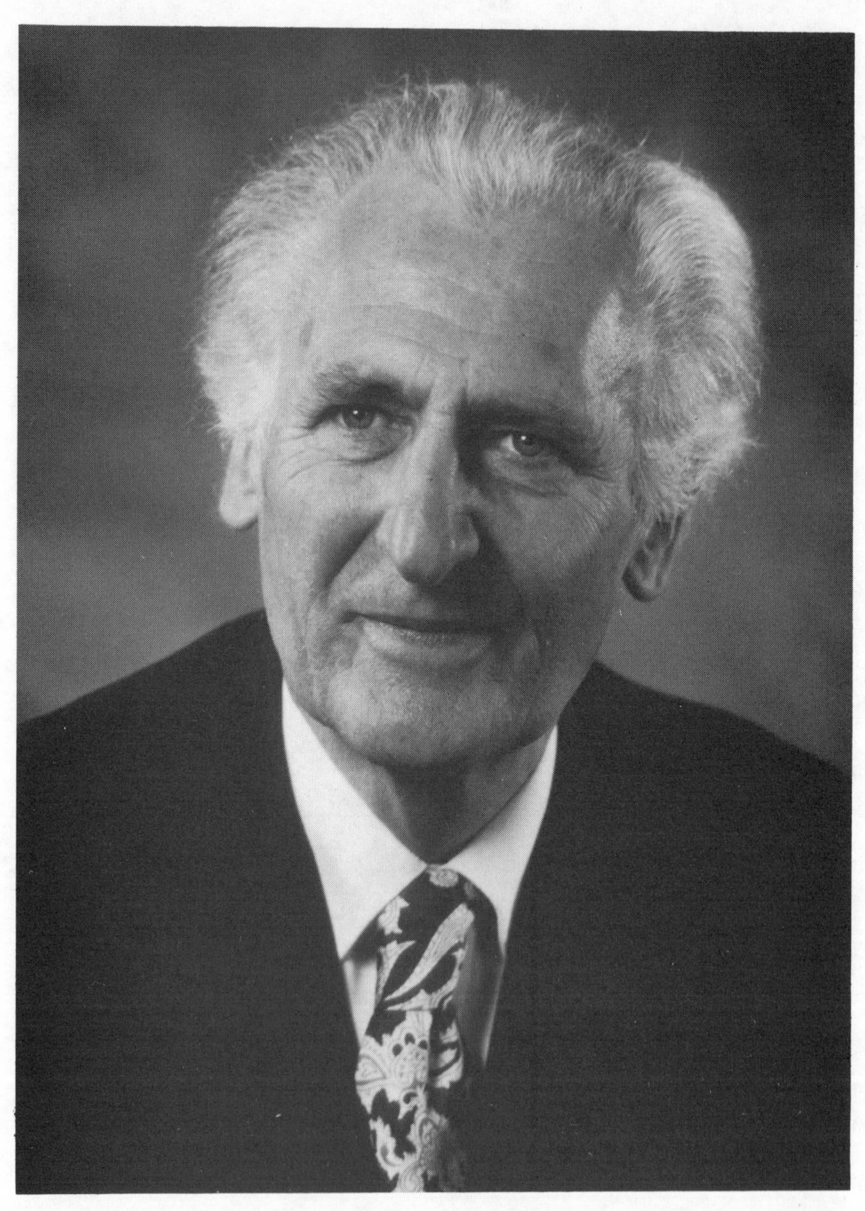

Sir Richard Doll

Cancer Risks and Prevention

Edited by

M. P. Vessey

Professor of Social and Community Medicine,
University of Oxford;
Fellow of St. Cross College, Oxford

and

Muir Gray

Community Physician,
Oxfordshire District Health Authority;
Fellow of Green College, Oxford

OXFORD NEW YORK TOKYO

OXFORD UNIVERSITY PRESS 1985

Oxford University Press, Walton Street, Oxford OX2 6DP

*Oxford New York Toronto
Delhi Bombay Calcutta Madras Karachi
Kuala Lumpur Singapore Hong Kong Tokyo
Nairobi Dar es Salaam Cape Town
Melbourne Auckland*

*and associated companies in
Beiruit Berlin Ibadan Nicosia*

British Library Cataloguing in Publication Data

*Cancer risks and prevention.— (Oxford medical publications)
1. Cancer 2. Epidemiology
I. Vessey, M. P. II. Gray, Muir
614.5'999 RA645.C3*

ISBN 0–19–261509–2

*Library of Congress Cataloging in Publication Data
Main entry under title:*

Cancer risks and prevention.

*(Oxford medical publication)
Includes bibliographies and index.
1. Cancer—Prevention. 2. Epidemiology. I. Vessey, M. P. (Martin P.) II. Gray, J. A. Muir (John Armstrong Muir) III. Series. [DNLM: 1. Neoplasms—etiology 2. Neoplasms—prevention & control.
QZ 200 C2173]
RC268.C367 1985 616.99'4'071 85–330
ISBN 0–19–261509–2*

*Set by Cambrian Typesetters, Frimley, Surrey,
Printed in Great Britain by
J. W. Arrowsmith Ltd, Bristol*

Preface

This series of essays was collected in honour of Richard and Joan Doll, on the occasion of Richard's retirement as Warden of Green College. The term 'retirement' with its connotations of rest and relaxation seems inappropriate: Richard's previous 'retirement' from the Regius Professorship of Medicine was followed by one of the busiest and most productive periods of his life during which he was responsible for establishing Green College. This retirement was in practice a transition from one occupation to another. Similarly Richard's 'retirement' from Green College is another transition, on this occasion to full-time cancer research. He still somehow finds time to listen to the theories of the youngest research workers with sincere interest, and is easily accessible in his office at Green College, or in the lunch-time bustle of the Radcliffe Infirmary canteen.

This *Festschrift*, therefore, is not in the British tradition, to mark the end of a distinguished career, but more in the tradition of Germany, where a *Festschrift* is often issued to honour someone on his birthday, looking both backwards and forwards. For this reason we chose to concentrate on cancer risks and cancer prevention, not only to cover a subject in which Richard has been pre-eminent but also to review a field in which he will continue to be a leader now that his change of occupation, following his second retirement, allows him once more to concentrate on research.

The contributors to this book constitute only a sample of the many people whose work has been influenced by Richard and the subjects covered comprise only a sample of the health problems which he studied during his career. The book is not intended to be a comprehensive text on cancer epidemiology and prevention; the topics have been selected to demonstrate some of the areas in which Richard's work has increased our knowledge about the aetiology of cancer and its prevention. The book does not, however, pay sufficient tribute to the other main impact of his epidemiological expertise: the influence his work has had on medical education and on the practice of medicine. The epidemiological approach is now employed in all areas of medicine and the mathematical techniques that were once the preserve of the statistician now form one of the foundations of clinical research and thus clinical practice.

Neither does the book directly pay tribute to the kindness that Richard and Joan have shown to so many students and colleagues. Our gratitude to them is best expressed, not in the compliments they deserve, but in the following discussion of one of the subjects they have done so much to advance – cancer risks and cancer prevention.

Oxford
December 1984

M.P.V.
M.G.

Contents

Contributors

Bruce Armstrong, DPhil, FRACP, Director, NH and MRC Research Unit in Epidemiology and Preventive Medicine, Department of Medicine, University of Western Australia.

Sir Francis Avery Jones, CBE, MD, FRCP, Consulting Physician, Central Middlesex Hospital, London; Consulting Gastroenterologist, St. Mark's Hospital, London; Emeritus Gastroenterologist to the Royal Navy.

Sir Austin Bradford Hill, CBE, DSc, FRS, Professor Emeritus of Medical Statistics, University of London. Formerly Honorary Director of the Statistical Research Unit of the Medical Research Council.

Paula Cook-Mozaffari, MA, BLitt, MRC External Scientific Staff, ICRF Cancer Epidemiology and Clinical Trials Unit, Radcliffe Infirmary, Oxford.

Charles Fletcher, CBE, MD, FRCP, FFCM, Professor Emeritus of Clinical Epidemiology, Royal Postgraduate Medical School, University of London.

Muir Gray, MD, MRCP(G), MRCGP, Specialist in Community Medicine, Oxfordshire Health Authority. Fellow of Green College, Oxford.

Nigel Gray, AM, MB, BS, FRACP, FRACMA, Director, Anti-Cancer Council of Victoria, East Melbourne, Australia.

Konrad Jamrozik, MB, BS, DPhil, Research Fellow in Clinical Epidemiology, University of Western Australia. Formerly Nuffield Dominions Scholar, University of Oxford.

Leo Kinlen, DPhil, FRCP, Director, CRC Cancer Epidemiology Unit, Medical School, Edinburgh.

Jim Mann, DM, PhD, FFCM, University Lecturer in Social and Community Medicine and Honorary Consultant Physician, Department of Community Medicine and General Practice, Radcliffe Infirmary, Oxford. Fellow of Wolfson College, Oxford.

Richard Peto, MA, MSc, ICRF Reader in Cancer Studies, Nuffield Department of Clinical Medicine, Radcliffe Infirmary, Oxford. Fellow of Green College, Oxford.

Malcolm Pike, PhD, Director, ICRF Cancer Epidemiology and Clinical Trials Unit, Radcliffe Infirmary, Oxford. Fellow of Green College, Oxford.

Rodolfo Saracci, MD, Chief, Unit of Analytical Epidemiology, International Agency for Research on Cancer, Lyon, France.

David Skegg, BMedSc, MB, ChB, DPhil, Professor, Department of Preventive and Social Medicine, University of Otago Medical School, Dunedin, New Zealand.

Peter Smith, DSc, Head, Tropical Epidemiology Unit, Department of Epidemiology, London School of Hygiene and Tropical Medicine, London.

Martin Vessey, MD, FRCP(Ed), FFCM, FRCGP, Professor, Department of Community Medicine and General Practice, Radcliffe Infirmary, Oxford. Fellow of St. Cross College, Oxford.

Nicholas Wald, MRCP, FFCM, Professor, Department of Environmental and Preventive Medicine, St. Bartholomew's Hospital Medical College, London.

Foreword

Sir Austin Bradford Hill, CBE, DSc, FRS,
Professor Emeritus of Medical Statistics, University of London

In 1945, at the end of the Second World War, I returned to the London School of Hygiene and Tropical Medicine. In succession to Professor Major Greenwood, I had been appointed Professor of Medical Statistics and Honorary Director of the group of statisticians on the staff of the Medical Research Council who had worked under him in the department. It was obvious that, in both teaching and research, a heavy load of work lay ahead.

On the academic side, many medical men and women released from war duties were anxious to be trained for work in the field of public health. The demand was so great that, for some time, the School had to run two parallel classes in the course for the University Diploma of Public Health. On the research side, I was, almost immediately, to be heavily involved in the Medical Research Council's trial of streptomycin in tuberculosis. This was the first randomized trial but with the rapid introduction of new drugs at that date it was clearly the precursor of many clinical trials. Running parallel were the large-scale trials of vaccines. Whooping cough was already on the doorstep; BCG and poliomyelitis were looming round the corner. Clinical and preventive medicine were changing and it was an exciting time.

To meet these requirements I had to rebuild my Department of Medical Statistics and Epidemiology and, hopefully, to develop the Medical Research Council group into a unit that could undertake its own researches and also give the statistical and epidemiological advice and collaboration that was likely to be called for on a growing scale.

In the later part of the war I had been working in the Medical Directorate of the Royal Air Force, ruled over by its vigorous and invigorating Director General of Medical Services, Sir Harold Whittingham. To work under my direction he had brought in a station medical officer from some distant aerodrome, Squadron-Leader Donald Reid. Reid had been doing some original work in measuring the stresses to which aircrew were subjected and their resulting health problems. The nature of this work and the interests it aroused in him led him, on demobilization, to consider specializing in psychiatric medicine. I was, however, able to attract him to epidemiology and he joined me at the London School of Hygiene and Tropical Medicine as a lecturer in my department. Somewhat later Peter Armitage, an accomplished statistician, joined my Medical Research Council staff. With these accessions the immediate pressures were reduced and I was able to give more time to a course of teaching (set up before the war) in which I took great interest. This was a brief course in statistical ideas and methods (on two days a week for three months). Non-medically qualified students were accepted along with the medically qualified. The former were usually statisticians (for example, Dr Austin Heady and Dr Peter Oldham) who sought to make their careers in the medical field. The object was to introduce them to examples of the types of problem they would meet, the methods needed to solve them, the nature of medical statistics, and the kind of medical know-how they should seek to be able to use them intelligently. With the medically qualified students the object was to give them a similar knowledge of the simple statistical methods they would find useful in research work but – still more – to make them *think* numerically and experimentally, e.g. of the problems of collecting and interpreting data, of presenting them, of avoiding and detecting bias, of sampling, and so on; in short, arithmetic, logic, and common sense.

To this course, in 1947, came Richard Doll and his wife-to-be Dr Joan Faulkner, who was then, and for many more years, a distinguished member of the Medical Research Council's Headquarters' Administrative Staff. I was already acquainted with Richard through his work on the aetiology of peptic ulcer. The Medical Research Council had set up a committee to supervise this study under the chairmanship of Professor John Ryle; and I was a member of this committee. I do know that Richard came to consult me, but nearly 40 years, and some 40 committees, later I cannot claim to have any reliable memory of this 'supervision'. But at least it must have been close enough to impress me with his grasp of the statistical aspects of the job and with his skills and persistence in carrying it out – to achieve, for instance, a response rate of nearly 100 per cent in some required group. Already he had clearly, perhaps intuitively, at heart my subsequent teaching that all the standard errors and chi-square tests in the world could not compensate for incomplete, imperfect, or biased data.

During his attendance at the short course at the London School of Hygiene and Tropical Medicine I had the opportunity to get to know Richard well. The numbers attending the course were usually in single figures, and much of the interest, on my side, lay in the close contact that I had with the younger medicos of the day who were thus showing an interest in 'sums'. What was their work? What were their aims?

It was this close contact and my judgement of his character that led me to invite Richard to join my staff, to investigate with me the aetiology of cancer of the lung. There had been, in 1947, a Medical Research Council conference to discuss the increased, and increasing, mortality from the disease, to which attention had been repeatedly drawn in the annual reports of the Registrar-General of England and Wales by that fine statistician Dr Percy Stocks, the Chief Medical Officer at the General Register Office. From the mortality returns – for town and country, and men and women – Stocks had argued effectively that the more accurate diagnosis of this cause of death was unlikely to be more than a contributory factor. An environmental cause was, therefore, to be sought and, initially, the obvious candidates were increasing air pollution (from the internal combustion engine) and the smoking of tobacco (with, in particular, the great increase in the smoking of cigarettes). Given funds and a medically qualified assistant, I was glad to accept the Council's invitation to undertake this research – with some initial aid and advice in its setting-up from Dr Percy Stocks and Sir Ernest Kennaway.

It was essential that my partner in the work should be *medically* qualified. There would be much organization involving hospitals, there would be much correspondence with doctors concerning their patients, over questions of diagnoses and the evidence upon which they were based. Owing to the First World War I had myself been unable to qualify in medicine and I had to seek someone willing to give medical support to an unqualified practitioner! I was, indeed, fortunate to have at hand Richard Doll and that he consented to play the role.

The inquiry, following the classical methods of epidemiology, was to be retrospective – in short, what were the characteristics and habits of patients with cancer of the lung in comparison with those of patients with other diseases? Smoking was only one fact. Deliberately, I widened the investigation. We sought information on many other personal features that might conceivably have a bearing on the problem – such as social class, occupational history, places of residence, specific or possible exposures to air pollution, forms of domestic heating in the home, and so on. All were brought into the final analysis. I decided also to include patients with cancer of some other sites, and their possible aetiological factors, in the hope that if we failed on the swings we might pick up a profit on the roundabouts.

On a grant from the Medical Research Council, Richard joined me at the beginning of 1948, and I soon realized how wise I had been in my choice. From twenty London hospitals we had a continuous flow of notifications of patients with cancer of the lung (and other selected sites); we had our own almoners visiting and interviewing these patients and also other patients whom they were instructed to choose (on closely defined rules) to serve as our 'controls'; we checked, after the discharge of each patient, the diagnosis of cancer and its basis – and we succeeded in doing so in 99.6 per cent – characteristic of Richard's persistent search for perfection and his capacity to persuade a host of doctors to respond to his requests; a monument to his administrative skills. Finally, he put the returns in order and, step by step, we jointly built up the statistical analysis of the data. We concluded that 'smoking is a factor, and an important factor, in the production of cancer of the lung'. This we published in the *British Medical Journal* in 1950.

Such a conclusion led, naturally, to a great deal of scientific controversy. Also, with important vested interests concerned, we were subject to much ill-informed and tendentious criticisms in the lay press. Coming of a legal family (downwards from an Attorney-General and a Judge of the High Court) I would send these on to my elder brother marked 'Query libellous?', but the invariable answer was 'No, vulgar abuse'.

Richard was clearly unmoved by all this, for in 1950 he became a whole-time member of my Statistical Research Unit. In other words, at this point he elected to make his career in medical statistics and epidemiology. At the same time he maintained his clinical attachment to the Central Middlesex Hospital. Of this I was strongly in favour as I believed that, whatever other interests he might have, nothing could keep the 'doctor' so happy as to have some patients in his care. It would also, as time was to show, allow him to develop his own clinical trials of treatments in gastroenterology. (But this is the province of Sir Francis Avery Jones and I must not trespass.)

Returning to cancer of the lung, we had embarked upon an extension of the retrospective inquiry. This had been confined to the London area. With certain modifications, we had extended it to some large provincial towns. Richard continued with the enormously heavy organizational task and the continual checking and thoughtful watching as the data flowed in. I was thus free of all fears that some data might be lacking in quantity or quality; and he had a remarkable capacity for working long hours at the most exacting tasks. When finally we called a halt we had the results of interviews with nearly 5000 patients, including nearly 1500 with cancer of the lung.

The results of our analysis of all this material confirmed those of our earlier paper, but with larger numbers, we were able to extend the analysis to the other features we had recorded. For instance, we were unable to implicate atmospheric pollution in itself as a cause of lung cancer (though conceivably it could act in conjunction with smoking). This second paper we published in the *British Medical Journal* in 1952.

While the work on this paper was in progress – I think it was in early 1951 – I suffered an attack of influenza. While I was convalescent, and had an unusual freedom from academic duties, I had time to think. And my thoughts were of a *prospective* inquiry. My choice of a population fell on the medical profession. This was based upon three beliefs: (1) that knowing the importance of the subject, medically qualified men and women would be sympathetic to such an inquiry; (2) that they would, therefore, be likely to reply on their smoking habits and history so long as the form was made short and simple; (3) that it would be possible to identify their subsequent deaths with the aid of the Registrars-General of the UK, since the medical qualification was likely to appear upon the death certificate.

On my return to the School I propounded this scheme to Richard and, at his suggestion, and as good experimentalists, we immediately put it to a preliminary test. We drew up a short and simple form and sent it to a small group of doctors drawn randomly from the medical register. The response was encouraging and so, in October 1951, we launched the full study. To this, we had finally some 40 000 responses and, as ever, Richard had their ordering and tabulating under full control.

I can remember opening many of those envelopes myself – not because we were short of clerical labour but because of my belief (which I still hold) that in such an investigation one should always get close to at least some of the original data if one is not to be misled subsequently by neat tabulations made by an assistant or, in these days, a computer.

We reported the results of this prospective inquiry in a brief paper in 1954 and more fully 2 years later, when a total of 1854 deaths from all causes had been reported to, or discovered by, us. They came not only from the returns made to us by the Registrars-General but from the General Medical Council and the British Medical Association and many other minor sources. In this Richard had again applied his customary assiduous search to ensure a complete record. For every one of the 88 deaths attributed to cancer of the lung he had sought confirmation, and the basis of the diagnosis, from doctor, consultant, or hospital. We accepted 84 as established. Once more, step by step, we jointly analysed these data and built up the statistical picture.

This is no place in which to discuss the results in detail and I shall confine myself to one paragraph from the summary to the paper (*British Medical Journal* 1956).

> From the retrospective studies . . . we concluded that if large groups of persons of different smoking habits were observed for a number of years they would reveal distinct differences in their rates of mortality from lung cancer. They would show, we believed, (1) a higher mortality in smokers than in non-smokers, (2) a higher mortality in heavy smokers than in light smokers, (3) a higher mortality in cigarette smokers than in pipe smokers, and (4) a higher mortality in those who continued to smoke than in those who gave it up. In each case the expected result has appeared in this prospective inquiry.

During these five years of the inquiry while we had to wait patiently (or impatiently) for the deaths to occur, Richard occupied himself with much other research (including his continued work on peptic ulcers). He examined the causes of death among gas workers with special reference to cancer of the lung. He made a similar study of asbestos workers. He collaborated with Peter Armitage in a study of the age distribution of human cancers and a multistage theory of carcinogenesis to explain it. He began his very fruitful association with Dr Court Brown, who was subsequently the Director of the Medical Research Council's Unit on Clinical and Population Cytogenetics. Together they studied the hazards of radiation and, in particular, the incidence of leukaemia in certain circumstances, e.g. in patients treated by irradiation for ankylosing spondylitis, in British radiologists, in geographical areas with varying levels of background radiation, in infants *in utero* whose mothers had been X-rayed during pregnancy.

In those five years 1951–55, while scoring up the deaths of British doctors, Richard published (alone or as a co-author) 26 papers – 9 dealing with gastroenterology, 13 with cancer, and 4 with miscellaneous subjects. Hardly time to squeeze in a dull moment! Equally I do not think we experienced many dull moments in the 10 years of continuous inquiry that we had now made into one subject – the aetiology of cancer of the lung. The intrinsic interest and the social importance of the subject were such that we were determined, throughout, to secure accurate data on a very large scale and covering every possible aetiological agent, to analyse them comprehensively and rigidly and, finally, to present them simply and clearly. Of course, we had long discussions on the analysis, and we made, no doubt, many adjustments in the ways of presentation to meet our individual viewpoints. But ultimately, as I recall, we never, over the whole 10 years, had a serious difference of opinion.

A few years later (1961) I decided to retire. To succeed me Donald Reid became Head of the Department of Medical Statistics and Epidemiology, Peter Armitage was appointed to the University Chair of Medical Statistics, and Richard, to my pleasure and great content, was appointed Director of the Statistical Research Unit. With him he took the prospective inquiry; with Malcolm Pike and Richard Peto, he continued it for a further 20 years. During this time he moved the unit to Oxford, on becoming the Regius Professor of Medicine. Though our paths occasionally crossed, e.g. in the work on the Committee on Safety of Medicines, in the main I could now only rejoice and admire from afar.

A recent major publication (with Richard Peto) was completed in 1981, not long before his own retirement. It was entitled *The causes of cancer*. He sent me a copy and this he had kindly inscribed: 'With continuing admiration and gratitude for your teaching, much of which is reflected in this book, and your friendship'.

In one's old age it is pleasant to have flattery and an assurance of the continued friendship which doubtless gives rise to it. Both serve to remind me of my good fortune – that a great many years ago I was in a position to initiate the distinguished career to which this present publication is a tribute.

Foreword

Sir Francis Avery Jones, CBE, MD, FRCP,
Consulting Physician, Central Middlesex Hospital, London;
Consulting Gastroenterologist, St. Mark's Hospital,
London.

Professor Richard Doll has become the leading epidemiologist of our time, contributing new concepts of Man's relationship with his environment and opening up new fields for scientific study. He has made numerous oustanding research contributions and at the same time encouraged and stimulated many around him in their own researches. One of the secrets of his success has been his great ability to organize both his own time and other peoples'. His research has covered a wide spectrum including smoking, radiation, drugs, diet, and infection in relation to cancer. He has defined a programme for prevention, particularly in relation to cancer and cardiovascular disease and signposted the way forward for scientists, educationalists and politicians. His has been a medical contribution of Harveian proportions.

In these two Forewords, Bradford Hill and I describe the foundations on which Richard's scientific career has been built. It was my good fortune to pave the way for his first major epidemiological study soon after the war, supported by the Medical Research Council and based at the Department of Gastroenterology at the Central Middlesex Hospital. Throughout the war I had been working as a physician and Deputy Medical Director under the direction of the Central Medical War Committee.

Being surrounded by a large industrial zone, and serving 300 000 people, the hospital had a busy and eventful war. At the beginning of the war, medical students from the Middlesex Hospital lived in the 'Central', where they continued their clinical training, and this was an important step in building up the Central Middlesex as the first District General Hospital to play a full role in undergraduate and postgraduate teaching and in research.

With the encouragement of the dynamic Medical Director, Dr Horace Joules, I was able to begin to establish a Department of Gastroenterology. Most of the patients admitted with peptic ulcer and its complications, together with the other main diseases affecting the gut, were cared for in my wards. Fortunately, having a tireless Czech assistant, Dr H. Pollak, it was possible for me to keep good records, particularly relating to gastric and duodenal ulcer and especially on patients who had bled. Links with the Invalid Kitchens of London, the forerunners of Meals on Wheels, enabled local factories to be stimulated to take a special interest in their dyspeptic workers. This brought me in touch with these cases, and a survey was arranged at the neighbouring Heinz factory to determine the prevalence of indigestion among their staff. The memorable figure of 57 per 1000 who had had or still had ulcer symptoms was recorded.

In the early post-war years plans were evolved to extend this work and an application was made to the Medical Research Council for support for a wide-scale study of occupational factors in the causation of gastric and duodenal ulcer. This project was accepted and sponsored by the Industrial Health Research Board of the Medical Research Council with a co-ordinating committee with Professor J.A. Ryle as Chairman, and Richard Doll was appointed to carry out the work. After a period of careful and detailed planning Richard tackled the field studies with great energy, covering a number of different occupations; a total of 6047 people were interviewed and assessed. The work took Richard to different parts of the country interviewing people at their places of work; his persistence knew no limits – he was prepared to climb to the top of a haystack if that was where a recalcitrant agricultural worker was to be found! It was a measure of his enthusiasm and good planning that as few as 1.6 per cent of those he wished to interview failed to come, a lapse rate remarkably small for this type of field inquiry.

The results of the survey were of great interest; among Londoners between the ages of 15 and 64 the prevalence of peptic ulcer was found to be 5.8 per cent for men and 1.9 per cent for women. This implied that over England and Wales the number of people with a peptic ulcer history was of the order of one and a half million and the number of men who had symptoms each year was over half a million. Foremen and others in positions of special responsibility in industry were found to be particualrly prone to peptic ulcer and agricultural workers particularly free from it. No confirmation was obtained of the widespread belief that bus drivers were especially liable to be sufferers. Anxiety at work, but not irregularity of meals or shift work, appeared to be aetiologically significant. Striking differences were observed between gastric and duodenal ulcers, notably in their social-class incidence, the former being more frequent among the labouring classes and rare among the professional, whereas duodenal ulcer was equally prevalent in all social classes.

Thanks to Richard's equally exhaustive library work and his skill in drafing, the Medical Research Council Report, Special Series No. 276 *Occupational factors in the aetiology of gastric and duodenal ulcer: with an estimate of their incidence in the general population* was published in 1951. This remains a classic study and proved to be an important guide for later field workers. At the time it demonstrated convincingly to the Medical Research Council that peptic ulcer with its high prevalence, its claim on hospital beds, and its unsolved aetiology made it worthy of further study. The report gave an academic hallmark to the Department of Gastroenterology at the Central Middlesex Hospital and was the first step towards the establishment within it of the MRC Gastroenterology Unit with Dr E.N. Rowlands as its Director.

Having finished this major study Richard retained a link with the Department of Gastroenterology but worked mainly at Gower Street under Professor Bradford Hill. During his clinical sessions at the Central he undertook a long-term study to discover whether any of the recognized treatments for gastric ulcer accelerated the rate of healing. Six beds were set aside for this study which continued for fourteen years. The work was of necessity slow as each clinical trial took approximately two years but by using a special factorial design he was able to acquire information about three different treatments during each trial. He studied the effects of bed rest in hospital, phenobarbitone, ascorbic acid, belladonna, cabbage juice, Robaden (a gastric tissue preparation), milk drip, milk drip with sodium bicarbonate, bland diet, normal diet, high fat diet, low fat diet, added bran, advice to stop smoking, and carbenoxolone sodium. He was able to identify only three factors which had a statistically significant beneficial effect on ulcer healing – bed rest in hospital, stopping smoking, and carbenoxolone sodium.

Hitherto, the medical treatment of peptic ulcer had been empirical, using anecdotal evidence. Now, for the first time a well-planned scientific study had produced real evidence. It was not surprising that it had not been done before as the numerous meticulous clinical observations that had to be made could not be combined with the heavy work load of a physician in charge of a department. For the first time the necessary conditions could be provided. Richard had the necessary statistical experience; he was able to establish an excellent rapport with patients, encouraging them to attend regularly his weekly outpatient clinic; he had the necessary in-patient facilities and was able to stimulate the continued and enthusiastic support of radiological colleagues; and above all he had quite remarkable critical faculties. He realized early on that nature had great healing abilities and the design of his studies eliminated the quick healers. Unfortunately, few subsequent workers have bothered to do so and this has accounted for the difficulty in interpreting so many later drug trials.

In 1964 Richard summarized the experience of his trials in an important major review on the medical treatment of gastric ulcer:

> It seems that we are now in a slightly better position to treat gastric ulcers scientifically than we were. The symptoms can usually be controlled by alkali without admission to hospital, but if they fail to respond to ambulant treatment they can always be relieved by bed rest with

continued intra-gastric drip containing a sufficient amount of sodium bicarbonate. Many ulcers will heal without any special treatment within a few weeks but can be assisted to heal by carbenoxolone. . . . Smokers should be advised to stop smoking but dieting apart from taking snacks between meals, is in my opinion not necessary.

Carbenoxolone, a liquorice derivative, proved to be an extraordinary preparation of great interest; it has no effect in reducing the aggressive anti-healing action of acid and pepsin in the stomach but instead it stimulates the defence mechanisms of the stomach, particularly increasing mucus secretion and in prolonging the life cycle of the gastric epithelial cell and so helping the repair mechanism. Having obtained good evidence of the benefit of carbenoxolone on gastric ulcer healing, to satisfy himself still further Richard embarked on a second trial of carbenoloxone which fully confirmed the earlier results. These trials stimulated the writing of over 600 scientific articles and for some years carbenoxolone was widely used in most countries around the world with the notable exception of the U.S. At that time it was the only effective drug treatment for peptic ulcer. It had one side-effect which was easily identified and treatable but unfortunately needed more supervision than most busy practitioners were prepared to give; this led to it being superseded by the H_2 receptor blocks which were no more effective but could be used without blood pressure and weight checks.

His observations on the role of diet have made life simpler for ulcer sufferers and have made yet another notable contribution to clinical practice. Only one observation failed to stand the test of time; antacids have since been shown to accelerate the healing of ulcers when given in large and clinically inconvenient amounts. Sodium carbonate, with its known effects as a mucolytic, may not have been the best choice.

Another important change in the clinical practice of gastroenterology came from his studies on the effect of smoking on the production and maintenance of gastric and duodenal ulcer. From his survey of the international scene it seemed unlikely that smoking was an important and direct cause of peptic ulcer. The distribution of gastric ulcer mortality throughout the world was quite unlike the distribution of tobacco smoking but nevertheless smoking could play a role in the production and maintenance of peptic ulcer. In his studies of doctors in Great Britain he found that the mortality from peptic ulcer was lowest among the non-smokers and this was confirmed by other studies in the U.S.A. and in this country. Part of the excess mortality was undoubtedly due to the greater risk of surgical intervention in individuals with chronic chest disease but the available evidence pointed strongly to smoking as having an anti-healing effect. The gastric ulcers that healed best in his trials were those in individuals who were advised to stop smoking and did so completely. A most interesting observation was the finding that the patients whose ulcers got bigger while having treatment were all heavy smokers. The possibility that smoking had a real adverse effect was further strengthened by the fact that those patients who were advised to stop smoking but only succeeded in reducing the amount smoked did better than the controls but not so well as those who stopped completely. The mechanism of the impairment of healing is uncertain, but it could be related to adverse effects of inhaled carbon monoxide. In encouraging patients to give up much-enjoyed life-long habits doctors have to be dogmatic and convincing. Richard's careful studies have enabled doctors to speak with real conviction.

As an Associate Physician in the Department of Gastroenterology he played a very active role in its research programme. His advice was invariably sought in the planning phase and this ensured that the work got off on the right lines. His strongly developed critical faculties with his ability to anticipate or detect fallacies, his easy approachability, his willingness if necessary to make a substantial personal contribution to the work made him a superb colleague. His collaborative studies within the department included work on the prognosis and management of acute perforated ulcers, on the risks of gastroscopy, gastric secretion in relation to subsequent dyspepsia, oestrogens, inheritance factors in peptic ulcer, the use of continuous intragastric milk drip, carbenoxolone in the treatment of gastric ulcer, and cortisone for ulcerative colitis. With his deepening interest in smoking and cancer it was natural that he should be involved in studies on cancer of the stomach and colon. He assessed the risk of neoplastic changes in simple gastric ulcer, drew attention to a possible link between liquid paraffin oil and cancer of the colon, and studied salivary thiocyanate in gastric cancer. He continued to develop an increasing interest and involvement in environmental factors associated with gastrointestinal cancer on a world scale. The World Organization of Gastroenterology (OMGE), founded in 1957 with Dr Henry L. Bockus as its first President, formed a Research Committee to organize co-operative studies among its member countries around the world. One of its first projects was to study the possible aetiological factors for cancer of the oesophagus, stomach, colon, and rectum. While acting as its first secretary I had great help from Richard in planning and later reporting this world-wide study. Subsequently, this subject remained one of his life-long interests, particularly in relation to diet and nutrition in different countries. These early international studies were indeed the springboard for the next phase of his incredibly productive career in epidemiology.

This Foreword gives me a most pleasing opportunity to acknowledge appreciatively the key role which Richard played in helping to build up the Department of Gastroenterology at Central Middlesex Hospital. He made a fundamental contribution to the emergence and recognition of gastroenterology as a specialty, a contribution reflected by his election to the honorary membership of the British Society of Gastroenterology.

1 The preventability of cancer

Richard Peto

Introduction

For perhaps a century or more, medicine has considered cancers arising from the various organs of the body as being in many respects completely different diseases, and over the past few decades it has emerged that not only their clinical manifestations and prognoses but also their causes may differ enormously. So, it makes as little sense to lump together cancers of the lung, stomach, and intestine when considering the causes of cancer as to lump together cholera, tuberculosis, and syphilis when considering infective diseases. In particular, it is not true that how one lives makes no difference to whether or not one gets cancer but merely determines where in the body the disease will be found. On the contrary, there is no general reason to expect that prevention of one type of cancer will cause any kind of compensatory increase in the onset rate of any unrelated type among people of a given age.

Although there are dozens of types and hundreds of sub-types of cancer, a few types predominate in each country. However, the particular types that predominate in different countries may differ. In both the U.S. and Britain cancer of the lung predominates (due chiefly to the effects of cigarettes), followed by cancers of the breast, large intestine, and (in Britain) stomach, none of which are much affected by tobacco. Together, these four types account for more than half of all cancer deaths. So, one chief aim of cancer research should be to devise practical measures for reducing the incidence of one or more of these particular four diseases, because even large reductions in minor types of cancer can have only minor effects on the total impact of cancer.

International differences: cancers must have causes

Of these four diseases (cancer of the lung, breast, large intestine, and stomach) only for lung cancer has an important cause been reliably identified. Despite this, each is known to be largely preventable. The evidence for their preventability is **first** that the onset rates of some of them are changing rapidly: among people of a given age there have been only minor fluctuations in disease-onset rates for cancers of the breast and of the large intestine in many European countries over the past few decades, but in almost all developed countries there have been vast increases in lung cancer – at least among smokers – and vast decreases in stomach cancer among both smokers and non-smokers. Every 20 or 30 years, lung cancer mortality has doubled in some countries, and every 20 or 30 years stomach cancer mortality has been halved in many countries, so – since there has been little change in the curability of these two diseases – large causes must exist.

Secondly, for these four and for many other types of cancer there are huge differences in the onset rates recorded in different countries. The international differences in lung and stomach cancer are not likely to be chiefly of genetic origin, and nor are those in the other two diseases. For, among people of a given age in different countries, strong correlations exist between certain dietary factors and the onset rates for cancers of the breast and large intestine (Fig. 1(a) and (b)). These striking correlations do not necessarily mean that the particular dietary factors used in Fig. 1 (fat or meat) must be among the important causes of these diseases: they may be causative, but reasonably good correlations can also be found with things like the number of telephones per head! But, what one can conclude from the existence of such strong correlations is that some important non-genetic cause(s) must exist for these two diseases, even though – unlike the other two diseases – their onset rates have been fairly steady for the past half century in many countries.

Thirdly, where migrants have been studied they generally develop internal cancer onset rates that are more similar to those of the population

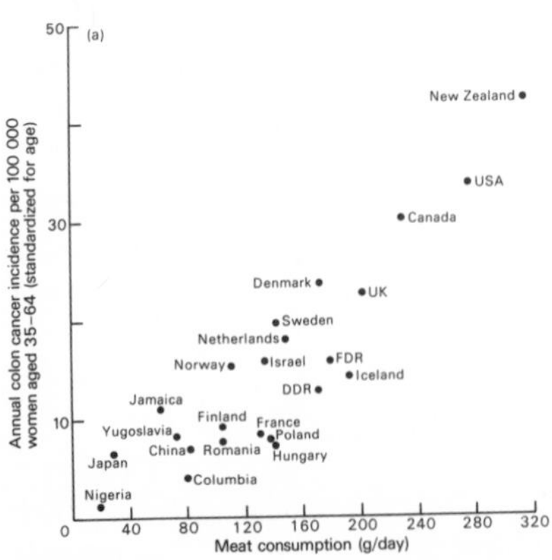

Fig. 1(a). Relationship between meat consumption in various countries and the risk, in those countries, of developing cancer of the colon.

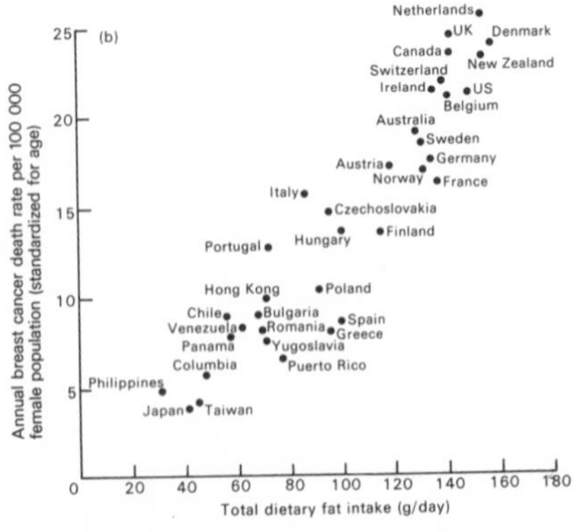

Fig. 1(b). Relationship between fat consumption in various countries and the risk, in those countries, of death from breast cancer.

they have joined than to those of the genetically similar population in their country of origin. Comparison of the cancer rates among blacks in the U.S. with those of blacks in West Africa, and comparison of cancer rates among Japanese Americans with those of Japanese in Japan, show huge differences. This has been particularly true for cancers of the breast and large intestine, which again confirms that these two are both largely avoidable diseases. For example, at any given age cancer of the large intestine is approximately equally common among American whites and blacks, yet it is only about one-tenth as common among West African blacks.

Arguments based on such international comparisons suggest that about 90 per cent of breast and large intestine cancer in Britain and America might be avoidable, and similar arguments for each other type of cancer suggest that in total at least 75 per cent of all cases of internal cancer could be avoided by means that some populations have already adopted. Since there are presumably preventive strategies that no population happens to have tried, perhaps over 75 per cent of cancer deaths in developed countries are in principle avoidable, although, apart from avoidance of tobacco, the important means of achieving this are far from being properly understood. The proportion of cancer deaths that will be found to be avoidable by *practicable* means is another question, of course, since there are many aspects of the lifestyle in impoverished countries that people in affluent ones will not willingly adopt. For example, it has proved difficult enough to control the effects of tobacco, and it may prove even more difficult to change any dietary factors that turn out to be important determinants of cancer – except, perhaps, if the change involves prescription of a healthy foodstuff rather than proscription of an unhealthy one.

Ancient or modern causes?

So, most cancers have causes. But what might they be? Are they chiefly new, or old, aspects of our lifestyle or environment? Cancer is certainly much more talked about nowadays than in previous decades, but this is not of itself evidence that cancer rates among non-smokers of a given age are rising. For, public awareness is influenced by the extensive media coverage of the growing body of cancer research; by the increasing willingness of cancer patients and their friends to discuss the disease openly rather than hush it up; by the substantial effects of tobacco on health and the publicity they receive; by the increasing numbers of people who live on into old age nowadays (cancer rates have always been far higher among the old than the young, so the more old people there are the more cancer deaths there will be, even if among people of a given age cancer onset rates were unchanged); and by the decrease in the toll taken by most other fatal diseases (as the percentage of deaths due to other diseases falls, even if the cancer rates do not change the percentage of deaths that are due to cancer must rise, and this will be noticed). For these and various other reasons, the increased public awareness of cancer and carcinogens cannot be taken as evidence for increasing cancer onset rates among people of a given age. More objective data must be sought.

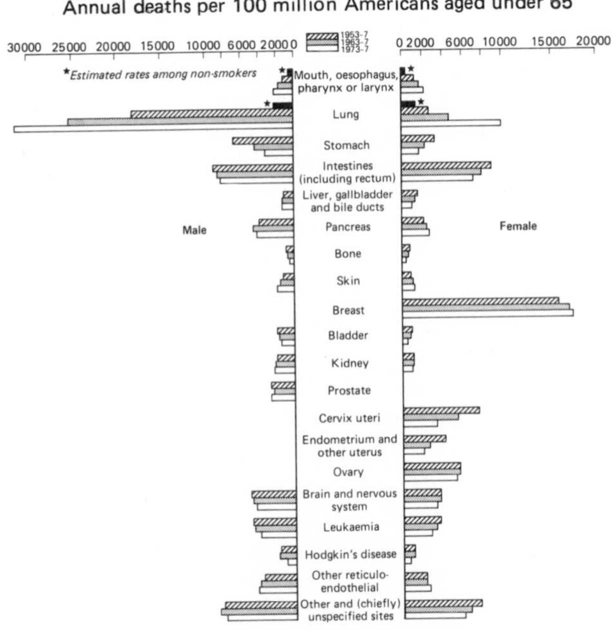

Fig. 2. Trends during the past quarter century in mortality from various types of cancer in the United States. Note the large increases in lung cancer mortality. Most of these trends (except for leukaemia and Hodgkin's disease) are not much affected by changes in treatment, for treatments for the common cancers were as likely to effect cure in the 1950s as in the 1970s. All these death certification rates are 'age standardized', that is, they are adjusted for any effects of changes in the age structure of the U.S. population. The cited rates are per 100 million people under 65; since there are at present about 100 million Americans of each sex aged under 65, the cited rates are similar to the actual numbers of middle-aged Americans that die of these diseases each year.

Unfortunately, none of the available data are entirely satisfactory for the assessment of trends in cancer onset rates. Changes in the numbers of new cases (fatal or non-fatal) of cancer that are recorded are affected not only by changes in cancer onset rates, but also by the changing degree of care with which non-fatal cancers are sought and their discovery recorded centrally. Likewise, changes in the numbers of deaths from cancer that are recorded are affected not only by changes in cancer onset rates and by the proportion of cancers that are cured, but also by the changing degree of care with which the causes of death – particularly of older people – are certified. Perhaps the best of the available data that bear on cancer onset rates are those relating to trends in *death* from various types of cancer during *middle* age, because although many cases of cancer are curable by surgery and radiotherapy, these treatments have both been widely available to middle-aged people for decades, and only for a few rather rare types of cancer have there been any large improvements demonstrated in curative treatment. For the common types of cancer, the likelihood of cure did not greatly improve between the 1950s and the early 1970s, and so in general the trends in mortality in Fig. 2 provide a fair indication of the corresponding real trends in disease onset rates.

Cancer among non-smokers

Among American men, the picture is dominated by the enormous and still increasing mortality from lung cancer, and there are also some small absolute increases in death from cancers of the mouth, throat, and larynx, which, for obvious reasons, are the other parts of the body where tobacco greatly increases the risk of cancer. Apart from this, however, there is no indication of any generalized increase in non-respiratory-tract cancer, and indeed at one site – the stomach – a steady decrease has continued for at least half a century.

Among American women a similar picture emerges, except that the absolute increases in lung cancer will not be as clearly evident as among men for another decade or two, and that mortality from cancer of the uterus is also decreasing. This latter decrease chiefly appears to involve mortality from cancer of the cervix rather than of the endometrium, but the former often gets confused with the latter on death certificates, causing what may be a largely artefactual decrease in endometrial cancer death certification rates.

It is known that the delayed effects of the adoption of cigarette smoking, which greatly increased during the Second World War in America, are the principal cause of the large current increases in lung cancer in that country. It is likely that improvements in genital hygiene, due to improved sanitation, have contributed to the decrease in cancer of the cervix, although in recent years cervical smears and prior hysterectomy have also helped. It is likely that some aspect of the modern American diet, possibly involving better food preservation, is chiefly responsible for the decrease in stomach cancer. However, apart from these changes there is, contrary to what many people imagine, no evidence of any generalized increase in cancer rates in the U.S. or Britain. Indeed, in Britain even the large increase in lung cancer in men due to the delayed effects of the switch to cigarettes is virtually complete, so total U.K. cancer rates (including lung) are now slowly decreasing.

The fact that present-day cancer rates do not exhibit any generalized increase (apart from the effects of smoking) does not, of course, guarantee that all, or nearly all, of the recently introduced new chemicals, pesticides, pollutants and habits are harmless. For it may be decades before any cancer-causing effects they may have become clearly evident. Yet it does guarantee that to concentrate on the scrutiny only of new environmental agents, to the exclusion of the investigation of long-established aspects of our way of life, is to ignore the possibility of preventing the continued occurrence of that mass of present-day cancers that are due to avoidable factors that must have characterized the lifestyle of much of the developed world at least throughout this century. Before discussing how we might set about investigating such factors, a review of what is already known about certain causes may be useful.

Common misapprehensions: infective and genetic factors

Although a few rare genetic conditions may strongly predispose to cancer, and some more common genetic conditions may less strongly predispose to cancer, there is no such thing as genetic immunity from cancer – although a remarkable number of smokers seem, at least in conversation, to believe they have it! In general, the fact that a few of his relatives have died of cancer should not cause anyone undue fears about his own safety. Conversely, the fact that his father or grandfather smoked 40 cigarettes a day until the age of 90 should not lull him into a false sense of security. Cancer arises from three things: nature, nurture and luck. In large populations nature and luck seem generally to average out and only nurture remains. So, study of cancer rates in relation to nurture tells us about the role of external factors, which is, both for government policy and for individual choices, the only thing of practical importance.

Tobacco

Observation of a few hundred thousand lifelong non-smokers for several years in the U.S. revealed very low lung cancer rates (Fig. 2). By contrast, in the U.S. as a whole some 95 000 people died of lung cancer in 1978. If the low lung cancer death rates among lifelong non-smokers had applied to the U.S. as a whole, only 12 000 would have died of the disease. Of course, the lifestyle of people who are lifelong non-smokers may also differ in other ways from that of the rest of the nation, but no such ways are known that are enormously relevant to lung cancer risk. So it is reasonable to infer that, but for the effects of tobacco, only 10 000–15 000 Americans would have died of lung cancer in 1978. Consequently, tobacco must have caused about 80 000–85 000 American lung cancer deaths in 1978 – a figure that can be regarded as quite reliable†. Similar arguments applied to other types of cancer that are affected by tobacco suggest that an additional 40 000 or so other American cancer deaths were caused by tobacco. The 1978 total of 120 000–125 000 American cancer deaths due to tobacco is extremely large, and this annual total is still increasing by about 4000 each year as the population ages and the delayed effects of past increases in cigarette use show up. Consequently, over 140 000 U.S. cancer deaths will have been caused by tobacco in 1984 – that is, about one third of all American cancer deaths. For most people, this number is so large as to be literally incomprehensible. When it is remembered that in addition tobacco probably kills even more people by respiratory and heart disease than by cancer, it becomes clear how urgent it is that some means be sought of reducing the enormous number of premature deaths due to tobacco – at least 300 000 per year, or 15 per cent of all American deaths.

One possibility that bypasses many political difficulties is to encourage, perhaps by prevention of the advertising of cigarettes with 10 or more mg of tar, the continuing switch to lower-tar cigarettes, because there is accumulating evidence that they are indeed somewhat less dangerous.

In Britain, where tobacco causes at least 100 000 out of our annual total of 600 000 deaths, an alternative strategy was, perhaps inadvertently, used in 1981 to increase the real cost of cigarettes. It has been estimated that recent price increases, due chiefly to the 1981 budget, have caused between one and two million people in Britain to stop smoking. This may well save some hundreds of thousands of lives in the long run, because:

(1) about a quarter of all regular cigarette smokers are killed before their time by tobacco;
(2) some of those killed would have died soon anyway, but others would have lived on for another 5, 10, 20, 30, or more years, the average being 10–15 years;
(3) those who stop smoking before they get cancer or serious heart or lung disease avoid nearly all their risk of dying from tobacco.

A final course of action that may help a little is to try to make ordinary people appreciate these three facts. However, so far it is the more-educated groups in Britain who have undergone the largest change in their

†It does not, however, include the 5000–10 000 Americans who, although actually dying of cigarette-induced lung cancer, were certified as having died of cancer of an 'unspecified' site of primary origin. These will be counted eventually among the other types of cancer affected by tobacco.

smoking habits since reliable evidence of the health hazards became available. In Britain in 1980, only 21 per cent of professional people reported using cigarettes, compared with 57 per cent of manual workers. In America too, cigarette smoking is coming to show the same inverse social gradient as in Britain, with heavy smoking by unskilled workers.

However, in marked contrast with recent decreases in Britain, the American cigarette industry had a record year in 1980/81 with the largest increase (2 per cent) in cigarette sales for some years. Commenting on this, the chairman of the largest American cigarette manufacturer was reported as saying that he thought the 'cancer problem' was no longer hitting sales as hard as before because 'so many things have been linked to cancer' that people were getting sceptical. He may well be right, because only a remarkably perceptive citizen would guess, from a typical year's media coverage, that tobacco caused one-third of all cancer deaths, a total ten times greater than the next most important reliably known cause – and, indeed, considerably greater than the number of deaths due to the total known effects of all other reliably known causes of cancer put together.

Alcohol

Alcohol too can cause cancer and probably accounts for about 12 000 cancer deaths every year in America. As an absolute number of people dying this too is large, but in comparison with the effects of tobacco it is much less significant. Expressed as a percentage alcohol accounts for only 3 per cent of all cancer deaths – chiefly, cancers of the mouth, throat, and larynx. Alcohol appears to act chiefly by augmenting the effects of tobacco on these diseases. So, one person's cancer may have had more than one cause, and most of the cancers caused by alcohol could also have been avoided by avoidance of tobacco. Alcohol also causes many accidental and violent deaths, plus some deaths from liver disease, yet moderate use of alcohol may perhaps (though there remains much doubt about this) prevent some deaths from heart disease. The net effects of alcohol on mortality are therefore substantially smaller – especially in view of the possible effect on heart disease – than those of tobacco.

Occupation

Dozens of occupations involve an excess risk of cancer, and probably many more occupational hazards still await discovery. As far as is known the worst such hazard is that due to asbestos dust, which, because of its wide distribution, currently causes perhaps 2 per cent of all U.S. cancer deaths. A tentative estimate may be made – by estimating for each sex the percentage of each type of cancer that is due to occupation – that occupational factors account for about 4 per cent of all American cancer deaths. But, until more systematic evidence is sought, there is a twofold uncertainty in this figure.

A growing source of difficulty in its estimation is the problem of making due allowance for the effects of tobacco. For example, single-handed general practitioners in Britain smoke more than hospital consultants, and get more lung cancer. Similarly, 10 years ago miners and quarrymen smoked nearly twice as much as administrators and managers, so the observation that they get nearly twice as much lung cancer is not evidence for any occupational hazard (except that of tobacco use). These contrasts will presumably be even greater in the future, because as public awareness of the hazards of tobacco has grown in Britain the professional classes have reduced their cigarette consumption considerably more than have the unskilled workers. So, in the past decade the ratio of the percentage of cigarette smokers among unskilled manual workers to that among professional workers has increased from twofold to threefold. (Moreover, at least in America, manual workers tend to smoke cigarettes with higher tar contents.)

Despite various such uncertainties, however, there is no foundation for recent suggestions that 20–40 per cent of all cancers are due to occupational factors. All these estimates appear to derive, directly or indirectly, from one unpublished American study which suffered from gross methodological defects that inflated the risk estimates by an order of magnitude. For example, its assumptions imply that, for two particular types of cancer, about 10 times more cases should in theory be being caused by occupational factors in America than are actually observed in the whole U.S. from all causes – occupational and other – of these two diseases! But, now that such rumours have begun to circulate, they may continue to do so, because they are the sort of thing that many people would rather like to believe of the modern world, and in addition they are useful ammunition for people who wish, perhaps for good reasons, to emphasize the need for stronger unions or stronger legislative controls.

Returning to the more reasonable estimate that 'only' a few per cent of cancer deaths are due to occupational factors, the question of what to do politically about such factors is still a difficult one. For, to control all occupational exposures to all chemicals is virtually impossible, while always to refuse to implement any controls until many workers have died and many more have had the seeds of future cancers implanted in them is barbarous. Laboratory tests must, despite the near-total quantitative uncertainty with which they predict human risk, somehow be used to help set priorities for the control of recent or future occupational exposure, but no wholly satisfactory way of utilizing them has yet evolved. In the mean time, we could adopt a more systematic way of linking records of various occupational circumstances with cancer occurrence some decades later. This would probably bring forward substantially the time of recognition (and hence reduction) of at least a few occupational hazards, either of cancer or of some other disease.

Although both in America and Britain the proportion of all cancer deaths due to occupational factors may be 'only' about 4 per cent, the detection of occupational hazards should have a greater priority in any programme of cancer research than their proportional importance might suggest. For, once identified, it is usually practicable greatly to reduce such hazards.

Environmental pollutants

The most important environmental pollutant has probably been urban air pollution by smoke, which may account – or have accounted – for as much as 1 per cent of all cancer deaths, chiefly by enhancing the effects of tobacco on lung cancer. Tobacco smoking also complicates estimation of the effects of urban pollution, because there is little or no difference between the lung cancer risks of urban and rural non-smokers, while the difference in risk between urban and rural smokers is approximately as great for unpolluted as for polluted cities. This is perhaps because urban smokers have been exposed to cigarette smoke more intensively, or for a greater proportion of their adult lives, than rural smokers have. Fortunately, the great reduction in smoke levels over the past 25 years in many of the more heavily polluted cities means that the future effects of present levels of air pollution by smoke will probably be smaller than the present estimate of 1 per cent, and on present evidence no other pollutants of air, food, or water seem likely to have any greater effects on current cancer rates. There is, however, too much uncertainty to justify complacency, especially about the hypothetical future effects of agents such as pesticides, herbicides, food preservatives, and sterilizants that must, of necessity, be used in biologically significant amounts.

Sexual activity

Cancer of the uterine cervix is far commoner among prostitutes than nuns, because it appears chiefly to be caused by some sexually transmitted infective agent – probably a virus. (The chief suspect used to be the type 2 herpes simplex virus, but with the recent discovery of several new types of human papilloma virus, one or more of these may be a more plausible candidate.) Conversely, cancer of the breast is far commoner among nuns than prostitutes, since the earlier a woman becomes pregnant the lower her breast cancer risks will be in middle and old age. Risks for this and many other types of cancer appear to be influenced, either favourably or otherwise, by hormonal factors, and deliberate favourable manipulation of such factors may ultimately be possible (see Chapters 8 and 9 in this book).

Radiation

The three chief sources of radiation to which humans are exposed are sunlight, natural background radiation from minerals and cosmic rays, and medical X-rays and radiotherapy. Assuming most skin cancer deaths are due to sunlight, and using current international estimates of radiation hazards, these three, together with the much smaller amounts from all other sources, probably account for about 3 per cent of all cancer deaths. But, only about 1 per cent could reasonably be described as 'avoidable' (those due to unnecessary medical procedures or to excessive exposure to sunlight).

Diet

Nutritional and other dietary factors are a chronic source of both frustration and excitement to epidemiologists. For many years there has been strong but indirect evidence that most of the types of cancer that are currently common could be substantially reduced by 'suitable' modification of national eating habits. This remains extremely plausible, but there is still no precise and reliable evidence to show exactly what dietary changes would be of major importance. The chief need is therefore simply for continued research rather than prophylactic action. However, on present evidence a switch in developed countries towards a diet lower in animal products, particularly certain types of fat, and higher in plant products, particularly certain types of fibre, might be prudent.

Various particular types of fat, various particular types of dietary fibre or other carbohydrates, and various vitamins, trace elements, and other micronutrients have been suspected of increasing or decreasing human cancer risks. Many of them can certainly have a profound effect on 'spontaneous' cancer risks among experimental animals, as well as on the response of such animals to cancer-causing agents. However, in humans the role of such nutrients remains uncertain, though this may perhaps simply be because nobody has yet looked at the human evidence in the right way.

Many dietary hypotheses await evaluation, some – such as the possible protective role of pentose-rich fibres – seeming already extremely promising. If the top 10 or 20 are evaluated really carefully, at least one or two ought to be confirmed, and it is reasonable to expect that dietary factors will eventually be found to have a major role in the avoidability of cancer. It is also, however, still quite reasonable to expect the opposite.

Current and developing knowledge of causes

Reasonable estimates and 'guestimates' of the likely roles of various factors discussed in this chapter are drawn together in Table 1. Table 1 is, however, not a summary of firm knowledge, but merely a prediction of what future research may reveal. If instead we were to tabulate what is reliably known (Table 2), the resulting picture would be very different and far less promising. If the perspective on the causes of cancer suggested by these two tables is at least approximately correct, then the chief need is to do something about smoking and to get reliable information about the effects of dietary, hormonal, and infective factors on human cancer – and, of course, on other human diseases. Towards this end, two rather opposite strategies may be envisaged, the *mechanistic* and the *black box* strategies.

Table 1 Future perfect
Estimate of the proportions of cancer deaths that will be found to be attributable to various factors‡

	Percentage of all U.S. or U.K. cancer deaths that might be avoidable	
	Best estimate	Range of acceptable estimates
Tobacco	30	25–40
Alcohol	3	2–4
Diet	35	10–70
Food additives	<1	−5†–2
Sexual behaviour	1	1
Yet-to-be-discovered hormonal analogues of reproductive factors	up to 6	0–12
Occupation	4	2–8
Pollution	2	1–5
Industrial products	<1	<1–2
Medicines and medical procedures	1	0.5–3
Geophysical factors (mostly natural background radiation and sunlight)	3	2–4
Infective processes	10?	1–?
Unknown	?‡	?
Total	200 or more‡	

† The net effects of food additives may be protective, e.g. against stomach cancer
‡ Since one cancer may have two or more causes, the grand total in such a table will probably, when more knowledge is available, greatly exceed 200. (It is merely a coincidence that the suggested figures in Table 1 happen to add up to about 100.)

Table 2 Present imperfect
Reliably established (as of 1981), practicable† ways of avoiding the onset of life-threatening cancer

	Percentage of all U.S. or U.K.cancer deaths known to be thus avoidable
Avoidance of tobacco smoke	30
Avoidance of alcoholic drinks or mouthwashes	3
Avoidance of obesity	2
Regular cervical screening and genital hygiene	1
Avoidance of inessential medical use of hormones or radiology	<1
Avoidance of unusual exposure to sunlight	<1
Avoidance of known effects of current levels of exposure to carcinogens (for which there is good epidemiological evidence of human hazard) in	
(i) occupational context	<1
(ii) food, water, or urban air	<1

† Excluding ways such as prophylactic prostatectomy, mastectomy, hysterectomy, oophorectomy, artificial menopause, or pregnancy

Research strategies: progress from ignorance?

The laboratory-based *mechanistic* strategy tries to find out how normal cells turn into cancer cells and what agents cause this, inhibit it or prevent the growth of the cancer. The trouble is, of course, that there may be many qualitatively different ways of turning normal cells into cancer cells, with the ones that matter being those that underlie the common cancers; and, there is no guarantee whatever that the mechanisms of cancerous change that are currently being investigated in the laboratory do not differ so greatly from those that importantly affect people as to make the related laboratory findings of no direct human relevance. To underline these difficulties, laboratory studies have thus far failed to identify reliably which are the important carcinogens and co-carcinogens in tobacco smoke, and have consistently failed to reproduce in animals the carcinogenic effects of alcohol in humans.

By contrast, the epidemiologically-based *black box* strategy tries to identify as many correlates, or inverse correlates, of human cancer risk as possible, without understanding exactly how cancer arises. Not all correlates point to true causes, of course. Indeed, most of them do not. But, having identified many correlates or inverse correlates, it is reasonable to hope that further investigation of them, probably in collaboration with laboratory scientists, will lead to identification of a few truly causative or truly protective factors with respect to which humans already differ.

Thus far the black box approach has yielded by far the most important findings, including both the role of tobacco (which was discovered before even the structure of DNA was known, let alone the agents or mechanisms by which DNA is damaged) and also the reasons for expecting that a few more large causes still await discovery. But, although epidemiology continues to yield a stream of discoveries of minor causes of human cancer, it seems to be rather bogged down in its search for major discoveries, except perhaps in poor countries. Indeed, in the quarter of a century since the discovery of the role of tobacco no other really major causes of cancer in developed countries have been reliably identified, although a major role of quid chewing in Asian oral cancer and of hepatitis B and, probably, aflatoxin in tropical liver cancer have been demonstrated. If dietary factors are as important as has been suggested, then perhaps the search for dietary correlates of cancer should progress from studies based, as in the past, chiefly on questionnaires to studies augmented by biochemical analyses of biological materials such as blood. Most dietary factors have measurable effects on the blood, and it would be interesting to discover which biochemical factors in apparently healthy people are correlated or inversely correlated with future cancer risks.

Somewhere there are undoubtedly major causes of cancer, and of many other diseases, awaiting discovery. All we need to do is ask the right questions in the right way in order to discover practicable ways of preventing the majority of the many deaths in middle age that still occur in developed countries. A search for biochemical correlates of disease is just one way of approaching such questions. Different scientists working in this area might have quite different views about the likely nature of future discoveries and therefore about which research activities should receive the greatest priority. This fissiparous range of divergent opinions should not be used as evidence that the scientific method is faltering. On the contrary, too great a consensus about where we should go would be dangerous. The sometimes acrimonious spectrum of opinion is one of the most valuable scientific assets when, as in the study of diet and cancer, all we know for certain is that we do not yet know very much for certain.

References

This chapter is largely a summary of two articles written with Sir Richard Doll, both of which are available through Oxford University Press (*The causes of cancer*, by Doll and Peto (1981) and our chapter in the *Oxford textbook of medicine*, ed. D.J. Weatherall *et al.* (1983)), or in *J. nat. Cancer Inst.* **66**, 1191–308. References to most of the assertions in the present chapter may be found in these articles.

2 The geography of cancer

Paula Cook-Mozaffari

It could be argued that the 'geography of cancer' and 'cancer epidemiology' are one and the same subject of study. Geography, which started as a mere descriptive listing of mountains, rivers, capes, and bays and of the principal products of exotic places, flowered into a phase, developed elegantly by Frenchmen such as Vidal de la Blache and De Mangeon (De Mangeon 1927), when it aimed at describing all aspects of the diverse regions of the world, fusing into a coherent whole the story of their natural resources – geology, topography, climate, soils, and vegetation – and building on this an understanding of the economic and other uses that man has made of his environment. Subsequently, from the sheer enormity of the task, the subject developed many specialities, with experts in such fields as 'the geography of plants', the 'geography of population', the 'geography of tourism', or the 'geography of hunger', who aimed first to describe the spatial pattern of their chosen subject and then to explain that particular pattern in terms of the variations observed for other phenomena – physical, biological, historical, or socio-economic. 'Medical geography' was recognized during the 1950s and 1960s and had enthusiastic proponents in Jaques May in the U.S. (1958) and Dudley Stamp in the U.K. (1964).

Viewed as a speciality of geography, 'the geography of cancer' encompasses the whole of cancer epidemiology so that the various working tools of the epidemiologist – the correlation, case-control, and cohort studies – provide information which can help to explain the spatial patterns of variation that occur for individual types of cancer. That being so, a comprehensive geography of cancer is not only clearly beyond the scope of this chapter but would also be impossible to write at the present stage of our knowledge of global incidence patterns and of underlying causes.† However, I will take a geographer's view of the geography of cancer as justification for presenting here not only a review of the advances that have been made in collecting and analysing data that reveal spatial patterns of incidence but also examples of epidemiological work in which spatial patterns have provided clues to causation, or have been the starting point in the search for causal hypotheses, or in which geographical comparisons

† A significant start has been made in the volume *Cancer epidemiology and prevention* (Schottenfeld and Fraumeni 1982)

have been used to test such hypotheses. The scope of the subject has long been appreciated by epidemiologists – a study group on methods of geographical pathology which met in Paris in 1957 summarized the aims as seeking to answer not only the questions 'who has *what* and *where*?' but as including also the question '*why*?' (Doll 1959) – and in the following quarter century epidemiologists have shown a great readiness to make use of a geographical approach wherever it has seemed appropriate.

Incidence and mortality data that reveal spatial patterns

No geographical studies are possible without a considerable body of data which will permit the description of spatial patterns. Cancer epidemiologists have been fortunate in this respect: there is a larger collection of morbidity data available for cancer studies than for the investigation of any other chronic disease. Cancer incidence data have become available from registries which had their inception in schemes planned during the 1930s in Europe and the U.S. In the U.K. registration was made initially by the Radium Commission which controlled the supply of radium to radiotherapy centres (Stocks 1950). It is slightly ironic that the desire to follow the fate of patients treated in hospital has been a strong promotor of cancer registration projects (Clemmensen 1965) when their value in distinguishing the work of different treatment regimens is limited, the latter being much better investigated by studies specifically designed for the purpose. However, the value of cancer registries as a source of information on incidence patterns has been considerable and has been immeasurably enhanced by the bringing together of morbidity and population data in a standard format in the four volumes of *Cancer incidence in five continents* (Doll *et al.* 1966, 1970; Waterhouse *et al.* 1976, 1982). Interest has accelerated with the appearance of each new volume and the number of registries that have been able to provide data of an adequate standard has increased with each successive volume. None the less, for the purpose of incidence surveys, data are only of value if they include virtually all cancer patients who are resident in a defined area during a prescribed period of time, and that exclude non-residents and duplicate entries. It is a complex and painstaking task to bring together records from all possible sources and there are still many regions, even in economically advanced countries, which are not covered by registration schemes sufficiently comprehensive to permit the calculation of reliable incidence rates. For example, cancer registration is carried out throughout England and Wales and annual reports are published which give tabulations of rate by region of residence (OPCS 1979–83). However considerable caution is required in interpreting patterns of regional variation from these figures in view of the variable standards of recording that apply in the different registries.

Mortality records provide an alternative source of data that can give an indication of incidence patterns, although at a Symposium on the Geographical Pathology of Cancer held in Oxford in 1950 (Clemmensen 1950), it was felt strongly that only incidence data were adequate in view of the biases that were beginning to affect mortality rates from the increasing efficiency of therapy and from the unequal availability of treatments in different regions and different countries. It remains a sad fact, more than 30 years later, that, for many types of cancer, effective treatment has still not been found and that mortality statistics remain a useful source of data for studying geographical variation in cancer frequency. National requirements for death certification, laid down by law, mean that mortality data are more extensively and more uniformly available than are incidence data, although completeness in this respect is, of course, offset by lower standards of diagnosis than are possible in the records of cancer registries. Within countries, mortality data have been used to prepare national atlases of the frequency of different types of cancer (Stocks 1936, 1937 and 1939; Howe 1970; Burbank 1971; Mason *et al.* 1975, 1976; Chen *et al.* 1979; Netherlands Centraal Bureau Vor de Statistiek 1980; Statistics Canada 1980; Chinese Academy of Medical Sciences 1981; Research Committee on Geographical Distribution of Diseases, Tokyo 1981; Gardner *et al.* 1983). For international comparisons, the WHO has published various digests of cancer deaths by age for different countries (for a listing see Waterhouse *et al.* 1976) and the late Dr Mitsuo Segi has calculated age-specific and age-standardized rates for these countries at different periods of time (culminating in Segi 1981). These in turn have been used to supplement incidence data in the production of world maps of cancer frequency (Doll 1967; Dunham and Bailar 1968) and estimated incidence rates have been published that comprise mortality rates adjusted for the average difference between incidence and mortality that was observed for areas where both sets of data were available (Doll 1969).

Indices that permit unbiased geographical comparisons

A development following the publication of international cancer incidence data has been the refinement of methods used for the comparison of rates in geographical studies. The need for the use of age-standardization, to allow for variations that occur for most types of cancer between populations of differing age-structure because of a sharp rise of incidence with age, has long been appreciated (Hill 1937). However, there have been a variety of approaches to the practice of standardization. The first three volumes of *Cancer incidence in five continents* appeared with age-standardized rates for each population calculated using three standard populations ('African', 'World', and 'European') in acknowledgement of the fact that use of a standard with a younger or older age structure alters the relative position of the different areas for which incidence data are available (Knowelden and Oettle 1962; Segi 1960). This occurs as a result of differences in the shape of the age curve for individual types of cancer in different parts of the world. However, much of the variation in the pattern of increase with age is restricted to the elderly (Doll and Cook 1967). If age-specific rates for the epithelial cancers, the cancers that make up almost 90 per cent of human malignancy in the Western world, are plotted on a graph with a double-logarithmic scale, the majority show an approximately linear increase with age up to the age of around 65. Among older people the rates tend to fall away at a less sharp rate of increase, although the upward linear trend continues to an older age in economically more prosperous parts of the world than it does in poorer areas. Since the slope of the increase tends to be characteristic for individual types of cancer (Cook *et al.* 1969) the age-specific rates from registries in different parts of the world appear as roughly parallel lines up to the age of around 65 and then diverge. The most likely reasons for the falling away of rates at older ages would seem to be: first, that the elderly are least able to make use of existing medical services (especially in poorer parts of the world where the distances to hospital are great and where the only means of transport may be for a relative to carry the patient on his back), and secondly that there tends to be a less thorough investigation of the deep-seated causes of ill health among the elderly (especially, again, in areas of the world where medical resources are scarce). Bearing this in mind, it seemed sensible to omit altogether from consideration incidence rates among those over the age of 65 (Doll and Cook, 1967). Such an omission could also be justified on the grounds that, since many human malignancies seem to have a long latent period, measured in decades rather than years, the factors that had been involved in the development of cancer among the elderly might long since have disappeared from the environment (Doll 1967). At the other end of the age-scale, for most types of cancer, the numbers are very low before the age of 35. 'Truncated rates' (for the age groups 35–64) were calculated from the age-specific rates in the first volume of *Cancer incidence in five continents* for the more common types of cancer (Doll 1967 (maps based on truncated rates); Doll 1969 (tabulation of rates)) and have appeared alongside the all-age incidence rates in the three subsequent volumes. In the latest volume, use of the 'African' and 'European' standards has been dropped.

A further refinement of the methods used to compare cancer incidence has come with the introduction of 'cumulative rates' (Day 1976) in which age-specific rates are summed, up to whatever age is considered the limit for reliable registration, and which give an indication of the proportion of the population (in the absence of other causes of death) who would have contracted a particular type of cancer before reaching that age. Cumulative rates have the advantage of being more directly comparable than are conventional incidence rates with the relative risk estimates that are obtained from case-control studies or from animal experiments. Cumulative rates for the age group 0–64 and 0–74 have appeared in the third and fourth volumes of *Cancer incidence in five continents*.

Despite the advantages of a single index for facilitating comprehension in geographical comparisons, more information may, of course, be forthcoming from a study of the way in which incidence changes with age. Breast cancer is unusual among epithelial cancers in that it shows a different pattern of age-specific incidence in different parts of the world (Day and Muir 1973). In high incidence areas in western Europe and the U.S. a break in the increase of incidence occurs at the time of the menopause followed by a continued increase with age. In low incidence areas such as Japan the age-specific rates decline after the age of 50. It has been suggested that the post menopausal 'Western' tumours could be associated with affluence, excessive food, and a resulting increase in oestrogen production (de Ward 1969). Primary liver cancer in Mozambique has an incidence in adolescents and young adults that is exceptional for any type of cancer anywhere in the world (Doll *et al*. 1966). Then between the ages of 25 and 55 the incidence rates are more or less constant, subsequently decreasing at older ages. This shape of age curve has been observed in a second region in Mozambique (van Rensburg *et al*. 1985) but occurs nowhere else in the world where figures are available. It is possible that the failure of the rates to increase with age indicates exhaustion of a pool of susceptible individuals.

Implications of the range of incidence for different types of cancer

Despite considerable progress in the accumulation of incidence data of a high standard, the coverage of the 'five continents' is still by no means complete since the numerous countries of South America, Africa, and much of Asia are represented by isolated centres in one or two territories. Unfortunately mortality data are also not available for most Third World countries; the scarcity of medical facilities in these territories may mean that even the fact of death goes unrecorded, let alone the cause. The few centres in such regions of the world that have made the very great effort to accumulate cancer incidence data of a high standard of completeness thus make a most important contribution to the study of cancer epidemiology. In particular, with the advent of the first reliable incidence figures it was possible to show (using truncated rates) that total cancer incidence in poorer parts of the world could be as high as that in the Western world (Cook 1968). Cali in Columbia was on a par with Liverpool in England or

New Brunswick in Canada. Lourenco Marques (now Maputo) in Mozambique had a very similar all-cancer rate to that in Slovenia, Yugoslavia or Miyaji, Japan or to that in New Zealand. Chinese in Singapore had higher all-cancer rates than did the population of Norway. This meant that the relative frequency studies from economically less developed countries that for several decades had shown high percentages for types of cancer that were rare in the West, such as cancer of the liver, cancer of the penis, or cancer of the nasopharynx, could be indicating genuinely higher rates and not merely showing a high proportion of a small total. It had long been suspected that this was the true situation by far-seeing observers such as Sir Albert Cook, a doctor who worked in Uganda from 1897 and who kept meticulous records of all cancers that he diagnosed. Sir Albert put forward the suggestion that the apparent rarity of cancer in Africa was merely an artefact resulting from the extreme frequency of infectious disease and from the absence of any mechanism whereby cancer patients are concentrated in referrals by general practitioners and clinics (Cook 1901). Another commonly held misconception about cancer in Africa was that cancer among 'natives' was not an indigenous disease but had been imported by the white man (Hollander 1923; Cameron Blair 1923). Analysis of the records for the period 1897 to 1965 from the hospital where Sir Albert had worked (Davies *et al.* 1964) showed that the proportional distribution of different types of cancer among Ugandan Africans had remained stable for over half a century from a period long before the local way of life had been distorted by European influences.

With the first gathering together of comparable international incidence and mortality figures during the 1960s it became possible to demonstrate the range of variation that exists for individual types of cancer between different parts of the world – with values that are much greater than the two- to three-fold range for the summed incidence of all malignancies. Many types of cancer are 10 or 20 times more common in areas of high than in areas of low incidence; cancer of the stomach appeared to be 30 times as common in Japan as in Uganda; cancer of the lung 40 times more common in Liverpool than in Nigeria; cancer of the penis 100 times more common in Jamaica than in Israel; cancer of the oesophagus 200 times more common in Kazakhstan than in Holland and cancer of the liver apparently 1000 times more common among young men in Lourenco Marques (now Maputo), Mozambique than in North America (Doll 1967). This quantification gave numerical expression to a realization that had been growing over previous decades (World Health Organization 1964) that, since for almost every cancer that was common in one country a region of the world could be found where it was very rare, the majority of human cancer must occur as a result of extrinsic factors and be potentially preventable. One estimate, for example, put the proportion that could be prevented at 80 per cent (Higginson 1969). That the geographical variations are not for the most part simply an expression of genetic differences between races has become apparent from migrant studies which indicate that people who have moved to a new country, as for example the Black, Chinese, and Japanese populations of the U.S., gradually acquire over several generations cancer patterns that are more similar to those of their host country than to those of the country of origin. For example, hepatocellular carcinoma which could be as much as 80 times more common in much of coastal China as among U.S. whites (Cook-Mozaffari and van Rensburg 1984) is 11 times more common among Chinese men who have emigrated to the U.S. than among white males but only 3 times as common among men of Chinese parentage born in the U.S. as among white males (King and Locke 1980). Similarly, black populations resident in the U.S. have incidence rates for cancers of the large intestine and prostate that are as high or higher than the incidence among U.S. whites (for whom these rank as two of the commonest malignancies) and yet cancer of the large intestine is practically unknown among black Africans and cancer of the prostate is only between a third to one-half as common as among American blacks (Doll *et al*. 1966, 1970; Waterhouse *et al*. 1976, 1982).

Migrant studies have been hampered in the past by a lack of detailed knowledge about regional incidence rates in the countries of origin of the migrants. The publication in recent years of cancer atlases from countries such as China or Japan permits more accurate comparison with the specific region of origin. For example, the study of Chinese immigrants to the U.S. indicated that the mortality rates for cancer of the oesophagus were lower among Chinese males in America than among Chinese in China (King and Locke 1980). However, in the absence of other data, the expected figures were calculated from rates for Taiwan whose people come for the most part from Fukien Province (a high-risk region in China), whereas U.S.-born Chinese had come mainly from the neighbouring Province of Kwantung where the incidence of oesophageal cancer was lower. It could be, therefore, that the apparent difference in frequency noted above was merely due to the limited comparisons that could be made and had nothing to do with migration to America (Ghadirian 1982).

Spread of geographical studies in areas of marked environmental contrast

The realization that a high proportion of human cancer must be caused by factors that are not inborn gave stimulus to the pursuit of both incidence and aetiological studies in less-developed parts of the world, on the grounds that it should be easier to isolate causes of tumour development in situations where people are much more dependent on, and less protected from, the physical and biololgical environments and where the customs and way of life developed over generations of isolation are still relatively unchanged.

Relative frequency and incidence surveys in Africa

A great deal has since been done to sketch in the outline of the cancer map, particularly in Africa, without waiting for the improvement in medical services that would be necessary for more conventional cancer registration. As anticipated, gradients of frequency have been found that are much sharper than are common in Europe or America. In 1962 Mr Denis Burkitt made a ten-week overland tour of hospitals in East, Central, and Southern Africa, so as to tap the experience of the many doctors who had worked for years in remote regions (Burkitt 1962a). With their help he established the limits of the lymphoma affecting children in Africa that has subsequently been given his name. Incidence was clearly related to temperature and rainfall with very few cases occurring in cold upland areas or in arid regions (Burkitt 1962b).

While Burkitt was undertaking his famous safari, the late Dr Ralph Burrell in Southern Africa was organizing a team of local technicians in the Transkei to gather information from each village on the incidence of cancer of the oesophagus. Initial reports had suggested that the disease was so common there that the symptoms had acquired a name in the local language, a situation most unusual for a malignant disease in a poor, rural area (Burrell 1962). He and subsequent workers have demonstrated a clear regional gradient within the Transkei from very common in the south to rare in the north (Rose 1973; Rose and McGlashan 1975; Rose and Fellingham 1981). Covering a wider area, the late Dr Georges Oettlé (1963) collected data on the occurrence of oesophageal cancer throughout Southern Africa, relating the number of cases diagnosed each year to the number of hospital beds, and indicating wide variations of frequency between different regions – differences that were striking enough to be apparent despite the limitations of the data. He also amassed evidence suggesting that over the past few decades there had been a great increase in the incidence of cancer of the oesophagus in areas where it was now common.

The following year Oettlé (1964) published an exhaustive compendium of the information available on the geographical distribution throughout sub-Saharan Africa of any cancer that was either unusually common (such as cancer of the liver or cancer of the oesophagus) or unusually rare (such as cancer of the large intestine) or distinctively African in its occurrence (such as Kaposi's sarcoma or Burkitt's lymphoma). Much of the information on which Oettlé was able to draw came from relative-frequency studies based on the data accumulated by histology laboratories and, as he was well aware, for many types of cancer these are of limited value in the African context. For superficial malignancies, such as cancer of the penis, which had been shown to be one of the commonest types of cancer diagnosed in Uganda while it was rarely seen among Kenyan Africans (Linsell and Martyn 1962; Dodge and Linsell 1963) histological series could give a reasonable indication of tumour incidence but, given the poor medical facilities of most rural areas, diagnoses of more deep-seated internal malignancies were often made without benefit of histological confirmation (Burkitt *et al.* 1968). Under these circumstances frequency studies based on histological series would both misrepresent the relative position of different types of cancer within the series and also, given variation in the biopsy rate between medical centres, misrepresent the geographical distribution of individual types of cancer. However, patients with cancer in Africa often present late with a massive tumour and clear clinical indications of the type of cancer. Bearing these factors in mind, and encouraged by the wealth of information that had been forthcoming during his initial tumour safari, Burkitt initiated a systematic recording of clinical experience in East and Central Africa, encouraging doctors in remote rural hospitals to send a monthly record over a period of years of the tumours that they had diagnosed during the previous month. Great stress was laid on the need to report all suspected malignancies and not just those with histological confirmation of diagnosis.

At the beginning of the survey information was requested only about some half-dozen types of cancer of particular interest so as to avoid asking too many questions of already overworked doctors, but subsequently all malignancies were included to provide a more stable denominator for asessing relative frequencies (Cook and Burkitt 1971). The observation noted above that the summed incidence of all types of cancer shows relatively little variation throughout the world (and even less between neighbouring territories) means that proportional frequencies based on all malignancies will give an approximately accurate representation of the relative incidence of particular cancers in different centres. This principle has therefore been exploited in the African survey (in a slightly modified form) to give estimates of age-standardized incidence rates that are adjusted for the inevitable under-reporting that has occurred (Cook-Mozaffari and Burkitt 1985). Total cancer incidence in each rural areas (minus some half-dozen sites that show particularly extreme geographical variations of incidence within short distances) has been linked to the average incidence observed in African cities that have cancer registries of a more conventional nature. Incidence rates for individual types of cancer have been adjusted accordingly.

The initial rural survey was subsequently extended to parts of West and Southern Africa and was supplemented by the establishment of registries in six cities in East and Central Africa. Use of the method of adjusting for under-reporting outlined above to cover also published relative frequency series from other parts of Africa has given, for some 70 regions throughout sub-Saharan Africa, estimated incidence rates that are approximately correctly placed on a scale of variation that can be used for international comparisons. For example, the incidence rates for cancer of the penis in the highest incidence regions of Uganda would seem to be five to ten times higher than the previously highest recorded rates in the Caribbean and South America. Cancer of the large intestine has a uniformly low incidence in all regions for which data are available (confirming the clinical impressions that led to promulgation of the low-fibre-diet hypothesis as a principal cause of the high incidence rates in Western populations (Oettlé 1967; Burkitt 1971). Gradients for incidence of cancer of the oesophagus exist between Kenya, Uganda, and northern Tanzania, or between southern Malawi and southern Tanzania, that are as striking as that which Burrell and his colleagues have demonstrated between the southern and northern regions of Transkei. Cancer of the nasopharynx in central Kenya has a moderate incidence, midway between the very low rates of Western populations and the high rates observed in southern China and in Eskimo populations (Lanier *et al.* 1976; Nielsen *et al.* 1977).

A further unusual data source that has been useful in indicating patterns of cancer incidence in Southern Africa are the records of the hospitals that serve the workers in the gold mines of Transvaal. Men are employed in the mines in large numbers not only from the provinces of South Africa but also from adjacent territories. Analyses of records over a period of 16 years have been made that, for example, confirm the very high incidence of cancer of the liver in Mozambique, and extend knowledge of the occurrence of tumours in the oesophagus, lung, and bladder (Harington *et al.* 1975; Bradshaw *et al.* 1982).

Aetiological investigations

Burkitt's lymphoma Aetiological investigations were quickly implemented in Africa to explore the meaning of the emerging patterns of incidence. The work on Burkitt's lymphoma is an outstanding case in point. Once the association of incidence with climate had been established, the obvious hypothesis was that some infective agent was involved in the development of the tumour. This was strengthened by realization that the disease occurred in areas where malaria was hyper- or holo-endemic (Burkitt 1969) and by fine-scale geographical studies in the West Nile District of Uganda that showed a clustering of cases in time and space (Pike *et al.* 1967; Williams *et al.* 1969). Perversely, subsequent studies in Tanzania and Ghana gave no evidence of space–time clustering (Brubaker *et al.* 1973;

Biggar and Nkrumah 1979; Morrow *et al.* 1977) but the occurrence of cases more frequently in homes that were overcrowded and poorly constructed (Morrow *et al.* 1974), a decline of incidence in the vicinity of the capital city of Uganda (an area of relative economic prosperity and with above-average access to medical facilities) (Morrow *et al.* 1976), and a relative deficiency of cases in large cities in West Africa (Biggar and Nkrumah 1979) were all consistent with an infective origin. Intensive investigations of the role of infection in the development of Burkitt's lymphoma (summarized by Morrow 1982) have suggested a three-stage model of pathogenesis in which infection by Epstein–Barr virus is followed by chronic malaria infection that increases the number and turnover of Epstein–Barr virus infected B-lymphocytes and thus opens the way for the emergence of malignant cytogenic change in the form of a chromosome-14 translocation that has regularly been found in biopsies of Burkitt's lymphoma. The logical conclusion of this train of investigation has been an attempt to change the geographical pattern of distribution. An intervention study is currently underway in northern Tanzania, planned to assess the effects of malaria control on the incidence of Burkitt's lymphoma (de Thé *et al.* 1978).

Primary liver cancer Studies of cancer of the liver in Africa have a particularly geographical flavour but, in this instance, the starting-point was not variation in incidence between different areas but the discovery that aflatoxin, occurring in Aspergillus moulds growing on foodstuffs, was highly carcinogenic in experimental animals (Sinnhuber *et al.* 1968; Butler 1970). A search was then made in Africa for gradients of incidence between adjacent regions where the climate changed markedly within a short distance and where different levels of Aspergillus growth could be anticipated. In each survey the expected variations of incidence were found (Tuyns *et al.* 1971; Alpert *et al.* 1971; Peers and Linsell 1973; Peers *et al.* 1976) and surveys of aflatoxin contamination in plate-samples of food or in crops brought to market for sale repeatedly showed a geographical association with incidence. The levels of contamination in Mozambique were so high that, if laboratory rats were fed the food consumed by the human population there, most would be expected to develop liver cancer within a year or two (van Rensburg *et al.* 1974).

Work that progressed contemporaneously on the role of hepatitis B virus has shown that carriers of hepatitis B virus are at particularly high risk for the development of primary liver cancer. Hepatitis B virus is widespread in Africa but surveys of prevalence among workers in the gold mines of South Africa (Bersohn *et al.* 1974) and in East Africa (Bagshawe *et al.* 1975) indicate no geographical association with incidence (van Rensburg 1982) and it seems likely that carriage of hepatitis B virus is a necessary conditioning factor in making the liver susceptible to the carcinogenic action of aflatoxin. The peculiar shape of age curve for primary liver cancer in Mozambique may indicate that the number of susceptible individuals in the population is insufficient to give full expression to the extraordinary levels of aflatoxin contamination that occur there.

The geography of cancer of the oesophagus, with particular reference to Iran

Aetiological studies with a geographical basis have been more extensive for cancer of the oesophagus than for any other type of cancer. It was suggested (Doll 1966, 1968, personal communication to Dr Janez Kmet of the IARC and to the author) that detailed investigation of the environment and way of life in a series of areas throughout the world where the frequency of cancer of the oesphagus showed the characteristic sharp gradient from high to low incidence (reported not just from Africa but also from France, the Soviet Union, China, and Iran (International Agency for Research on Cancer 1968)) would be the approach most likely to yield new aetiological clues, and to lift epidemiological research on this front from the stalemate of case-control studies that had shown an association with the consumption of alcohol and tobacco within areas of high, moderate, and low incidence but which gave no explanation of the great differences in incidence between such regions (Doll 1967). Work progressed furthest along these lines in Iran where Dr Kmet fought for a programme of international and multidisciplinary cooperation that would mobilize skills on a sufficient scale to yield unambiguous results.

Mapping of incidence in Iran

An initial journey through the north of Iran to question doctors about the frequency with which they diagnosed different types of cancer had indicated that to the east of the Caspian Sea the incidence of oesophageal cancer was very high (Kmet, Internal Report to the IARC 1966), perhaps as high as in the neighbouring Soviet Republics of Kazakhstan and Turkmenistan (Merkova *et al.* 1963), where incidence rates higher than those from any other region of the world had been reported (Doll 1969). Three hundred miles to the west, in the densely populated coastal region to the south-west of the Caspian, the disease was rarely seen. The most obvious environmental difference between the regions of high and low incidence was the change from a very dry climate to one of abundant rainfall. The climatic variation was in turn reflected in a host of differences in soil types, natural vegetation, and crop patterns (Kmet and Mahboubi 1972). In 1968 a cancer registry was established in order to check the initial impressions of incidence. In the absence of large hospitals or of any standard system of record-keeping, technicians were sent every few weeks to collect notification forms from some 600 doctors (including general practitioners as well as surgeons and radiologists†). Information concerning *all* malignancies was requested so as to permit assessment of any regional variation in the level of recording for cancer of the oesophagus.

The first three years of registration showed a level of incidence in some regions to the east of the Caspian that were outstandingly high for any type of cancer anywhere in the world (Mahboubi *et al*. 1973), the equivalent, for example, of the rates for bronchial carcinoma among lifelong heavy smokers in London (Dr N.E. Day, personal communication). A request for details of the ethnic composition of each village from the technicians of the Malaria Eradication Organization showed that the highest incidence rates occurred among Turkomans but that the patterns of incidence seemed to cut across, rather than simply reflect, ethnic differences and that both high and lower rates were being recorded for Persian, Turkoman, and Turkish groups resident in the area.

Significance of the sex ratio in different regions of the world

It was possible to define some nine regions of differing incidence patterns in the north of Iran and this diversity made feasible the plan that had been emerging for a large-scale population investigation to be carried out within Iran. Geographical comparisons of just two areas yield an unmanageable host of differences; marked variation of incidence between a number of areas of contrasting environment offers the possibility of eliminating irrelevancies. This was the philosophy of the original plan of looking at areas of sharp incidence gradients throughout the world, but as work progressed in Iran it became clear that there were major aetiological differences between regions where cancer of the oesophagus was very much a disease of men, for example in East Africa and France, and where factors in the social environment, such as alcohol or tobacco, could be assumed to have a dominant role, and the situation in Iran where alcohol was forbidden by religion and where in the areas of highest incidence women were even slightly more at risk than men. Subsequent work in Africa has suggested that the consumption of beer made from maize and the smoking of tobacco pipes are involved as risk factors there (Cook 1971; Schonland and Bradshaw 1969; Bradshaw *et al*. 1983) while in France a case-control study has indicated that most of the excess risk within

† The only pathologist working in the area was established at the Caspian Cancer Registry in the Teheran Institute of Public Health, who together with the IARC were responsible for inauguration of the Registry.

Normandy and Brittany can be explained in a multiplicative effect of smoking and drinking although there is an additional risk related to apple brandy and cider (Tuyns *et al.* 1977, 1979).

Preliminary environmental studies in Iran

A foundation of knowledge concerning the environment and way of life in the north of Iran was built-up from maps available from various university and government research institutes in Teheran and by preparation of numerous agricultural and economic maps from statistics published by the National Census Office. With these began the process of eliminating less-promising hypotheses. For example, visits to the areas of high incidence had suggested that the wide stretches of saline soil to be found there might have some aetiological implication, perhaps through their interference with the uptake of zinc by plants which could in turn exacerbate the problems of zinc loss by heavy sweating that had been noted in the dry regions of Iran (Prasad and Oberleas 1974). Detailed study of the soil and vegetation maps, however, showed neighbouring Turkoman areas, also of very high incidence, where Brown Forest soils with no salinity had developed under the original cover of thick deciduous woodland.

The population survey

Visual inspection of the many maps accumulated showed that the closest correlation with incidence remained the negative association with rainfall that had been observed originally. The need was quickly felt for information on variables that were closer to man and that had greater physiological significance than mean annual rainfall, on dietary intake, for example and on the origin, storage, and preparation of foodstuffs. However, very little information had previously been collected by other investigators on the geographical distribution of such variables and a population survey was planned to supply the deficiencies (Iran–International Agency for Cancer Research Joint Study Group 1977). The environmental knowledge that had already been acquired was used for the construction of a sampling frame in which regions, defined by incidence, were subdivided by contrasting environmental factors. Villages were chosen at random from within each region and field teams moved from village to village during the course of a year, living in tents to facilitate access to remote regions and to encourage co-operation among the interviewees – who appreciated a willingness to share something of the hardships to which they were accustomed. The survey was restricted to rural areas and thus excluded some 20 or 30 small towns where social and economic changes had been rapid over the past few decades and where it was possible that the conditions which had produced the high incidence levels for cancer of the oesophagus had already partly disappeared. A quantitative dietary intake survey was completed for each village together with detailed questioning about the origin and preparation of the foodstuffs consumed. In addition a questionnaire was administered to obtain information on various economic activities such as carpet-making, common in areas of high incidence and possibly involving the use of harmful dyestuffs, and on the division of economic tasks between men and women. Questions were also included concerning the consumption of tobacco, opium, and alcohol – the latter to explore further the conflict between its free availability in all the small towns of the north of Iran and the taboo of sin surrounding its consumption. The dietary and socio-economic questionnaires were backed by physiological measurements on a sample of the population to assess, for example, various serum indicators of dietary deficiency, and to measure the level of morphine metabolites in the urine. Chemical analyses of plate samples of prepared foodstuffs were made to look for known carcinogenic agents.

This phase of investigations in Iran marked a massive clearing of the ground of negative results. There was no difference between regions, for example, in the occurrence of nitrosamines, polycyclic hydrocarbons, aflatoxins, or other mycotoxins, and only low levels of each of these contaminants were observed. Hypotheses that had arisen from a partial knowledge of the customs of the region, concerning the scattering of poppy seeds on bread, the use of dung balls for fuel, or the consumption of salt fish, were dropped from further consideration when the true pattern of their use was more accurately established. Certain habits and economic practices that were peculiar to the areas of high incidence – the consumption of 'majoveh' (a special food made of crushed pomegranate seeds and black pepper that was craved by pregnant women), the chewing of 'nass' (a mixture of tobacco, lime, and woodash), and the making of carpets and felts – were found to be activities confined strictly to one sex and were thus unlikely to be involved in the development of a disease that was so widespread in both men and women. (Men never ate 'majoveh', women did not chew 'nass', and men had no part in any of the stages of carpet-making once the sheep had been sheared.)

Diet

The outstanding features of the diet of the areas of highest incidence were a very low intake of fruit and vegetables and derivation of a high proportion of protein and other nutrients from home-baked, unrefined wheat bread. The Turkomans of the driest areas were semi-nomadic pastoralists who kept sheep, goats, and camels. Grain for bread was mostly obtained by trading, since the steppeland – parched brown during most of the year – often fails to yield a crop, and agriculture, even when possible, is regarded as a poor alternative to the wealth of great flocks. Further to the south, where Turkomans had settled many generations previously in the more fertile regions of the Brown Forest soils, they had retained the dietary practices of the steppeland and had not increased their consumption of fruit and vegetables. To the west, in the Persian areas of lower incidence, the staple grain was rice; deciduous and citrus fruits were abundant and green vegetables were both gathered from the forest and grown in gardens in all the villages. The measured-intake survey showed that the diet in the highest incidence regions had very low levels of animal protein, vitamin A, riboflavin, and vitamin C (Hormozdiari *et al.* 1975). However, poverty and poor diet were found also in certain areas of the western regions and it took a subsequent case-control study to confirm that a lifelong low intake of fruit and vegetables was particularly characteristic of the patients with cancer of the oesophagus and that, even in the generally poor rural communities of northern Iran, it is the lowest socio-economic group that is worst affected (Cook-Mozaffari *et al.* 1979). Clinical and biochemical examination of schoolchildren in the region of highest incidence showed little evidence of low vitamin A intake but widespread riboflavin deficiency (Kmet *et al.* 1980).

The case-control study also investigated certain variables that had shown a geographical association with incidence in the population survey such as the consumption of sheep's milk and yoghurt, the use of sesame oil for cooking, and the consumption of bread. None showed a raised intake among patients. However, the possibility of an aetiological role for bread remained, either through the contamination of grain by mycotoxins during storage in the underground pits characteristic of the high-incidence areas (none were found (Lacey and Booth 1980)) or by contamination with extraneous seeds that were abundant in wheat samples from these areas. Seeds were found containing shikimik acid, which has been associated with tumour development in cattle (Jarrett *et al.* 1978), and many abrasive seeds were present that are known to cause gastric disturbances when they are included in cattle feed (Day 1980). Also there were seeds with finely pointed silica fibres that could act as a stimulant to cell growth if lodged in the oesophagus (O'Neill *et al.* 1980).

Opium dross

A further positive result of the population survey was that the few urine samples that it had been possible to collect had indicated a high intake of opium in the regions of highest incidence. Subsequently it was noted that in these regions opium was taken mainly as dross scraped from the inside of the opium pipe and was often swallowed. Dross was found to be mutagenic whereas raw opium was not (Hewer *et al.* 1978). In the same paper a parallel situation was reported from Transkei in South Africa where dottle is swallowed from the stem of tobacco pipes. Enquiry about opium intake in the Iranian Province of Kerman where consumption was believed to be high and yet where relative frequency studies had indicated a rather low incidence for cancer of the oesophagus showed that opium was so abundant in this area that dross was hardly ever used but was exported instead to other parts of the country (Ghadirian 1982). A survey of abnormal pathology in oesophageal tissue in Turkoman villages showed very high levels of oesophagitis in adults of all ages. There was, however, no indication of higher levels among opium addicts than in the rest of the population and it is unlikely that opium consumption is the initiating factor for the development of the oesophagitis (Crespi *et al.* 1979).

Aetiological implications

Further investigations were planned for Iran, of opium consumption and of the effect of the administration of vitamin supplements on the occurrence of oesophagitis in particular, but also on the precise patterns of occurrence within different ethnic groups (the latter to look more at the possibility of a Turko–Mongolian susceptibility to the disease). However, the international programme of research was cut short by political events in 1979. Fortunately, work had already been sufficiently extensive to indicate both the probable circumstances that account for much of the exceptionally high level of incidence within Iran and to point the way to the common aetiological threads that link the apparently disparate areas of high incidence in different regions of the world. An initial requirement would seem to be a weakening of the oesophageal mucosa by a diet that is low in certain essential nutrients. Studies of serum vitamin levels in high incidence areas of China have shown a low intake of both riboflavin and retinol (Muños 1982) and oesophagitis is also common there (Muños *et al.* 1982). An intervention study is now underway to assess the effect of vitamin supplements. In Washington D.C. in the U.S. a case-control study among black males, for whom alcohol consumption was the dominant risk factor, also showed an underlying history of a low intake of fruit, vegetables, and animal protein (Pottern *et al.* 1981). Clearly the nutritional imbalances engendered by a heavy consumption of alcohol may further exacerbate the effects of poor dietary status. This could be of particular relevance in those parts of Africa where maize is the staple foodstuff, giving a diet that is only marginally adequate for cetain essential nutrients (van Rensburg 1981).

In addition to the debilitating effects of poor diet, physical trauma also seems to play some part in further weakening the structure of the oesophagus. In Iran this is provided by the repeated intake of dry scratchy bread and perhaps by the consumption of hot tea. Studies elsewhere in the world have pointed to hot, spicy, and abrasive foods as possible risk factors (Martinez 1969; DeJong *et al.* 1974; Hirayama 1971; Segi 1975; Kolycheva 1980).

Acting on tissues made susceptible in these ways would seem to be a variety of weak carcinogens, perhaps from opium dross or seeds contaminating wheat in Iran, from pipe dottle and home-brewed maize beer in Africa, from tobacco smoke and home distilled apple brandy in Normandy and Brittany and from 'pickled' vegetables and steamed maize bread in China (Kaplan and Tsichitani 1978). The latter is stored for several weeks before consumption and fungal mould is apparently widespread and relished as the preferred taste of bread. 'Pickled' vegetables and mouldy bread are suspected sources of nitrosamines and nitrosamine precursors in China that may be present at higher levels than have been found elsewhere. In other parts of the world low levels of nitrosamines have been found in home-made beers and spirits and in foodstuffs, but would seem to be ubiquitous and not confined to areas of high incidence for cancer of the oesophagus (International Agency for Research on Cancer 1975, 1976). Tobacco smoke, which is mostly inhaled rather than swallowed, or grains of opium dross swallowed swiftly with tea (to avoid the bitter taste) can also offer only a weakly carcinogenic stimulus to the oesophagus. However, it has been suggested that alcohol (Doll 1971) and perhaps also hot tea (Day and Muños 1980) might act as solvents, facilitating the passage of carcinogens to the basal layers of the oesophagus. In Iran, China, and Southern Africa a further factor may be the lodgement of silica fibres or particles in the oesophageal tissues, so providing an anchorage for the spread of tumour cells (Bhatt *et al.* 1984).

It seems that where several of the factors that have been outlined above occur together in one region they act multiplicatively to produce a very high incidence of cancer of the oesophagus, and that the disappearance of any single factor from adjacent areas has a far more dramatic effect in lowering incidence than would occur if that variable were acting alone. This it has been suggested is the explanation of the sharp gradients of frequency that are so characteristic of the occurrence of cancer of the oesophagus but which do not occur in the world map of, say, cancer of the lung, where a single risk factor is dominant (Day *et al.* 1982).

Maps and computers

The foundation of the Iran studies was a correlation approach. The wide range of incidence within short distances and the broad regional changes involving only some nine permutations of incidence meant that in the initial stages of the search for hypotheses, comparison with environmental and socio-economic variables could be done by visual inspection of maps. This approach is unlikely to be of use in generating hypotheses, or for eliminating unrelated variables, with the far more complex patterns of incidence that are apparent in the various national atlases of cancer mortality, based on rates in hundreds or thousands of areas. These distribution patterns require more sophisticated statistical and computational techniques to isolate related variables. Such was the path of investigation that led to discovery of work with asbestos in World War II shipyards as the cause of the unexpected concentrations of high incidence for lung cancer in coastal Georgia, shown in the atlas maps (Blot *et al.* 1979; Mason *et al.* 1975). As in Iran, the geographical correlations were part of a larger programme. They first paved the way for a search of death certificates and for informed case-control studies, and later provided confirmation of correlation once suspicion had fallen on the shipyards.

The spread of familiarity with computing techniques among epidemiologists means that detailed exploration of the occurrence of different types of cancer in terms of environmental and socio-economic variables can more routinely take its place as part of any sequence of aetiological investigations and that atlases can become a starting-point and not, as they have tended to be in the past, a conclusion, with the compilers falling exhausted on the shore from the effort of producing the maps. Great credit is due to early research workers such as Dr Percy Stocks who, in a pre-computer era, not only mapped but also explored the meaning of his maps in studies, for example, of the aetiology of gastric cancer in North Wales, Cornwall, and Devon (Stocks 1936, 1957; Stocks and Davies 1964).

Areal case-control studies

Another geographical approach that has received an impetus with the computerization of mortality data has been the use of what can be termed 'areal case-control' studies, set up to help confirm or refute the presence of a suspected carcinogenic hazard. When claims were made that fluroide added to drinking water was causing excess cancer in the U.S., studies were mounted in which counties or cities with a high natural or artificial fluoride content in their water supplies were matched with control areas so that comparisons of cancer death rates could be made (Hoover *et al.* 1976; Erickson 1978; Rogot *et al.* 1978). Allowance was made for socio-economic and demographic variables that were known to be geographically associated with incidence, and no evidence was found for a carcinogenic role of fluoride, either in these studies or in a series of smaller areal-case-control investigations conducted elsewhere in the world (Kinlen 1975; Goodhall and Foster 1980; Cook-Mozaffari *et al.* 1981). A similar approach is being used to search for any possible indication of increased cancer risk in the vicinity of nuclear establishments (other than Sellafield) in England and Wales (Baron 1984; Cook-Mozaffari *et al.* 1985). The work that has already been done around Sellafield is enigmatic in that geographical analyses of mortality and incidence data suggest that there may be an increased rate of leukaemia amoung persons under the age of 25 (Yorkshire Television 1983; Gardner and Winter 1984). On the other hand, accumulated knowledge of the amount of radiation necessary to cause an excess incidence, together with generous estimation of the exposure levels that could have been received by children in the area, suggest that discharges from the reprocessing plant could not have been responsible for an increase (Black 1984).

The way forward

In the above partial account I have attempted to illustrate how the spread of geographical knowledge of the diverse patterns of cancer incidence, made possible both by painstaking record-keeping by medical staff throughout the world and by advances in skills for eliminating spurious variations caused by different levels of medical care or different fashions of diagnosis, has made a dual contribution to the progress of cancer research. The constant posing of the question, 'Why this distribution pattern?' has stimulated fruitful hypotheses of causation, and the background knowledge of 'what is happening where?' has helped in the elimination of ill-conceived theories. Although there is now a certain predictability in the cancer patterns that will emerge for different territories, there is scope still for further contributions to knowledge of incidence patterns. Much of the Middle East, India, South-East Asia and South America are still uncharted territory. For the Soviet Union data are available only for selected types of cancer and only for whole Republics (Napalkov *et al.* 1982).

It is clear from the history of cancer registration that the combined effort of a few enthusiasts serving a particular community can in the space of a few years put another point on the cancer map. The work in Uganda during the 1950s and 1960s is an outstanding example of what can be done in this respect (Templeton 1973). The work elsewhere in Africa and in Iran shows that useful information can be forthcoming without waiting for the improvements in medical services necessary for conventional cancer registration. Almost certainly, foci of high incidence remain to be discovered in many parts of the world; foci such as those that occur for cancers of the renal pelvis and ureter in Bulgaria, Yugoslavia, and Rumania in association with Balkan nephropathy and whose origin is still under investigation (Radovanovic 1979; Radovanovic and Peric 1979) or such as the foci for pleural mesotheliomas that occur among villagers in Turkey who are exposed to zeolite fibres from stone dust in houses hewn from the local rocks (Baris *et al.* 1981).

In countries where relatively good data already exist there is still a need for it to be made more accessible and for making it yield more abundantly. For example, the postcoding of addresses on death certificates or incidence files in England and Wales may facilitate the delineation of regions that maximize incidence differences for particular types of cancer rather than reflecting the arbitrary division of the countryside by administrators and planners. In conjunction, demographic and socio-economic data from the most recent national census can be marshalled into almost any regional framework, although a number of 'interfaces' remain before this can be done at the push of a button. This possibility of recombining cancer data and demographic and socio-economic data into new groupings should be of value in highlighting unsuspected risks, perhaps of industrial origin, by making it possible to answer with greater specificity 'Why this pattern of occurrence?'.

In the search for aetiological hypotheses to explain the patterns of distribution that have been observed, the greater emphasis in recent years on quantification of variables that closely affect human populations or that have expression in physiological markers may mean that it is increasingly difficult to find ready-made data sources that give information for the comparisons that are considered desirable. Nonetheless, certain broad inter-country correlations of this kind have been possible (Armstrong and Doll 1975; Gray *et al.* 1979) and the International Agency for Research on Cancer has launched programmes to ensure optimal use of such information as is available by collecting together and computerizing the results of dietary intake surveys from different parts of the world (Agthe 1981) and by establishing the whereabouts of existing collections of human biological material that could be used for international comparisons (Lenoir *et al.* 1983). However, existing data sources may well have defects that limit their usefulness. They are likely, for example, to have been collected for a population group, such as blood donors, that is not typical of the general population. Under these circumstances, the only fruitful approach may be to conduct surveys that are specifically designed to investigate population differences in areas of differing incidence. The report of the population surveys conducted in Iran (Iran – International Agency for Research on Cancer Joint Study Group 1977) was subtitled 'a prodrome', pointing the way, it was hoped, to the kind of breadth of knowledge that it is desirable to acquire as a preliminary to more specific case-control or cohort studies.

In the exploitation of geographical differences to test particular hypotheses, the study of sample population groups is gradually becoming an established epidemiological technique. A detailed investigation has been made, for example, on the extent to which the known risk factors (age at menarche, age at first full-term pregnancy, age at menopause, and postmenopausal weight) could explain the large differences in breast cancer incidence between women in Japan and U.S. white women (Pike *et al*. 1983). Population studies are continuing to be used to explore the roles of aflatoxin consumption and hepatitis B infection in the aetiology of primary liver cancer, with a survey, for example, in regions of differing incidence in Swaziland (Muños and Peers 1983), while for gastric cancer, studies have been taking place to assess dietary intake, and, in particular, the intake of nitrates, in areas of high and low incidence in Japan (Kamiyama 1983), and in England and Wales (Forman *et al*. 1984).

References

Agthe, C. (1981). *Surveillance of environmental aspects related to cancer in humans* (SEARCH), pp. 49–50. IARC Annual Report. IARC, Lyon.

Alpert, M.E., Hutt, M.S.R., Wogan, G.N., *et al*. (1971). Association between aflatoxin content of food and hepatoma frequency in Uganda. *Cancer* **28**, 253–60.

Armstrong, B. and Doll, R. (1975). Environmental factors and cancer incidence and mortality in different countries, with special reference to dietary practices. *Int. J. Cancer* **15**, 617–31.

Bagshawe, A.F., Gacengi, D.M., Cameron, C.H., Dorman, J., and Dane, D.S. (1975). Hepatitis Bs antigen and liver cancer. *Brit. J. Cancer* **31**, 581–4.

Baris, Y., Saracci, R., Simonato, L., Skidmore, J., and Artvinli, M. (1981). An epidemiological and environmental investigation of malignant mesothelioma and radiological chest abnormalities in two villages of central Turkey. *Lancet* **i**, 984–7.

Baron, J. (1984). Cancer mortality in small areas around nuclear facilities in England and Wales. *Brit. J. Cancer* **50**, 815–24.

Bersohn, I., Mcnab, G.M., Pyzikowska, J., and Kew, M.C. (1974). The prevalence of hepatitis B (Australia) antigen in southern Africa. *S. Afr. med. J.* **48**, 941–4.

Bhatt, T., Coombs, M., and O'Neill, C. (1984). Biogenic silica fibre promotes carcinogenesis in mouse skin. *Int. J. Cancer* **34**, 519–28.

Biggar, R.J. and Nkrumah, F.K. (1979). Burkitt's lymphoma in Ghana: urban-rural distrbution, time-space clustering and seasonality. *Int. J. Cancer* **23**, 330–6.

Black, Sir Douglas (1984). *Investigation of the possible increased incidence of cancer in West Cumbria*. Report of the Independent Advisory Group. HMSO, London.

Blot, W.J., Fraumeni, J.F., Mason, T.J., and Hoover, R.N. (1979). Developing clues to environmental cancer: a stepwise approach with the use of cancer mortality data. *Environ. Hlth Perspec.* **32**, 53–8.

Bradshaw, E., McGlashan, N.D., Fitzgerald, D., and Harington, J.S. (1982). Analyses of cancer incidence in black gold miners from Southern Africa. (1964–79). *Brit. J. Cancer* **46**, 737–48.

Bradshaw, E., McGlashan, N.D., and Harington, J.S. (1983). *Oesophageal cancer: smoking and drinking in Transkei*. Occasional paper No. 27, Institute for Social and Economic Research, Rhodes University, Grahamstown, South Africa.

Brubaker, G., Geser, A., and Pike, M.C. (1973). Burkitt's lymphoma in the North Mara District of Tanzania 1964–70; failure to find evidence of time-space clustering in a high-risk isolated rural area. *Brit. J. Cancer* **28**, 469–72.

Burbank, F. (1971). *Patterns in cancer mortality in the United States 1950–67.* National Cancer Institute Monograph Vol. 33: NCI, Washington DC.

Burkitt, D.P. (1962a). A 'tumour safari' in East and Central Africa. *Brit. J. Cancer* **16**, 379–86.

Burkitt, D.P. (1962b). Determining the climatic limits of a children's cancer common in Africa. *Brit. med. J.* **ii**, 1019–23.

Burkitt, D.P. (1969). Etiology of Burkitt's lymphoma. An alternative hypothesis to a vectored virus. *J. nat. Cancer Inst.* **42**, 19–28.

Burkitt, D.P. (1971). Epidemiology of cancer of the colon and rectum. *Cancer* **28**, 1–13.

Burkitt, D.P., Hutt, M.S.R., and Slavin, G. (1968). Clinicopathological studies of cancer distribution in Africa. *Brit. J. Cancer* **22**, 1–6.

Burrell, R.J.W. (1962). Esophageal cancer among Bantu in the Transkei. *J. nat. Cancer Inst.* **28**, 495–514.

Butler, W.H. (1970). Liver injury induced by aflatoxin. *Prog. Liv. Dis.* **3**, 408–18.

Cameron Blair, M. (1923). Freedom of Negro Races from Cancer (letter). *Brit. med. J.* **ii**, 130–1.

Canadian Government Publishing Centre (1980). *Mortality atlas of Canada*, Vol. 1: *Cancer*.

Chen, K-P., Wu, H-Y., Yen, C-C., and Cheng, Y.J. (1979). *Colour atlas of cancer mortality by administrative and other classified districts in Taiwan area; 1968–76.* National Science Council Special Publication No. 3, Taiwan.

Chinese Academy of Medical Sciences (1981). *Atlas of cancer mortality in the People's Republic of China*. China Map Press, Beijing.

Clemmensen, J. (1950). Conference on Geographical Pathology and Demography of Cancer, Oxford, 1950. Preliminary Report. *J. nat. Cancer Inst.* **11**, 627–62.

Clemmensen, J. (1965). *Statistical Studies in the Aetiology of Malignant Neoplasms*, Vol. 1: *Review and Results*. Munksgaard, Copenhagen.

Cook, A.R. (1901). Disease patterns in Uganda. *J. trop. Med. Hyg.* **4**, 175–8.

Cook, P. (1968). 'The setting up of new cancer registries'. Paper presented at a meeting on Sources of Cancer Statistics, IARC, Lyon.

Cook, P. (1971). Cancer of the oesophagus in Africa. *Brit. J. Cancer* **25**, 853–880.

Cook, P.J. and Burkitt, D.P. (1971). Cancer in Africa. *Brit. med. Bull.* **27**, 14–20.

Cook-Mozaffari, P. and Burkitt, D.P. (1985). Cancer in Africa. (In preparation.)

Cook-Mozaffari, P. and van Rensburg, Schalk. (1984). Cancer of the liver. *Brit. med. Bull.* **40**, 342–5.

Cook-Mozaffari, P.J., Azordegan, F., Day, N.E., Ressicaud, A., Sabai, C., and Aramesh, B. (1979). Oesophageal cancer studies in the Caspian Littoral of Iran: results of a case-control study. *Brit. J. Cancer* **39**, 293–309.

Cook-Mozaffari, P., Bulusu, L., and Doll, R. (1981). Fluoridation of water supplies and cancer mortality I: a search for an effect in the U.K. on risk of death from cancer. *J. Epidemiol. Comm. Hlth* **35**, 227–32.

Cook-Mozaffari, P.J., Alderson, M.R., Forster, F., *et al.* (1985). An investigation of cancer incidence and mortality in the vicinity of nuclear establishments in England and Wales. (In preparation.)

Cook, P.J., Doll, R., and Fellingham, S.A. (1969). A mathematical model for the age distribution of cancer in man. *Int. J. Cancer* **4**, 93–112.

Crespi, M., Muños, N., Garsii, A., Aramesh, B., Amiri, G., Mojtakai, A., and Casale, V. (1979). Oesophageal lesions in northern Iran: a pre-malignant condition. *Lancet* **ii**, 217–22.

Davies, J.N.P., Elmes, S., Hutt, M.S.R., Mtimavalye, L.A.R., Owor, R., and Shaper, L. (1964). Cancer in an African community, 1897–1956. An analysis of the records of Mengo Hospital, Kampala, Uganda. *Brit. med. J.* **1**, 259–64.

Day, N.E. (1976). A new measure of standardised incidence, the cumulative rate. In: Waterhouse *et al.* (1976) (*op. cit.*), pp. 443–5.

Day, N.E. (1980) (ed.). Contaminants of wheat samples from the Turkoman area of Iran. In *Etiology of oesophageal cancer in the Caspian Littoral of Iran*, pp. 15–17, Annex 1. Final Report to the NCI (Contract No. NCI CP 71048). IARC, Lyon.

Day, N.E. and Muir, C.S. (1973). Aetiological clues from epidemiology. *Modern trends in oncology* (ed. R.W. Raven), Vol. 1, Butterworths, London.

Day, N.E. and Muños, N. (1982). Esophagus. In Schottenfeld and Fraumeni (*op. cit*), pp. 596–623.

Day, N.E., Muños, N., and Ghadirian, P. (1982). Epidemiology of oesophageal cancer; a review. In *Epidemiology of cancer of the digestive tract* (ed. P. Correa and W. Haenzel). Martinus Nyhoff, The Hague.

de Jong, U.W., Breslow, N., Goh Ewe Hong, J., Sridharan, M., and Shannugaratnam, K. (1974). Aetiological factors in oesophageal cancer in Singapore Chinese. *Int. J. Cancer* **13**, 291–303.

de Mangeon, A. (1927). *Iles Brittaniques*. In *Geographie universelle*, 1er Tome. Libraire Armand Colin, Paris.

de Thé, G., Geser, A., Day, N.E. *et al.* (1982). Epidemiological evidence for a causal relationship between Epstein–Barr virus and Burkitt's lymphoma from Ugandan prospective study. *Nature, Lond.* **274**, 756–61.

de Waard, F. (1969). The epidemiology of breast cancer; review and prospects. *Int. J. Cancer* **4**, 577–86.

Dodge, O.G. and Linsell, C.A. (1963). Carcinoma of the penis in Uganda and Kenya Africans. *Cancer* **16**, 1255–63.

Doll, R. (1959) (ed.) *Methods of geographical pathology*. Blackwell Scientific Publications, Oxford.

Doll, R. (1967). *Prevention of cancer: pointers from epidemiology*. The Nuffield Provincial Hospitals Trust.

Doll, R. (1969). The geographical distribution of cancer. *Brit. J. Cancer* **23**, 1–8.

Doll, R. (1971). Oesophageal cancer: a preventable disease? International Seminar on Epidemiology of Oesophageal Cancer, Bangalore, India, sponsored by the Indian Cancer Society and the International Union against Cancer.

Doll, R. and Cook, P. (1967). Summarising indices for comparison of cancer incidence data. *Int. J. Cancer* **2**, 269–79.

Doll, R., Payne, P., and Waterhouse, J. (1966) (eds). *Cancer incidence in five continents*, Vol. I. Springer-Verlag, Berlin.

Doll, R., Muir, C., and Waterhouse, J. (1970) (eds). *Cancer incidence in five continents*, Vol II. Springer-Verlag, Berlin.

Dunham, L.J. and Bailar, J.C. (1968). World maps of cancer mortality rates and frequency ratios. *J. nat. Cancer Inst.* **41**, 155–203.

Erickson, J.D. (1978). Mortality in selected cities with fluoridated and non-fluoridated water supplies. *New Engl. J. Med.* **298**, 1112–6.

Forman, D., Al Dabbagh, S., and Doll, R. (1985). Nitrates, nitrites and gastric cancer in Great Britain. *Nature, Lond.* **313**, 620–5.

Gardner, M.J. and Winter, P.D. (1984). Mortality in Cumberland during 1959–78 with reference to cancer in young people around Windscale. *Lancet* **i**, 216–17.

Gardner, M.J., Winter, P.D., Taylor, C.P., and Acheson, E.D. (1983). *Atlas of cancer mortality in England and Wales, 1968–78*. Wiley, Chichester.

Ghadirian, P. (1982). An epidemiological study of oesophageal cancer with particular reference to northern Iran. PhD. Thesis, University of London.

Goodhall, C.M. and Foster, F.H. (1980). Fluoridation and cancer mortality in New Zealand. *New Zealand med. J.* **92**, 164–7.

Gray, G.E., Pike, M.C., and Henderson, B.E. (1979). Breast cancer incidence and mortality rates in different countries in relation to known risk factors and dietary practices. *Brit. J. Cancer* **39**, 1–7.

Harington, J.S., McGlashan, N.D., Bradshaw, E., Geddes, E.W., and Purves, L.R. (1975). A spatial and temporal analysis of four cancers in African gold miners from southern Africa. *Brit. J. Cancer* **31**, 665–78.

Hewer, T., Rose, E., Ghadirian, P., Castegnaro, H., Melveille, C., Bartsch, H., and Day, N.E. (1978). Ingested mutagens from opium and tobacco pyrolysis products and cancer of the oesophagus. *Lancet* **ii**, 494–6.

Higginson, J. (1969). Present trends in cancer epidemiology. In *Proceedings on the eighth Canadian Cancer Research Conference, Ontario 1968* (ed. J.F. Morgan), pp. 40–75. Pergamon Press, Oxford.

Hill, A.B. (1937). *Principles of medical statistics. The Lancet*, London.

Hirayama, T. (1971). An epidemiological study of cancer of the oesophagus in Japan, with special reference to the combined effect of selected environmental factors. International Seminar on Epidemiology of Oesphageal Cancer, Bangalore, India, sponsored by the Indian Cancer Society and the International Union against Cancer.

Hollander, B. (1923). Freedom of Negro Races from cancer (letter). *Brit. med. J.* **ii**, 46.

Hoover, R.N., McKay, F.W., and Fraumeni, J.F. (1976). Fluoridated drinking water and the occurrence of cancer. *J. nat. Cancer Inst.* **57**, 757–68.

Hormozdiari, H., Day, N.E., Aramesh, B., and Mahboubi, E. (1975). Dietary factors and oesophageal cancer in the Caspian Littoral of Iran. *Cancer Res.* **35**, 3493–8.

Howe, G.M. (1970). *National atlas of disease mortality in the United Kingdom* (2nd edn). Royal Geographical Society, Nelson, London.

International Agency for Research on Cancer (1968). Internal report of a conference held to discuss future plans for research into the aetiology of cancer in the oesophagus.

International Agency for Research on Cancer (1975). *Annual report*. IARC, Lyon.

International Agency for Research on Cancer (1976). *Annual report*. IARC, Lyon.

Iran – International Agency for Reseach on Cancer Joint Study Group (1977). Oesophageal cancer studies in the Caspian Littoral of Iran: results of population studies – a prodrome. *J. nat. Cancer Inst.* **59**, 1127–38.

Jarrett, W.F., McNeil, P.E., Grimshaw, W.T., Selman, I.E., and McIntyre, W.I. (1978). High incidence area of cattle cancer with a possible interaction between an environmental carcinogen and a papilloma virus. *Nature, Lond.* **274**, 215–7.

Kamiyama, S. (1983). *Regional differences in stomach cancer mortality and dietary mutagenicity. Directory of on-going research in cancer epidemiology*, IARC Scientific Publications No. 50. IARC, Lyon.

Kaplan, H.S. and Tsuchitani, P.J. (1978) (eds). *Cancer in China*. Alan R. Liss, New York.

King, H. and Locke, F.B. (1980). Cancer mortality among Chinese in the United States. *J. nat. Cancer Inst.* **65**, 1141–8.

Kinlen, L. (1975). Cancer incidence in relation to fluoride level in water supplies.

Brit. dent. J. **138**, 221–4.

Kmet, J. and Mahboubi, E. (1972). Oesophageal cancer in the Caspian Littoral of Iran: initial studies. *Science, N.Y.* **175**, 846–53.

Kmet, J., McLaren, D.S., and Siassi, F. (1980). Epidemiology of oesophageal cancer with specific reference to nutritional studies among Turkoman of Iran. In *Advances in modern human nutrition*, Vol. 1, pp. 343–65 (ed. R.B. Tobin and M.A. Mehlman). Pathotox, Ill., U.S.A.

Knowelden, J. and Oettlé, A.G. (1962). *Report of the African sub-committee on geographic pathology of the International Union Against Cancer.* UICC, cited by Davies, J.N.P., Wilson, B.A., and Knowelden, J. (1962). Cancer Incidence of the African population of Kyadondo (Uganda). *Lancet* **ii**, 328–30.

Kolycheva, N.I. (1980). Epidemiology of oesophageal cancer in the U.S.S.R. In *Cancer epidemiology in the U.S.A. and U.S.S.R.* (ed. D. Levin) pp. 191–7. NIH Publication No. 80–2044. Department of Health and Human Services, Washington.

Lacey, J. and Booth, C. (1980). Microbiological studies of cereal grains and other foodstuffs. In *Etiology of esophageal cancer in the Caspian Littoral of Iran* (ed. N.E. Day). Final Report to the NCI Annex G. (Contract No. NCI-CP-71048). IARC, Lyon.

Lanier, A.P., Bender, T.R., Blot, W.J. *et al.* (1976). Cancer incidence in Alaskan natives. *Int. J. Cancer* **18**, 409–12.

Lenoir, G., Walker, A., Sohier, R., and Tulinius, H. (1983). *Survey of existing collections of human biological material*, pp.122–3. IARC Annual Report. IARC, Lyon.

Linsell, C.A. and Martyn, R. (1962). The Kenya Cancer Registry. *E. Afr. med. J.* **39**, 642–8.

Mahboubi, E., Kmet, J., Cook, P.J. *et al.* (1973). Oesophageal cancer studies in the Caspian Littoral of Iran: the Caspian Cancer Registry. *Brit. J. Cancer* **28**, 192–214.

Martinez, I. (1969). Factors associated with cancer of the oesophagus, mouth and pharynx in Puerto Rico. *J. nat. Cancer Inst.* **42**, 1069–94.

Mason, T.J., McKay, F.W., Hoover, R., Blot, W.J., and Fraumeni, J.F. (1975). *Atlas of cancer mortality for U.S. counties 1950–69.* DHEW Publication No. 75–780. U.S. Government Printing Office, Washington.

Mason, T.J., McKay, F.W., Hoover, R., Blot, W.J., and Fraumeni, J.F. (1976). *Atlas of cancer mortality studies among U.S. non-whites: 1950–1969.* DHEW Publication No. 76–1204. U.S. Government Printing Office, Washington.

May, J.M. (1958). *The ecology of human disease.* MD Publications Inc., New York.

Merkova, A.M., Tserkovnogo, G.F., and Kaufman, B.D. (1963). *Morbidity and mortality from malignant neoplasms in the U.S.S.R.* English edn. (ed. J.G. Dean). Pitman Medical, London.

Morrow, R.H. (1982). Burkitt's lymphoma. In Schottenfeld and Fraumeni (1982). (*op. cit.*), pp. 779–94.

Morrow, R.H., Kisuule, A., and Mafigiri, J. (1974). Socio-economic factors in Burkitt's lymphoma. *Cancer Res.* **34**, 1212.

Morrow, R.H., Kisuule, A., Pike, M.C. *et al.* (1976). Burkitt's lymphoma in the Mengo Districts of Uganda. Epidemiologic features and their relationship to malaria. *J. nat. Cancer Inst.* **56**, 479–83.

Morrow, R.H., Pike, M.C. and Smith, P.G. (1977). Further studies of space-time clustering of Burkitt's lymphoma in Uganda. *Brit. J. Cancer* **35**, 668–73.

Muños, N. (1982). Oesophageal cancer. In *Annual report*. IARC, Lyon.

Muños, N., Crespi, M., Grassi, A., Qinq, W.G., Qiong, S., and Cai, L.Z. (1982). Precursor lesions of oesophageal cancer in high-risk populations in Iran and China. *Lancet* **i**, 876–9.

Muños, N. and Peers, F.G. (1983). *Aflatoxin and hepatitis B studies in Swaziland*, pp. 48–9. IARC Annual Report. IARC, Lyon.

Napalkov, N.P., Tserkovny, G.F., Merabishviti, V.M., Parkin, D.M., Smans, M., and Muir, C.S. (1982). *Cancer incidence in the U.S.S.R.* IARC Scientific Publications No. 48. IARC, Lyon.

Netherlands Centraal Bureau voor de Statistiek. (1980). *Atlas of cancer mortality in the Netherlands*. Netherlands Central Bureau of Statistics, The Hague.

Nielsen, N.H., Mikkelsen, F., and Hensen, J.P.H. (1977). Nasopharyngeal carcinoma in Greenland. The incidence in an artic Eskimo population. *Acta pathol. microbiol. Scand.* **85A**, 850–8.

Oettlé, A.G. (1963). Regional variations in the frequency of Bantu oesophageal cancer cases admitted to hospitals in South Africa. *S. Afr. med. J.* **37**, 434–9.

Oettlé, A.G. (1964). Cancer in Africa, especially in regions south of the Sahara. *J. nat. Cancer Inst.* **33**, 383–437.

Oettlé, A.G. (1967). Primary neoplasms of the alimentary canal in Whites and Bantu of the Transvaal, 1949–53. In *Tumours of the alimentary tract in Africans*. National Cancer Institute Monograph, Vol. 25, pp. 97–110. NCI, Washington.

O'Neill, C.H., Hodges, G.M., Riddle, P.N., Jordan, P.N., Newman, R.H., Flood, R.J., and Toulson, E.C. (1980). A fine fibrous silica contaminant of flour in the high oesophageal cancer area of northern Iran. *Int. J. Cancer* **26**, 617–28.

Office of Population Censuses and Surveys (1979–83). *Cancer statistics, registrations*. Series MBI, Nos 1–12. HMSO, London.

Peers, F.G., Gilman, G.A., and Linsell, C.A. (1976). Dietary aflatoxin and human liver cancer. A study in Swaziland. *Int. J. Cancer* **17**, 167–76.

Peers, F.G. and Linsell, C.A. (1973). Dietary aflatoxins and liver cancer. A population-based study in Kenya. *Brit. J. Cancer* **27**, 473–84.

Pike, M.C., Williams, E.H., and Wright, B. (1967). Burkitt's tumour in the West Nile District of Uganda, 1961–65. *Brit. med. J.* **ii**, 395–9.

Pike, M.C., Krailo, M.D., Henderson, B.E., Casagrande, J.T., and Hoel, D.G. (1983). 'Hormonal' risk factors, 'breast tissue age' and the incidence of breast cancer. *Nature, Lond.* **303**, 767–70.

Pottern, L.M., Morris, L.E., Blot, W.J., Zieglar, R.G., and Fraumeni, J.F. (1981). Oesophageal cancer among black men in Washington, D.C. 1 – Alcohol tobacco and other risk factors. *J. nat. Cancer Inst.* **67**, 777–83.

Prasad, A.S. and Oberleas, D. (1974). Zinc deficiency in man. *Lancet* **i**, 463–4.

Radovanovic, Z. (1979). Topographical distribution of Balkan endemic nephropathy in Serbia (Yugoslavia). *Trop. geogr. Med.* **31**, 185–9.

Radovanovic, Z. and Peric, J. (1979). Hydrogeological characteristics of endemic nephropathy foci. *Publ. Hlth Lond.* **93**, 76–81.

Research Committee on Geographical Distribution of Diseases (1981). *National atlas of major disease mortalities in cities, towns and villages in Japan.* Jiji Press, Tokyo.

Rogot, E., Sharrett, A.R., Feinleib, M., and Fabitz, R.R. (1978). Trends in urban mortality in relation to fluoridation levels. *Amer. J. Epidemiol.* **107**, 104–12.

Rose, E.F. (1973). Esophageal cancer in Transkei: 1955–69. *J. nat. Cancer Inst.* **51**, 7–16.

Rose, E.F., and McGlashan, N.D. (1975). The spatial distribution of oesophageal carcinoma in the Transkei, South Africa. *Brit. J. Cancer* **31**, 197–206.

Rose, E.F. and Fellingham, S.A. (1981). Cancer patterns in Transkei. *S. Afr. J. Science* **77**, 555–61.

Schonland, M. and Bradshaw, E. (1969). Oesophageal cancer in Natal Bantu: a review of 516 cases. *S. Afr. med. J.* **43**, 1029–31.

Schottenfeld, D. and Fraumeni, J.F. (1982) (eds). *Cancer epidemiology and prevention.* Saunders, Philadelphia.

Segi, M. (1960). *Cancer mortality for selected sites in 24 countries: 1950–57.* Department of Public Health, Tohuku University School of Medicine, Sendai.

Segi, M. (1975). Tea gruel as a possible factor for cancer of the oesophagus. *Gann* **66**, 199–202.

Segi, M. (1981). *Age adjusted death rates for cancer for selected sites (A-Classification) in 40 countries in 1976.* Segi Institute of Cancer Epidemiology, Nagoya.

Sinnhuber, R.O., Wales, J.H., Ayres, J.L. *et al.* (1968). Dietary factors and hepatoma in rainbow trout (*Salmo gardneiri*). 1. Aflatoxins in vegetable protein foodstuffs. *J. nat. Cancer Inst.* **41**, 711–18.

Stamp, D. (1964). *Some aspects of medical geography.* Oxford University Press, London.

Stocks, P. (1936). *Distribution in England and Wales of cancer in various organs,* pp. 239–80. Thirteenth Annual Report of the British Empire Cancer Campaign.

Stocks, P. (1937). *Distribution in England and Wales of cancer of various organs,* pp. 198–223. Fourteenth Annual Report of the British Empire Cancer Campaign.

Stocks, P. (1939). *Distribution in England and Wales of cancer of various organs,* pp. 308–343. Sixteenth Annual Report of the British Empire Cancer Campaign.

Stocks, P. (1950). *Cancer registration in England and Wales: an enquiry into treatment and its results.* General Register Office: Studies on Medical and Population Subjects, No. 3. HMSO, London.

Stocks, P. (1957). *Cancer incidence in North Wales and Liverpool regions in relation to habits and environment,* Supplement 11, pp. 1–156. British Empire Cancer Campaign Annual Report.

Stocks, P. and Davies, R.I. (1964). Zinc and copper content of soils associated with the incidence of cancer of the stomach and other organs. *Brit. J. Cancer* **18**, 14.

Templeton, A.C. (1973) (ed.). *Tumours in a tropical country: a survey of Uganda, 1964–68.* Springer-Verlag, New York.

Tuyns, A.J., Loubiere, R., and Duvernet-Battest, F. (1971). Regional variations in primary liver cancer in Ivory Coast. *J. nat. Cancer Inst.* **47**, 131–5.

Tuyns, A.J., Pequignat, G., and Jensen, O.M. (1977). Le cancer de l'oesophage en Ile et Vilaine en function de niveaus de consummation d'alcohol et de tabac. Des risques qui se multiplient. *Bull. Cancer* **64**, 45–60.

Tuyns, A.J., Pequignat, G., and Abbatucci, J.S. (1979). Oesophageal cancer and alcohol consumption: importance of type of beverage. *Inst. J. Cancer* **23**, 443–7.

van Rensburg, S.J. (1981). Epidemiologic and dietary evidence for a specific nutritional predisposition to esophageal cancer. *J. nat. Cancer Inst.* **67**, 243–51.

van Rensburg, S.J. (1982). Perspectives on risk factors for hepatocellular carcinoma. In: *Proceedings of the Thirteenth International Cancer Congress,* p. 341. UICC, Seattle.

van Rensburg, S.J., Cook-Mozaffari, P., van Schalkwyk, D.J., van der Watt, J.J.

Vincent, T.J., and Purchase, I.F.H. (1985). Hepatocellular carcinoma and dietary aflatoxin in Mozambique and Transkei.

van Rensburg, S.J., van der Watt, J.J., and Purchase, I.F.H. (1974). Primary liver cancer rate and aflatoxin intake in a high cancer area. *S. Afr. med. J.* **48**, 2508 a–d.

Waterhouse, J., Muir, C., Correa, P., and Powell, J. (1976) (eds). *Cancer incidence in five continents*, Vol. III. IARC Scientific Publications, No. 15, IARC, Lyon.

Waterhouse, J., Muir, C., Shanmugaratnam, K., and Powell, J. (1982) (eds). *Cancer incidence in five Continents*, Vol. IV. IARC Scientific Publications No. 42. IARC, Lyon.

Williams, E.H., Spit, P., and Pike, M.C. (1969). Further evidence of space-time clustering of Burkitt's lymphoma patients in the West Nile District of Uganda. *Brit. J. Cancer* **23**, 235–46.

World Health Organization (1964). *Prevention of Cancer*. World Health Organization Technical Report Series No. 276. WHO, Geneva.

Yorkshire Television. (1983). Windscale – the Nuclear Laundry. Programme shown on ITV on 1 November.

3 Smoking

N. J. Wald

Introduction

Cigarette smoking is securely established as the principal cause of lung cancer in Western countries and it is also becoming the leading cause of lung cancer in an increasing number of economically less developed countries. The basic mechanism by which a normal cell becomes malignant is still unknown. But it is remarkable that so much coherent scientific information about the relationship between smoking and lung cancer has emerged from what can only be a very crude estimate of the extent to which smoke components are deposited on the bronchial epithelium – that is by asking people how many cigarettes they smoke each day.

Epidemiological enquiry has yielded comprehensive information on the dose–response relationship between the amount smoked and the risk of lung cancer, on the effects of duration of exposure assessed independently of the amount smoked, and on the interaction with other pulmonary carcinogens such as asbestos and ionizing radiation. Our knowledge of smoking habits can explain nearly all the differences in the pattern of lung cancer in different communities, between the sexes, and across different age groups and birth cohorts. The evidence incriminating smoking as an important cause of disease has resulted in action which has led to the decline of smoking as a popular habit in the U.K. The epidemic of lung cancer is, as a result, now gradually abating.

In this chapter I make no attempt to review the enormous volume of evidence about cigarette smoking and cancer, which is already well documented. Instead, I have chosen to focus on the trends in cigarette smoking and in mortality from two smoking-associated diseases (lung cancer and coronary heart disease) and to describe some research which I pursued while working with Sir Richard Doll in Oxford. Arising from this description I have tried to draw conclusions that are relevant to future public health policy – particularly concerning whether low-tar cigarettes are less harmful than high-tar cigarettes.

Trends in cigarette smoking in the U.K.

Fig. 1 shows the annual average consumption of manufactured cigarettes

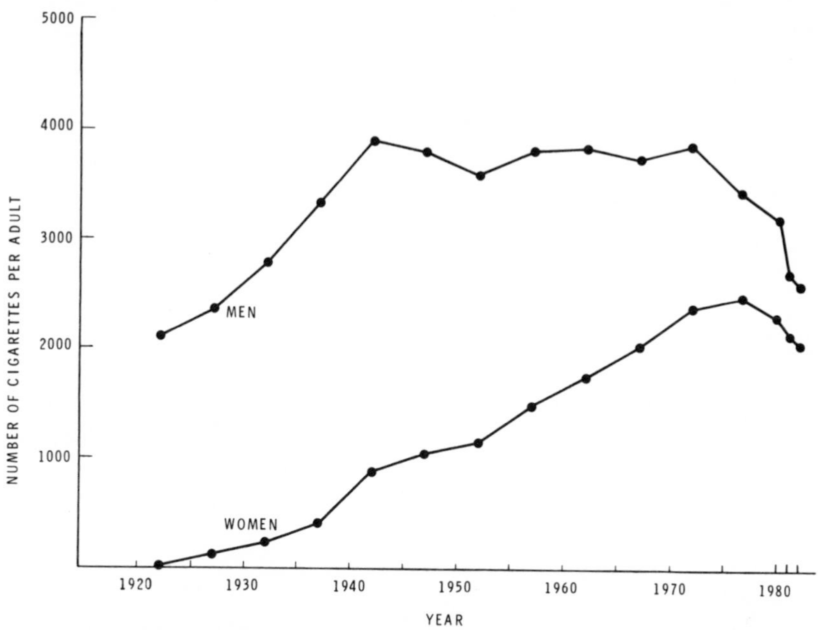

Fig. 1. Annual consumption of cigarettes per adult in the U.K. (data from Tobacco Advisory Council).

per adult in the U.K. from 1920 to 1982. Cigarette consumption among men reached a peak in 1941 (4420 cigarettes per adult male per year), and did not change materially until about 1973 (3980). Thereafter it declined more rapidly to 2600 in 1982 – a fall of 35 per cent. Among women, cigarette consumption increased to a maximum in 1974 (2630 cigarettes per adult female per year) and thereafter declined to 2050 in 1982, a decrease of 22 per cent between 1974 and 1982.

Fig. 2 shows the percentage of smokers of manufactured cigarettes between 1948 and 1982. During this period the proportion of male smokers of manufactured cigarettes declined from 65 per cent to 35 per cent. Among women the percentage rose from 41 per cent to a peak of 45 per cent in 1966, and declined gradually thereafter to 35 per cent in 1982.

Fig. 3 shows the changes in the tar, nicotine, and carbon monoxide yields of U.K.-manufactured cigarettes from 1934 to 1982. The most notable change is the halving in the tar yield over this period. Nicotine yields have declined also, but to a lesser extent, while carbon monoxide yields have not changed much. There is a striking relationship between the prevalence of smoking and social class (see Table 1) and, among smokers, between the smoking of relatively high-tar cigarettes and low social class. In 1980, 20 per cent of men in social groups A and B (professional and managerial)

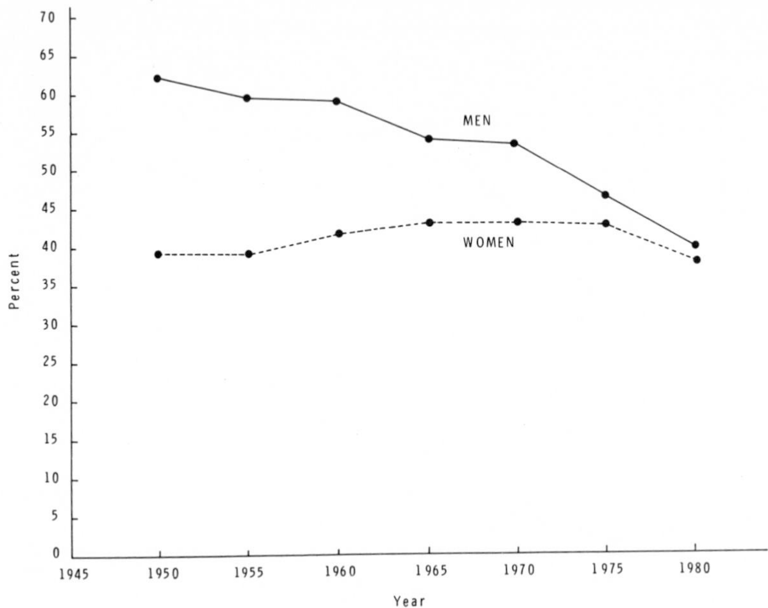

Fig. 2. Prevalence of manufactured-cigarette smoking in the U.K. among adult men and women (data from Tobacco Advisory Council).

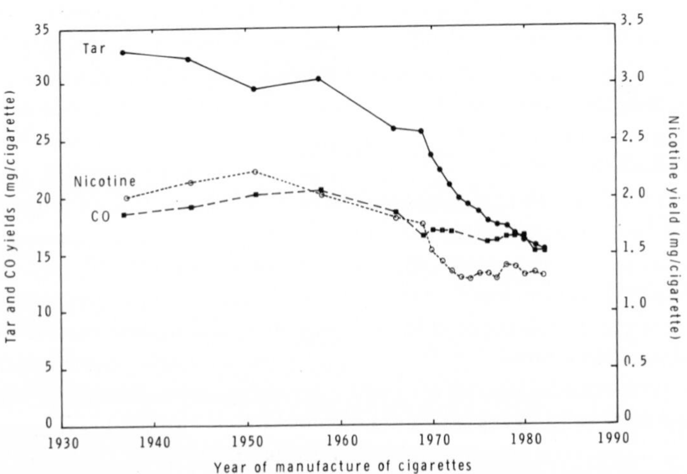

Fig. 3. Sales-weighted tar, nicotine, and carbon monoxide yields of U.K. cigarettes (from Wald *et al.* 1981a).

Table 1. Percentage of adults (16 or more years of age) smoking cigarettes in Britain in 1980 according to social group† and tar yield (source: DHSS)

	Men				Women			
Tar yield per cigarette	AB	C1	C2	DE	AB	C1	C2	DE
⩾ 16 mg	12	26	33	35	14	16	23	26
< 16 mg	6	8	7	8	10	12	13	12
Not known or hand-rolled	2	6	8	12	3	1	1	2
Total	20	40	48	55	27	29	37	40

† Key to social groups:
AB = Higher/intermediate managerial administrative or professional
C1 = Supervisory or clinical and junior managerial, administrative or professional
C2 = Skilled manual workers
DE = Semi- and unskilled manual workers, State pensioners or widows and casual workers

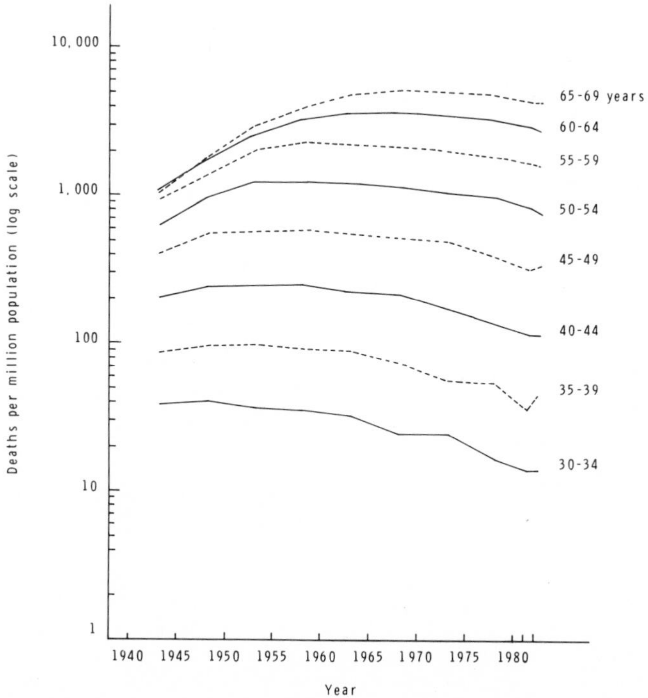

Fig. 4. Lung cancer annual mortality in men in England and Wales: five-year averages except for 1980, 1981, and 1982, which show rates for individual years (from OPCS).

smoked compared with about 55 per cent in social groups D and E (semi- and unskilled workers and unemployed) – the proportion among high-tar cigarettes (⩾ 16 mg) were about 12 per cent and 35 per cent respectively. Similar trends were apparent for women.

Trends in lung cancer mortality in England and Wales

Fig. 4 shows that male lung cancer mortality in England and Wales is now declining in all age groups from 30 to 69 years. Among the younger men, who in recent years have smoked fewer cigarettes and cigarettes yielding less tar than men of the same age in earlier years, the decline has been substantial – about 50 per cent. Lung cancer mortality has increased and is continuing to increase in women aged 55 years or more (see Fig. 5) – the rate more than doubling over the last 30 years. Lung cancer has however, declined in younger women whose consumption has decreased in recent years, both in terms of number of cigarettes smoked and tar delivery. The

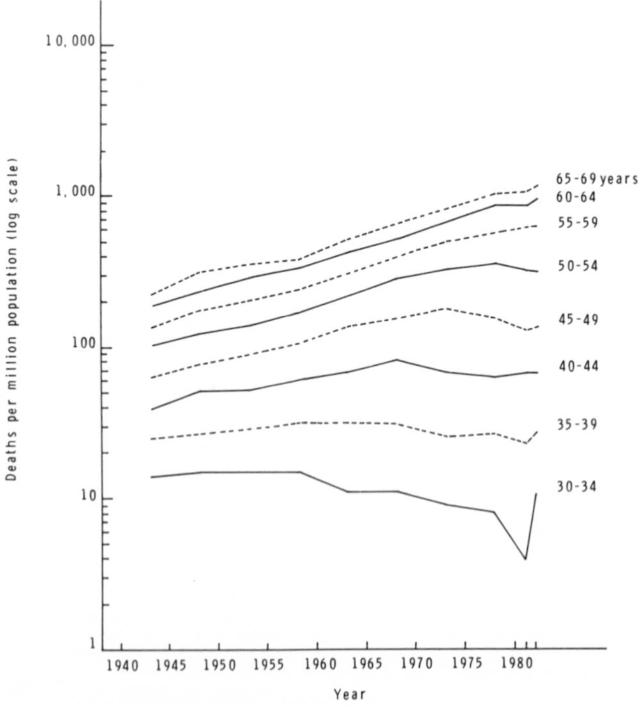

Fig. 5. Lung cancer annual mortality in women in England and Wales: five-year averages except for 1980, 1981, and 1982, which show rates for individual years (from OPCS).

decline started, as it did in men, earlier in younger than in older age groups. (A small 'dip' in the lung cancer rates for 1981 illustrated in Figs. 4 and 5 is unlikely to represent a real change in the mortality rate. It was almost certainly due to industrial action by registration officers in 1981 which meant that some of the information normally requested to aid cause of death coding was unavailable. As a result more deaths than usual were assigned to other categories.)

Trends in coronary heart disease mortality in England and Wales

Figs. 6 and 7 show the mortality rates due to coronary heart disease among men and women in England and Wales from 1955 to 1982. There was an increase in the rates in most age groups until the 1970s and thereafter, perhaps a small decline in both sexes.

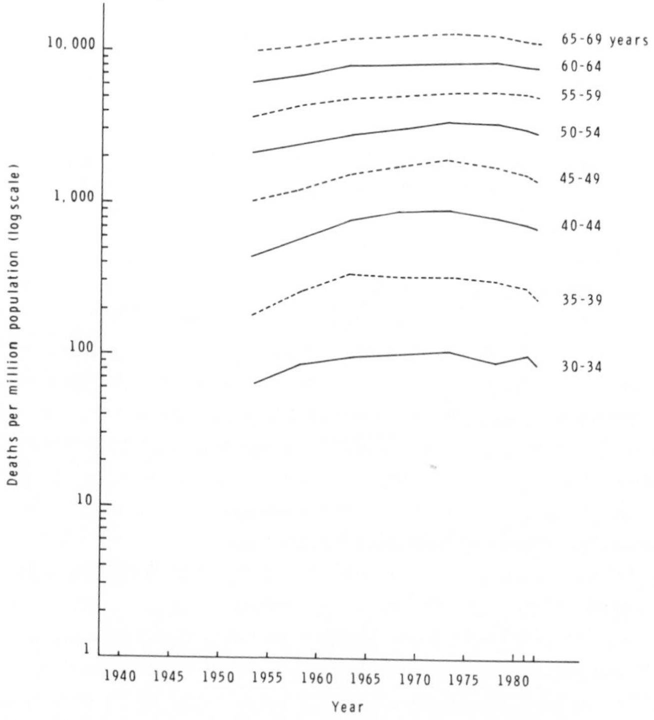

Fig. 6. Coronary heart disease annual mortality in men in England and Wales: five-year averages except for 1980, 1981, and 1982, which shows rates for individual years (from OPCS).

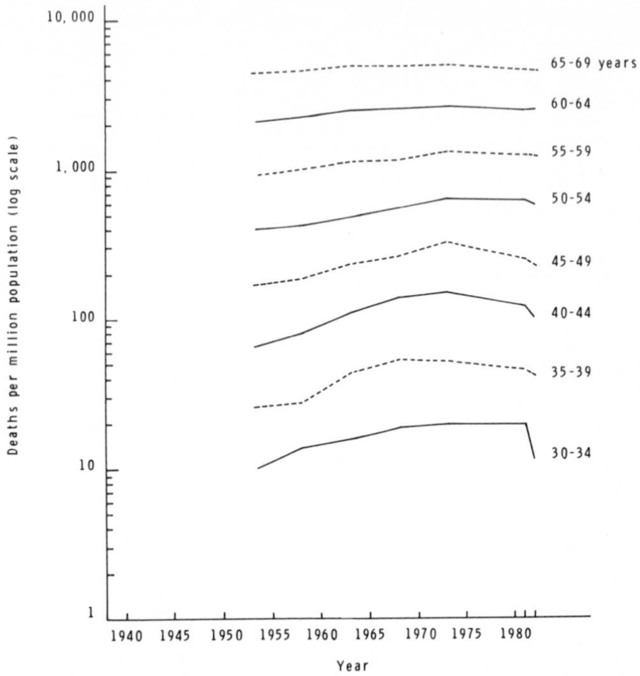

Fig. 7. Coronary heart disease annual mortality in women in England and Wales: five-year averages except for 1980, 1981, and 1982, which show rates for individual years (from OPCS).

National trends in coronary heart disease mortality in England and Wales are not readily interpreted in the light of trends in cigarette consumption but, *overall*, they would not be expected to be so. Unlike the position with lung cancer, smoking is only a contributory cause of coronary heart disease, accounting for a relatively small proportion of the *total* deaths from this condition. It is only in the younger age groups, say, under the age of about 50 years, in which death rates are comparatively low, that the relative risk is high (see Fig. 8). Among persons aged under 50 years coronary heart disease mortality has changed in a way that has to some extent reflected smoking habits; it has increased in parallel with changes in smoking habits in the past and in recent years has declined with them too (Figs 1 and 6). There has not, however, been a reduction in coronary heart disease rates in relation to the decline in sales-weighted tar and nicotine yields. In so far as carbon monoxide yields of cigarettes did not decline appreciably in past decades, and have only done so in recent years, the trends in coronary heart disease mortality among young adults appear to reflect trends in the carbon monoxide yield of cigarettes better than they reflect trends in tar or nicotine yields. However, this evidence incriminating carbon monoxide is weak.

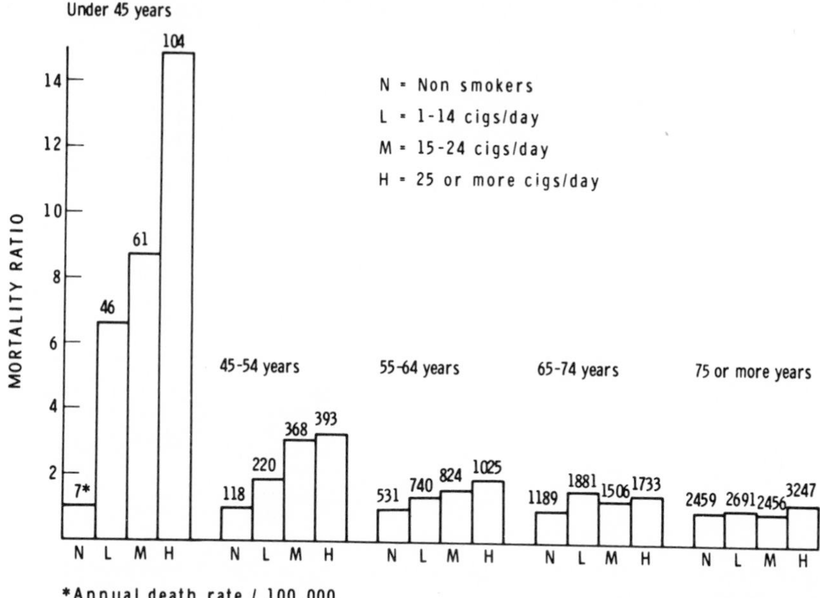

Fig. 8. Coronary heart disease mortality in cigarette smokers compared with coronary heart disease mortality in non-smokers among British male doctors (from Wald 1978).

What component of cigarette smoke causes coronary heart disease?

Data have recently been obtained that tend to exclude nicotine as the toxic agent in cigarette smoke that causes coronary heart disease. Serum levels of cotinine (a principle metabolite of nicotine) in pipe smokers are as high as in cigarette smokers (Fig. 9). Urinary nicotine measurements are also high in pipe smokers (Fig. 10). It is evident therefore that pipe smokers have high systemic nicotine concentrations and since large prospective studies have shown that pipe smokers have no material excess risk of coronary heart disease, but cigarette smokers do, we can be reasonably confident that exposure to high systemic concentrations of nicotine is not an important cause of coronary heart disease. The results cannot however, exclude the possibility that nicotine might exert a toxic effect on the cardiovascular system by a 'pulse' effect – that is through the occurrence of sudden high levels of nicotine as a result of the inhalation of cigarette smoke.

The probable exclusion of nicotine as the major cause of cardiovascular disease in smokers does not mean that the other component of cigarette smoke most often suggested as being involved, carbon monoxide, is the

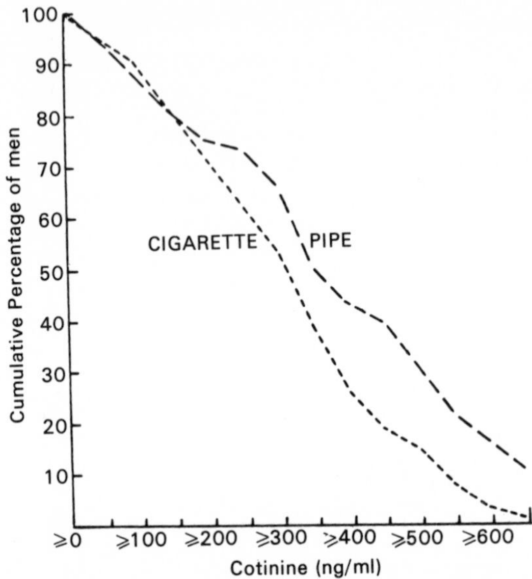

Fig. 9. Distribution of serum cotinine concentrations in cigarette and pipe smokers (from Wald *et al.* 1981b).

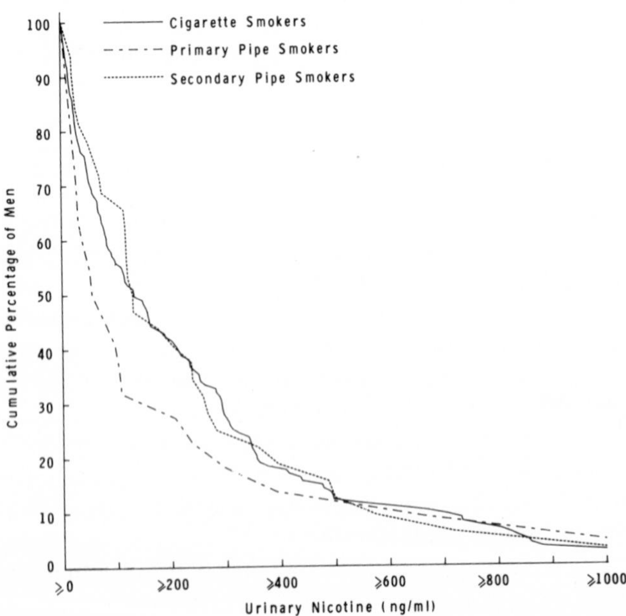

Fig. 10. Distribution of urinary nicotine concentrations in cigarette and pipe smokers. The pipe smokers were classified according to whether they had never smoked cigarettes (primary) or whether they had previously smoked cigarettes (secondary) (from Wald *et al.* 1984c).

cause. The identification of the component of cigarette smoke responsible for the excess risk is one of the most important outstanding questions in the field of smoking research.

Do people smoke to obtain nicotine?

The initiation and maintenance of the smoking habit is a complex process. There is a continuing debate between those who emphasize the social and psychological factors on the one hand, and those who emphasize the pharmacological factors on the other. There is obviously a complex interaction between both groups of factors, but the importance of nicotine in determining national smoking habits may have been exaggerated. Nicotine certainly has a role and perhaps the best recent evidence comes from the randomized clinical trials of the use of nicotine chewing-gum in programmes designed to help people give up smoking. In virtually all of these, the nicotine gum was more effective (and satisfying) than the placebo (Table 2). However, the effect overall appears to be modest and restricted to a relatively small proportion of smokers.

Table 2. Results of randomized controlled trials of nicotine chewing-gum (from Jamrozik *et al.* 1984).

Principal author	Number of subjects	Odds ratio (in favour of nicotine gum)	95 per cent confidence limits
Placebo-controlled studies			
Axelsson	812	0.90	0.66 – 1.23
Puska	229	1.42	0.82 – 2.46
Malcolm	136	4.92	1.53 –15.88
Fagerstrom	100	2.17	0.95 – 4.91
Fee	352	1.53	0.77 – 3.05
Jarvis	116	3.34	1.47 – 7.57
British Thoracic Association	802	0.84	0.53 – 1.31
Schneider	60	1.71	0.52 – 5.62
Hjalmarson	206	2.14	1.09 – 4.20
Jamrozik	200	1.25	0.47 – 3.31
Studies using counselled patients as controls			
Malcolm	137	1.83	0.74 – 4.47
British Thoracic Association	777	1.16	0.71 – 1.90
Russell	1354	2.24	1.41 – 3.55

The trials that have shown the greatest effects have been those performed in special clinics attracting, perhaps, the more pharmacologically dependent smokers whereas, by contrast, in studies performed in general practice the effect was much smaller.

In the U.S. as well as in the U.K., sales-weighted nicotine yields of cigarettes have declined. If nicotine were a major factor influencing national smoking habits one would have expected cigarette consumption to have increased. In fact, in recent years, both in the U.S. and in the U.K., cigarette consumption has declined. In the U.S., more so than in the U.K., a large proportion of smokers now smoke cigarettes with low nicotine deliveries and presumably find them acceptable.

Many studies in the past which focused on nicotine as the substance influencing smoking habits failed to control for the delivery of other cigarette components, such as tar; effects that were observed were often interpreted as being due to nicotine. In fact they could equally well have been due to other factors, such as tar, which were correlated with the nicotine yield of the cigarettes.

Interestingly, in a recent investigation, the inhaling habits of smokers could be no better explained by the nicotine yield of cigarettes than by their tar yield (Wald *et al.* 1981c), and two other investigations have suggested that the tar yield of a cigarette influences the manner of smoking more than the nicotine yield (Sutton *et al.* 1982; Stepney 1981).

The conclusion that emerges from these investigations is that the control of nicotine yields is not critical in the control of cigarette consumption in the community. This means that any policy which advocates maintaining the nicotine yields of cigarettes in order to make them more acceptable may not be necessary. Certainly such a policy of deliberately maintaining nicotine yields at a relatively high level should not be accepted automatically without further supporting evidence. There may, in any case, be a disadvantage in such a policy; maintaining any pharmacological dependence provided by nicotine will make it more difficult for smokers to give up the habit.

Whatever the merits, or otherwise, of maintaining the nicotine yields of cigarettes, consumption can be effectively controlled by public education and by increasing the real price of cigarettes. The latter is widely accepted as being an effective measure, but it is one that has not been effectively implemented. Although in monetary terms cigarettes are now more expensive than in the past (Fig. 11) after taking inflation into account, in 1980 they were at about their cheapest level ever (Fig. 12). Recent tax increases on cigarettes have begun to reverse this trend.

Compensatory smoking

As a result of a productive scientific cooperation with the British United Provident Association (BUPA), who run a screening centre in London,

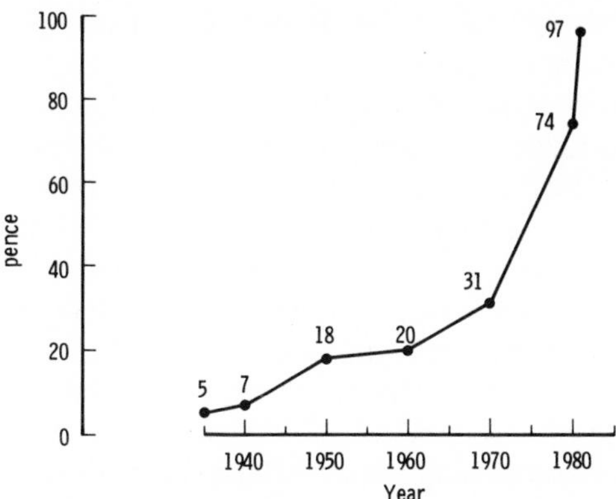

Fig. 11. Price of 20 U.K. cigarettes from 1935 to 1980 (from the Tobacco Advisory Council and *The Times* 1982).

various questions relating to smoking and health have been investigated on a scale which would not otherwise have been possible without incurring great cost (Wald *et al.* 1984a). The smoking habits of men attending the centre were studied by questionnaire and biochemical means (measuring carbon monoxide in breath and blood and nicotine and cotinine levels in blood and urine). The men smoked outside the laboratory, thereby avoiding the imposition of special constraints on smoking habits which

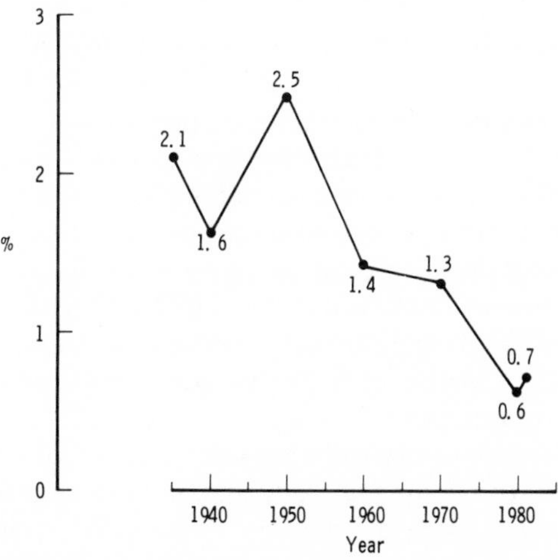

Fig. 12. Price of 20 U.K. cigarettes as a percentage of the contemporary average weekly earnings (men) (from *The Times*, 1982).

might have invalidated the results. Recent data from this work demonstrated clearly the phenomenon of 'compensatory smoking' – that is the intake of cigarette smoke was adjusted sufficiently to provide similar amounts of nicotine/carbon monoxide regardless of the nicotine/carbon monoxide yield of the cigarette (Table 3). It was not, however, significantly increased to achieve a similar intake of tar as the tar yield of the cigarette decreased. If, therefore, carbon monoxide or nicotine (or some other constituent of tobacco smoke which is correlated with the yield of either) is the cause of the excess risk of heart disease in smokers, one would expect smokers of cigarettes with relatively low yields to have about the same excess risk of heart disease as smokers of cigarettes with higher yields. On the other hand, the risk of lung cancer, which is generally regarded as being related to the tar yield of the cigarette, is likely to be lower in smokers of low tar cigarettes than in smokers of high tar cigarettes.

Table 3. Relative intake of tar, nicotine, and carbon monoxide (CO) according to quintile of tar, nicotine, and CO yield of cigarette (2455 smokers) (based on Wald *et al.* 1984a and later correction)

	Quintile of cigarette yield				
Yield	1st (lowest)	2nd	3rd	4th	5th (highest)
Tar	68	84	87	93	100
Nicotine	86	86	89	96	100
CO	97	86	96	97	100

These 'predictions' from the study of compensatory smoking are indeed borne out by the results of epidemiological studies. Tables 4–8 show data from five different studies on the risk of coronary heart disease associated with cigarette smoking, classified according to yield or type of cigarette (plain or filter – the plain cigarette having higher average tar yields than the filter cigarettes). None of the studies shows any material influence of the tar/nicotine yield on the risk of coronary heart disease.

Tables 4, 5, 9 10, and 11 show data from different studies on the risk of lung cancer according to cigarette yield and type. In all the studies the risk is lower in smokers of low tar or filter cigarettes compared with smokers of high tar or plain cigarettes.

The study on compensatory smoking referred to above also shows that although the extent of inhaling was adjusted to achieve a similar intake of nicotine and carbon monoxide regardless of the yield of the cigarette, the intake of carbon monoxide among smokers of cigarettes with unventilated filters (the usual type, without perforations in the paper around the filter tip) was greater than that among smokers of plain cigarettes (Table 12).

Table 4. Mortality ratio for current cigarette smokers according to cause and tar yield of cigarette matched for age and cigarette consumption (American Cancer Society Study; Hammond *et al.* 1976).

	Tar yield of cigarettes (no. of deaths in brackets)		
Disease	H	L vs. H	M vs. H
Lung cancer			
Men	1.00	0.81 (384)	0.96 (414)
Women	1.00	0.60 (169)	0.78 (190)
Coronary heart disease			
Men	1.00	0.89 (1952)	0.95 (2011)
Women	1.00	0.81 (1057)	0.86 (1090)
All cause mortality			
Men	1.00	0.85 (4589)	0.93 (4786)
Women	1.00	0.83 (4137)	0.88 (4249)

Key: H = > 26 mg tar; M = 18–26 mg tar; L = < 18 mg tar

Table 5. Mortality ratio for current cigarette smokers according to cause and type of cigarette standardized for age, and cigarette consumption (West Central Scotland Study; Hawthorne and Fry 1978)

	Type of cigarette	
Disease	Plain	Filter
Ischaemic heart disease	1.00	1.05
Cerebrovascular disease	1.00	1.73
Lung cancer	1.00	0.83
Chronic bronchitis	1.00	0.72
All causes	1.00	1.02

Table 6. Mortality ratio for specified coronary heart disease outcomes among men aged less than 55 years according to smoking habits (Framingham Study; Castelli *et al.* 1981)

		Type of cigarette	
	Non-smoker	Filter	Plain
Myocardial infarction	1.00 (20)	2.31 (40)	1.90 (24)
Coronary heart disease death	1.00 (9)	2.15 (17)	1.56 (9)
Total coronary heart disease	1.00 (40)	1.76 (62)	1.73 (44)

Table 7. Coronary heart disease mortality ratio (relative to life-long non-smokers of cigarettes) according to cigarette consumption and to tar yield: ratio standardized for age and employment grade (Whitehall Study; Higgenbottam *et al.* 1982) (Coronary heart disease death rate for life-long non-smokers of cigarettes = 275/100 000/year.)

	No. of cigarettes smoked per day (no. of deaths in brackets)		
Tar yield (mg/cigarette)	1–9	10–19	⩾20
18–23	1.20 (28)	2.00 (88)	2.37 (121)
24–32	1.16 (10)	2.61 (40)	2.16 (42)
⩾33	2.57 (27)	2.29 (41)	2.85 (10)
Total	1.47 (65)	2.16 (169)	2.31 (173)

Table 8. Relative risk of myocardial infarction according to nicotine yield of cigarettes smoked (Drug Epidemiology Unit Study; Wald and Doll 1983) (based on 390 cases and 589 controls)

		Approx. quintile of cigarette yield				
	Non-smoker	1st	2nd	3rd	4th	5th
Nicotine	1.0	3.8	4.1	3.4	2.4	3.2
CO	1.0	3.5	4.4	3.2	2.9	3.3

Limits of quintiles:
Nicotine <0.8, 0.8–0.9, 1.0–1.1, 1.2–1.4, ⩾1.5 mg/cigarette
CO <10, 10–14, 15–17, 18, ⩾19 mg/cigarette

Table 9. Lung cancer mortality ratio according to type of cigarette and sex (Wynder and Hoffmann 1979)

	n	Plain cigarettes	Filter cigarettes
Men	333	1.00	0.76
Women	63	1.00	0.75

This result raises a difficulty, since if carbon monoxide is implicated in causing heart disease and, as we know, tar is related to lung cancer, present cigarettes on the market which are least harmful with respect to one disease are not least harmful with respect to the other. Unfortunately, studying this directly, in terms of the mortality experience of smokers

Table 10. Lung cancer relative risk adjusted for age, years of smoking, and number of cigarettes smoked per day according to sex and tar yield of cigarette (high tar = 100) (Vienna Study: Kunze and Vutuc 1980; Vutuc and Kunze 1982)

	Number of cases of lung cancer	Tar yield (mg/cigarette)		
		>24	15–24	<15
Men	252	100	66	30
Women	297	100	49	29

Table 11. Lung cancer mortality ratio (relative to life-long non-smokers of cigarettes) according to cigarette consumption and to tar yield: ratio standardized for age and employment grade (Whitehall Study: Higenbottam *et al.* 1982). (No. of deaths shown in brackets; lung cancer death rate for life-long non-smokers of cigarettes = 20/100 000/year)

	No. of cigarettes smoked per day		
Tar yield (mg/cigarette)	1–9	10–19	⩾20
18–23	4.25 (6)	7.10 (24)	10.70 (42)
24–32	2.65 (1)	7.50 (10)	17.80 (22)
⩾33 mg	7.65 (15)	8.90 (59)	17.05 (5)
Total	4.15 (15)	8.90 (59)	11.80 (69)

Table 12. Relative intake of tar, nicotine, and CO according to type of cigarette; 2455 smokers (based on Wald *et al.* 1984a)

	Type of cigarette		
Yield	Plain	Unventilated filter	Ventilated filter
Tar	100	98	80
Nicotine	100	92	97
CO	100	162	163

smoking plain and filter cigarettes, will now be difficult because only a very small proportion of smokers use plain cigarettes.

Most of the work on compensatory smoking performed in collaboration with BUPA has been based on one marker of tobacco smoke absorption, namely carbon monoxide. While this will not perfectly reflect the absorption of all other tobacco smoke components (for example, tar, on the bronchial epithelium) it will better reflect others (such as nicotine) which are absorbed through the pulmonary alveoli. Indeed the results using carbon monoxide compare well with those from studies using other markers such as nicotine. Perhaps the best validation is that the results have led to the formulation of predictions regarding the risk of heart disease and lung cancer in smokers that appear to be evident in practice.

The inhaling anomaly

Lung cancer is less common among heavy smokers who say that they inhale than it is among those who say that they do not inhale. This observation was the only substantial point put forward by Sir Ronald Fisher in support of his contention that smoking was not a cause of lung cancer, but that it was associated with the disease through sharing a common cause, such as a particular genetic constitution (Fisher 1959). The basis for this surprising observation is sound. Three retrospective studies have demonstrated the anomaly (see Table 13) as well as three prospective studies (see Table 14). All six studies are consistent in showing that the risk of lung cancer was higher among self-described inhalers than among self-described non-inhalers in light smokers, but that the opposite was true in heavy smokers.

Using the absorption of carbon monoxide from cigarette smoke as an index of the extent of inhaling it was possible to investigate the inhaling

Table 13. Proportions of subjects who reported that they inhaled tobacco smoke among patients with lung cancer and control patients by cigarette consumption (from Wald and Doll (1976 and 1983): summary of data from three retrospective studies)

	Reported inhalers (%)					
	Doll and Hill		Schwartz *et al.*		Spicer	
No. of cigarettes/day	Patients with lung cancer	Control patients	Patients with lung cancer	Control patients	Patients with lung cancer	Control patients
1–4	50	48	50 (1–9)	29 (1–9)	58	38
5–9	81 (5–14)	79 (5–14)			79 (5–14)	81 (5–14)
10–14			59 (10–24)	46 (10–24)		
15–19	72 (15–24)	82 (15–24)			75 (15–24)	83 (15–24)
20–24						
25+	62	71	60	72	68	81

Table 14. Lung cancer mortality ratio according to self-described inhaling and cigarette consumption (from three prospective studies) (number of deaths shown in brackets)

Cigarette consumption†	Self-described inhaling status					
	Doctor's study (Doll and Peto 1976)		Whitehall study (Higenbottam *et al.* 1982)		Migrants study (Higenbottam *et al.* 1982)	
	Yes	No	Yes	No	Yes	No
Light	1.00 (8)	1.81 (18)	1.00 (5)	1.16 (10)	1.00 (3)	1.00 (6)
Moderate	1.00 (9)	1.51 (29)	1.00 (12)	1.02 (47)	1.00 (8)	1.00 (38)
Heavy	1.00 (29)	0.44 (32)	1.00 (18)	0.71 (51)	1.00 (51)	0.54 (35)

† Definition of smoking categories (cigarettes/day). Light, moderate, and heavy given respectively: Doctors' study: 1–14, 15–24, 25 or more; Whitehall study: 1–9, 10–19, 20 or more; Migrants study: 1–9, 10–19, 20 or more.

anomaly and test an explanation for it. The explanation for the anomaly may be illustrated by reference to Fig. 13. The top of the Figure compares the presumed extent of inhaling of a light smoker who says that he does not inhale (A) with that of a light smoker who says that he does (B). On average, (A) transfers little of the smoke taken in to his mouth beyond the larynx, while (B) transfers the smoke further along the respiratory tract so that much of it reaches the main bronchi. The bottom of the Figure illustrates the presumed extent of inhaling in a heavy smoker (A) who says that he does not inhale compared with that in heavy smoker (B) who says that he does. (A) deposits much of the smoke taken in through the mouth as far into his lungs as the main bronchi, but (B) transfers much of the smoke further, into the peripheral parts of the lungs. If allowance is made for the total amount smoked, and bearing in mind the principal target site for the carcinoma is the epithelium of the main bronchi, it would be expected that among light smokers the inhaler (B) would have a higher risk of lung cancer than the non inhaler (A), but that among heavy smokers the non-inhaler (A) would have a higher risk of lung cancer than the inhaler (B).

The explanation for this anomaly is therefore based upon two propositions: (1) that self-described inhaling reflects a systematically different extent of inhaling among light and heavy smokers, and (2) that heavy smokers who inhale deeply deposit less of the smoke condensate on their main bronchi and thereby to some extent protect themselves against the risk of developing tumours at this site. The first proposition is borne out by the data given in Table 15 which show the extent of alveolar inhaling according to amount smoked and self-described inhaling habits, and the second by data reported by Doll and Hill (1952). They found that a higher

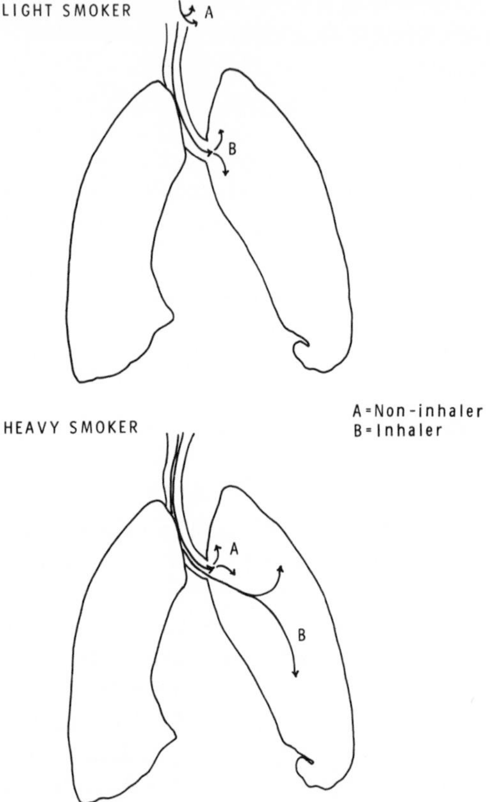

Fig. 13. Possible inhaling pattern of self-described non-inhaler (A) and self-described inhaler (B) according to cigarette consumption. Arrows indicate main site of tobacco smoke deposition in respiratory tract that might occur in each of the four examples. (Light smoker < 20 and heavy smoker > 20 cigarettes a day) (from Wald *et al.* 1983).

Table 15. Relative index of inhaling based on carbon monoxyhaemoglobin levels according to cigarette consumption and self-described inhaling catgory (from Wald *et al.* 1983)

Self-described inhaling category	Cigarette consumption	
	<20 per day	⩾20 per day
Non-inhaler	100	136
Inhaler	136	157

proportion of smokers with *peripheral* lung cancers said that they inhale compared with smokers having *central* tumours (63 per cent vs. 52 per cent) a statistically highly significant difference, although there was no significant difference in cigarette consumption. What was once seen as an objection to smoking as a cause of lung cancer can be explained and is consistent with smoking being a cause of the disease.

Breathing other people's smoke

The relationship between the number of cigarettes a person smokes each day and his risk of lung cancer is approximately linear, without any suggestion of a threshold below which there is no increase in the risk. It follows, therefore, that exposure to tobacco smoke at low concentrations will cause an increased risk of lung cancer, although the risk may be small. Widespread interest in the risk of lung cancer associated with breathing other people's smoke arose from the publication of studies in which a crude measure of exposure, namely enquiry about the smoking habits of the spouses of non-smokers, was associated with an increased risk of lung cancer. The results of the four studies published by 1983 are illustrated in Fig. 14. All the results are consistent with the summary estimate of an increased risk of lung cancer of about 50 per cent.

An uncertainty in the interpretation of the results from these studies arises from doubt about whether information on the smoking habits of the spouses of non-smokers provides valid information about a person's exposure to other people's smoke. To investigate this further, cotinine, a metabolite of nicotine, was measured in the urine of non-smokers to see whether it would be a useful marker of exposure to other people's smoke. The results (see Table 16) showed that there was a good correlation between a person's urinary cotinine concentration and the estimated exposure to other people's tobacco smoke over the past seven days. It was also found that urinary cotinine levels in non-smoking men who were married to women who smoked were significantly higher than the mean concentration in men with non-smoking wives (see Table 17). As would be expected, the mean exposure to other people's smoke by these two groups was also different (median 21.2 and 6.5 hours respectively). Interestingly there was also a difference in the number of hours of exposure to other people's smoke outside the home (median 10.7 and 6.0 respectively) suggesting that living with a smoking wife indicates a tolerance to other people's smoke and a willingness to be exposed to it, outside as well as within the home.

The chief importance of these biochemical data is that they validate the use of a spouse's smoking history as a method of indicating exposure to other people's tobacco smoke. The validity of the estimate of the

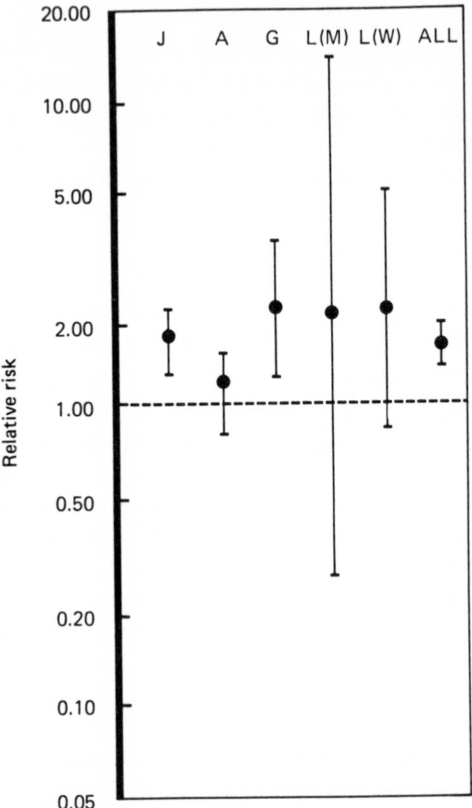

Fig. 14. The relative risk (point estimate and 95 per cent confidence interval) of lung cancer in non-smokers whose spouses smoke compared with non-smokers whose spouses do not smoke. Results from four studies (J = Japanese Study (Hiryama 1981), A = American Cancer Society Study (Garfinkel 1981), G = Greek Study (Trichopolous *et al.* 1983), L = Louisiana Study (Correa *et al.* 1983), M = men, W = women) and all studies combined (all).

magnitude of the risk from any individual study would require a direct measure of exposure, such as urinary cotinine, from a sample of the individuals studied.

Estimates of the risk of lung cancer from 'passive smoking' which can be derived from urinary cotinine and lung cancer risk in smokers and non-smokers are reasonably similar to the average estimate derived from the studies based on enquiries into the smoking habits of spouses of non-smokers and illustrated in Fig. 14. The differences in the estimates of the relative risk between each of the four studies have raised doubts about the validity of the studies, but, in fact, the differences are small and could have been due to chance (see the confidence intervals shown in Fig. 14). They

Table 16. Urinary cotinine in non-smokers according to number of reported hours of exposure to other people's tobacco smoke within the past seven days (including day urine sample was collected) (from Wald *et al.* 1984b)

Duration of exposure			Urinary cotinine (ng/ml) mean† ± S.D.
Quintile	Limits (h)	No.	
1st	0.0–	43	2.8±3.0
2nd	1.5–	47	3.4±2.7
3rd	4.5–	43	5.3±4.3
4th	8.6–	43	14.7±19.5
5th	20.0–80.0	45	29.6±73.7
All	0.0–80.0	221	11.2±35.6

† Trend with increasing exposure was significant ($p<0.001$).

Table 17. Urinary cotinine concentration and number of reported hours of exposure to other people's tobacco smoke within the past seven days in non-smoking married men according to smoking habits of their wives (from Wald *et al.* unpublished)

Smoking category wife	No.	Urinary cotinine concentration (ng/ml)			Exposure to other people's smoke in preceding week (h)					
					Total			Outside home		
		Mean	(S.E.)	Median	Mean	(S.E.)	Median	Mean	(S.E.)	Median
Non-smoker	101	8.54	(1.31)	5.00	11.01	(1.20)	6.53	9.97	(1.16)	6.00
Smoker	20	25.15	(14.83)	9.00	23.18	(4.14)	21.17	16.45	(3.29)	10.71

could also be due to differences in the extent of exposure and, expressed as a relative risk rather than an absolute excess risk, they would be expected to vary somewhat according to the background rate of lung cancer in non-smokers. Indeed, given the sources of variation, the similarity in results between the studies is more remarkable than their differences.

Conclusions

Cigarette smoking is a habit which is now declining steadily in Britain. Although there is much that we do not know about the specific toxic components of cigarette smoke, the reduction in tar yields and the reduction in cigarette smoking have produced a notable decline in lung cancer. Coronary heart disease has not changed in the same way. Biochemical studies on compensatory smoking suggest that the intake of smoke components, particularly nicotine and carbon monoxide, has not decreased as much as had previously been expected and this may explain the failure to observe an effect of low tar cigarettes on coronary heart disease mortality.

Recent data on biochemical estimates of exposure to other people's smoke predict a risk of lung cancer that is of a similar order of magnitude to the risk observed in non-smokers living with smoking spouses. The risk is small, but nonetheless real, and places smoking in a category comparable to other environmental and occupational carcinogens – also deserving social, political and legislative strategies to reduce its effects in the community.

Acknowledgements

I thank the following for help in obtaining some of the data referred to in this chapter: Dr Jillian Boreham, Dr Helen Van Vunakis, the British United Provident Association, the Laboratory of the Government Chemist, the Foundation for Blood Research, and the Tobacco Advisory Council. I also thank the Imperial Cancer Research Fund and the Medical Research Council for their financial support.

References

Castelli, W.P. *et al.* (1981). The filter cigarette and coronary heart disease: the Framingham study. *Lancet* **ii**, 109–13.

Correa, P., Williams Pickle, L., Fontham, E., Lin, Y., and Haenszel, W. (1983). Passive smoking and lung cancer. *Lancet* **ii**, 595–7.

Doll, R. and Hill, A.B. (1952). The study of the aetiology of carcinoma of the lung. *Brit. med. J.* **ii**, 1271–86.

Doll, R. and Peto, R. (1976). Mortality in relation to smoking: 20 years' observations on male British doctors. *Brit. med. J.* **ii**, 1525–36.

Fisher, R.A. (1959). *Smoking: the cancer controversy.* Oliver and Boyd, Edinburgh and London.

Garfinkel, L. (1981). Time trends in lung cancer mortality among non-smokers and a note on passive smoking. *J. nat. Cancer Inst.* **66**, 1061–6.

Hammond, E.C., Garfinkel, L., Seidman, H., and Lew, E.A. (1976). 'Tar' and nicotine content of cigarette smoke in relation to death rates. *Environ. Res.* **12**, 263–74.

Hawthorne, V.M. and Fry, J.S. (1978). Smoking and health; cardiorespiratory disease, mortality, and smoking behaviour in West Central Scotland. *J. Epidemiol. comm. Hlth* **32**, 260–6.

Higenbottam, T., Shipley, M.J., and Rose, G. (1982). Cigarettes, lung cancer, and coronary heart disease: the effects of inhalation and tar yield. *J. Epidemiol. comm. Hlth* **26**, 113–7.

Jamrozik, K., Fowler, G., Vessey, M., and Wald, N. (1984). Placebo controlled trial of nicotine chewing gum in general practice. *Brit. med. J.* **289**, 794–7.

Kunze, M. and Vutuc, C. (1980). Threshold of tar exposure: Analysis of smoking history of male lung cancer cases and controls. In *Banbury Report No. 3: A safe cigarette?* (ed. G. Gori and F. Bock), pp. 26–9. Cold Spring Harbor Laboratory, New York.

Stepney, R. (1981). Would a medium-nicotine, low-tar cigarette be less hazardous to health? *Brit. med. J.* **283**, 1292–6.

Sutton, R.S., Russell, M.A.H., Iyer, R., Feyerabend, C., and Saloojee, Y. (1982). Relationship betwen cigarette yields, puffing patterns, and smoke intake: evidence for tar compensation? *Brit. med. J.* **286**, 600–3.

Trichopolous, D., Kalandid, A., Sparios, L., and MacMahon, B. (1983). Lung cancer and passive smoking: conclusion of Greek study. *Lancet* **ii**, 677–8.

Vutuc, C. and Kunze, M. (1982). Lung cancer risk in women in relation to tar yield of cigarettes. A short report. *Preventive Med.* **11**, 713–6.

Wald, N.J. (1978). Smoking in relation to lung cancer and coronary heart disease. *Bull. int. Union Against Tuberc.* **53**, 325–33.

Wald, N.J. and Doll, R. (1983). Epidemiology of lung cancer. In *Lung cancer* (ed. E.L. Wynder and S. Hecht). UICC Tech. Rep. Ser. **25**(3). UICC, Geneva.

Wald, N.J., Doll. R., and Copeland, G. (1981a). Trends in tar, nicotine, and carbon monoxide yields of U.K. cigarettes manufactured since 1934. *Brit. med. J.* **282**, 763–5.

Wald, N.J., Idle, M., Boreham, J., Bailey, A., and Van Vunakis, H. (1981b). Serum cotinine levels in pipe smokers: evidence against nicotine as cause of coronary heart disease. *Lancet* **ii**, 775–7.

Wald, N.J., Idle, M., Boreham, J., and Bailey, A. (1981c) The importance of tar and nicotine in determining cigarette smoking habits. *J. Epidemiol. comm. Hlth* **35**(1), 23–4.

Wald, N.J., Idle, M., Boreham, J., and Bailey, A. (1983). Inhaling and lung cancer: an anomaly explained. *Brit. med. J.* **287**, 1273–5.

Wald, N.J., Boreham, J., and Bailey, A. (1984a). Relative intake of tar, nicotine and carbon monoxide from cigarettes of different yields. *Thorax* **39**, 361–4.

Wald, N.J., Boreham, J., Bailey, A., Ritchie, C., Haddow, J.E., and Knight, G. (1984b). Urinary cotinine as marker of breathing other people's smoke. *Lancet* **i**, 230–1.

Wald, N.J., Idle, M., Boreham, J., Bailey, A., and Van Vunakis, H. (1984c). Urinary nicotine in cigarette and pipe smokers. *Thorax* **39**, 365–8.

Wynder, E.L. and Hoffmann, D. (1979). Tobacco and health: a societal challenge. *New Engl. J. Med.* **300**(16), 894–903.

4 Diet

B.K. Armstrong and J.I. Mann

The concept that diet may influence cancer risk is probably as old as recognition of cancer itself. Indeed, with reference to 'Ye Ge' (difficulty with swallowing), presumed to be the ancient equivalent of the modern problem of oesophageal cancer in parts of China, Yong-He Yan stated in his pharmacopoeia (Ji Sheng Fang) of the Song Dynasty (960–1279 AD) '. . . eat and drink in moderation (not in excess, not at a rapid rate, foods not too hot and not overly hard), maintain an even temperament, eat a good diet and Ye Ge will not develop' (Li, 1982).

It is doubtful whether such statements were based on any empirical data; rather they most likely arose from the theoretical, or philosophical, belief that food was fundamental to many human disorders. Such was probably also the basis of Jonathan Hutchinson's fourth general aphorism on cancer: 'Anything which disturbs the forces of nutrition may give proclivity to cancerous processes or methods of growth' (Hutchinson 1892).

Empirical data on the association between diet and cancer first began to be collected in the first half of this century with actuarial studies relating obesity to cancer, experimental studies of food restriction and cancer, observations of the effects of wartime famine on cancer rates, and some early case-control studies (McCoy 1959; Stocks and Kay 1933; Tannenbaum 1940). From a historical viewpoint, the study of Stocks and Kay (1933) is remarkable. It was a matched case-control study covering 462 cases of cancer of different types. Dietary information was elicited by means of a simple food-frequency questionnaire. The main positive results were the apparent protective effect of wholemeal bread, vegetables (turnips, carrots, cauliflower, onions, beetroot, watercress, and cabbage), and fresh milk, and an apparent harmful effect of beer, particularly on cancer of the upper alimentary tract. In commenting on the result for beer, Stocks and Kay (1933) drew attention to the greater than two-fold excess mortality from cancer of the upper alimentary tract in barmen and waiters as seen in the Registrar General's Decennial Supplement for England and Wales (1921). They noted also that falls in per caput beer consumption in Britain after 1915 had been followed, after 1926, by a fall in mortality from cancer of the upper alimentary tract. On this same subject Clemmesen reported, in 1946, that variation in mortality from cancer of the oesophagus between Switzerland, England, and Denmark was consistent with variation in alcohol consumption between these three countries (cited by Stocks 1947).

By 1950 there was a substantial body of observations relating diet to human cancer. In addition to the above studies referring to wholemeal bread, vegetables, milk, and alcohol, a number of investigations described high rates of cancer in obese subjects, particularly cancers of the liver, gall bladder, intestines, and urogenital organs (McCoy 1959); there was much speculation on the relationship between dietary deficiency and liver cancer in malnourished populations (McCoy 1959); and links had been made between iron deficiency, Plummer-Vinson syndrome and upper alimentary cancer, and iodine deficiency, goitre, and thyroid cancer (Stocks 1916/17; Ahlbom 1936; McCoy 1959).

The renewed interest in diet and human cancer developing since the 1960s may be attributed mainly to recognition of the geographic variability of cancer incidence and its correlation for many cancer sites with variation in patterns of food and nutrient intake (Armstrong and Doll 1975). Descriptive and analytical epidemiological studies of diet and cancer have proliferated and the arguably new discipline of metabolic epidemiology has developed. The latter combines metabolic studies, in epidemiological investigations, with exposure and disease variables to add credence to, or subtract credence from, supposed associations and to elucidate the mechanisms which may lead from dietary (or other) causes to disease effects.

A number of recent reviews have catalogued by food, nutrient, cancer site, or supposed mechanism the various associations between diet and cancer (see, for example, Doll 1979; Armstrong *et al.* 1982; and Committee on Diet, Nutrition and Cancer 1982). We have chosen therefore, in this chapter, to take a different approach. We shall describe the ways in which the various epidemiological methods, descriptive and analytical, have been applied to the study of diet and cancer. We shall refer to selected empirical observations for the purpose of illustration only and assess critically the contributions which each method has made and, perhaps, has yet to make.

Descriptive epidemiology

Descriptive epidemiology is the description of disease frequency according to the characteristics of populations, particularly geographic location (place), era of observation (time), and the personal characteristics of population subgroups such as sex, occupation, place of birth, religion, and socioeconomic status (person). The term ‘ecological studies’ has been used for descriptive studies in which disease frequency is correlated with some measure of aggregate exposure to a supposed agent of disease in population strata defined by place, time, or person variables. Ecological studies have been used extensively in the study of diet and cancer.

Geographic correlation

Fat and breast cancer Lea (1967) first described the strong correlation between fat intake and breast cancer mortality in 33 countries. There were, in addition, strong positive correlations between breast cancer mortality and consumption of sugar, animal protein, eggs, and milk (fish was the only other dietary variable studied). Similar results have since been published by a number of other workers (see Table 1) studying different

Table 1. Geographical correlation studies showing association between breast cancer frequency and measures of fat intake

Author	Measure of breast cancer frequency	Correlation units	No. of exposure variables	Most highly correlated variable
Between countries				
Lea 1967	Mortality 1964	33 countries	6	?
Carroll *et al.* 1968	Mortality 1952–3	22 countries	2	Total fat
Hems 1970	Mortality 1962–6	22 countries	8	Sugar
Drasar and Irving 1973a	Incidence 1960–2	37 countries	12	Total fat
Armstrong and Doll	Mortality 1964–5	32 countries	22	Total fat
1975	Incidence 1959–66	23 countries	22	Gross national product
Knox 1977	Mortality 1970	20 countries	58	Total fat
Maruchi *et al.* 1977	Mortality 1966–7	18 developed countries	11	Sugar
Hems 1978	Mortality 1970	41 countries	13	Total fat
Gray *et al.* 1979	Mortality 1964–5	26 countries	8	Total fat
	Incidence 1959–66	20 countries	8	Animal protein
Within a single country				
Stocks 1970	Mortality 1954–63	9 regions of England & Wales	7	Butter and cheese
Maruchi *et al.* 1977	Mortality 1969–71	46 prefectures of Japan	11	Milk and dairy products
Hirayama 1978	Mortality 1970	12 districts of of Japan	39	Pork
Gaskill *et al.* 1979	Mortality 1969–71	48 contiguous United States	30	Age of first marriage

although sometimes overlapping sets of countries, or regions within a single country, different sets of variables, and carrying the analysis to different levels of sophistication. In almost all studies total fat intake or a dietary variable closely correlated with it has shown the strongest correlation with frequency of breast cancer. An example of the strength of correlation seen is shown in Fig. 1.

As shown in Table 1, most studies have considered a number of possible explanatory variables for the geographic variation of breast cancer frequency. Of particular importance are those which have considered non-dietary variables associated with breast cancer. Hems (1978) concluded that strong associations observed between breast cancer mortality and intake of fat, animal protein, and animal calories were independent of all other dietary variables studied and childbearing, which was measured as completed family size. The effects, however, of fat, animal protein, and

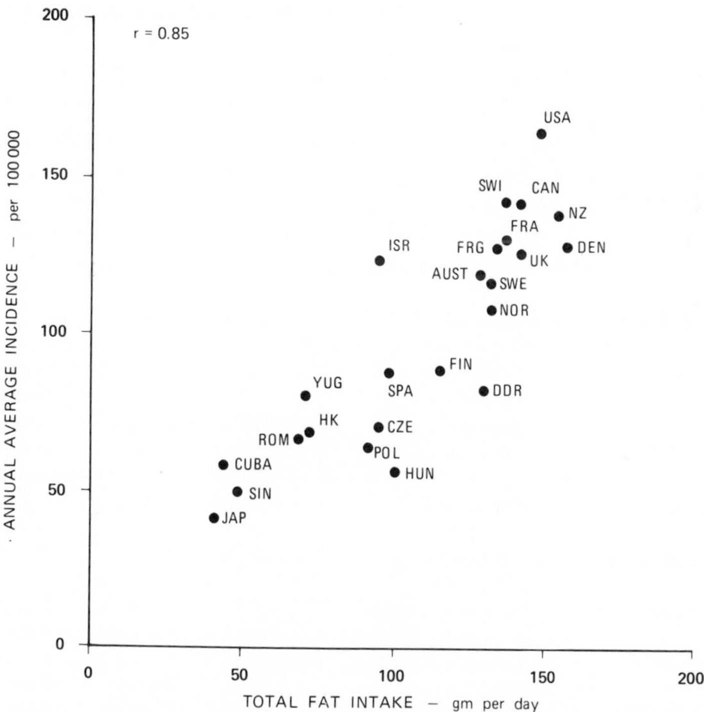

Fig. 1. Correlation of age-standardized incidence of breast cancer in women aged 35–64 years in 1972–1977 in 25 countries with estimated per caput daily fat consumption in 1964–1966. Incidence data are those reasonably representative of whole countries given by Doll and Smith (1982). Data on fat consumption from Food and Agriculture Organization (1971).

animal calories could not be distinguished from one another because of their close intercorrelation. Refined sugar had an independent correlation with breast cancer mortality. Gray *et al.* (1979) concluded that correlations between breast cancer mortality and fat and animal protein intake were independent of effects of body height and weight and age at menarche, for which they also had data. In contrast, however, Gaskill *et al.* (1979) noted that positive correlations between breast cancer mortality and total fats and total protein in the 43 contiguous United States became insignificant when age at first marriage or median income were taken into account. In commenting on this finding they observed: 'The variation in diet from one state to another within the United States may be indequate for one to detect significant differences in specific dietary components, particularly in one that is difficult to measure with accuracy or for which only incomplete data are available.'

Fibre and colorectal cancer International correlation studies of some measure of fibre intake and frequency of colorectal cancer have almost uniformly showed an apparent protective effect (Table 2). Wherever they have been examined, however, there have been stronger correlations with fat, meat, or animal protein intake which could explain the apparent protective effect of fibre (see, for example, Armstrong and Doll 1975; Liu *et al.* 1979). Estimates of fibre intake in these studies, however, have been far from satisfactory (Cummings 1981) and the question arises whether the apparent weakness of the fibre effect could be due to measurement error.

Table 2. Geographical correlation studies showing association between frequency of colorectal cancer and measures of fibre intake

Author	Measure of frequency of colorectal cancer	Correlation units	Definition of fibre	Nature of apparent association
Drasar & Irving 1973a	Estimated incidence	37 countries	Crude fibre†	No association
Drasar & Irving 1973b	Estimated incidence	37 countries	Cereals	Protective
Armstrong & Doll 1975	Mortality 1964–5	32 countries	Cereals	Protective
	Incidence 1959–65	23 countries	Cereals	Protective
Howell 1975	Mortality 1964–5	37 countries	Cereals	Protective
			Pulses	Protective
Schrauzer 1976	Mortality 1964–5	16 countries	Cereals	Protective
Liu *et al.* 1979	Mortality 1967–73	20 industrial countries	Fibre‡	Protective

† Estimated from cereals, potatoes, other starchy foods, pulses, nuts and seeds, vegetables, fruit

‡ Sum of fruits, vegetables, grains, and legumes

That this may be true is suggested by the results of studies in fewer population units in which accurate estimates of fibre intake have been made. Bingham *et al.* (1979) were able to correlate estimates of per caput intake of fibre and its components with mortality from cancer of the colon in nine regions of England, Wales, and Scotland. Total dietary fibre was not significantly correlated with mortality from cancer of the colon but pentose fibre was highly correlated negatively ($r = -0.96$; apparent protective effect). Fat intake was also uncorrelated with colon cancer mortality. The pentose fraction of fibre is the fraction with the greatest effect on large-bowel function (Cummings *et al.* 1978).

Studies which have compared fibre intake in two regions of Scandinavia with substantially different rates of colon cancer – rural Finland (low) and urban Denmark (high) – also suggest a correlation of fibre with colon cancer independent of fat intake. MacLennan *et al.* (1978) found a high total fibre intake (30.9 g/day) in Finland and a low intake (17.2 g/day) in Denmark. Fat intake did not differ significantly between the two populations but meat intake was higher in Denmark than Finland. The distributions of fibre fractions were similar in the two populations. Similar results were obtained in a second study incorporating two additional areas, urban Finland and rural Denmark, of intermediate risk of bowel cancer (Jensen *et al.* 1982). In this study the difference in total fibre intake was mainly due to differences in pentosan and cellulose intake.

Analysis of trends over time

Trends in cancer incidence or mortality over time in relation to dietary variables have been studied comparatively rarely. This is due in part, at least, to a lack of the necessary time series data. Figs 2 and 3 show trends in mortality from colorectal and breast cancer in the U.S. and Australia and the corresponding trends in total fat and meat consumption and several variables which might be taken as indicators of fibre intake.

Over the periods studied there were fluctuations in mortality from both cancers which could be related to environmental variables. For breast cancer the fluctuations were small; a recent upturn in the U.S. and Australia occurred in parallel with a rising fat intake but in other respects the trends were not parallel. Other explanations, particularly change in age at first birth and parity, have been advanced for the recent changes in breast cancer rates (Armstrong 1976; Fleming *et al.* 1981).

For colorectal cancer the trends are even less like those which might have been expected. In the U.S. recent falls in mortality, particularly in women, occurred in parallel with falls in intake of fruit and vegetables, cereal products, and crude fibre. Over the same period, meat intake and fat intake were rising. These are the opposite of dietary changes which

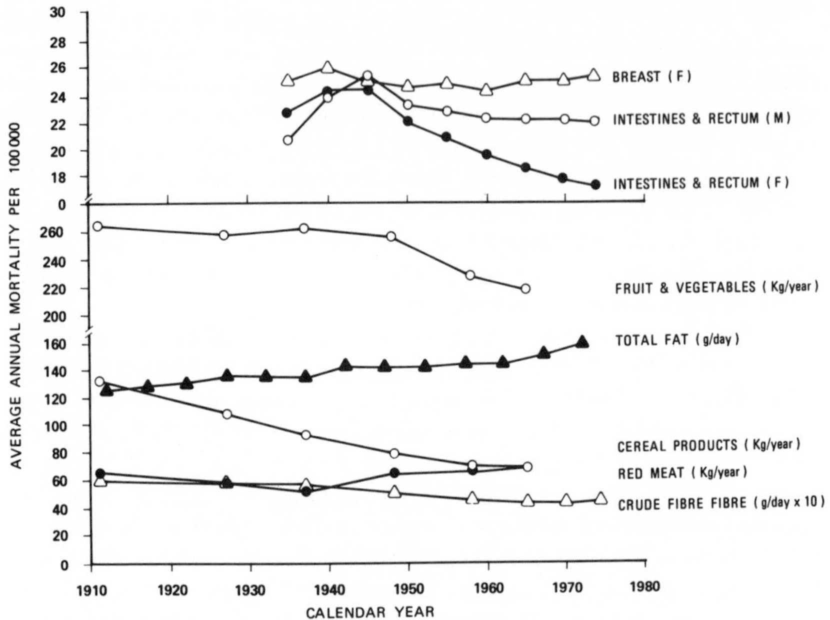

Fig. 2. Trends in mortality from cancer of the breast, intestines, and rectum in the U.S. in relation to trends in apparent intake of fat, meat, cereals, fruit and vegetables, and crude fibre. Data from Friend (1967), Gortner (1975), and Devesa and Silverman (1978).

might have been expected to produce falls in mortality from colorectal cancer. Males in Australia showed a recent rise in mortality from colorectal cancer in a period of rising fat intake but also rising intake of fruit and vegetables. Increasing alcohol intake has been ventured as an alternative explanation for this trend (McMichael 1979).

These data serve to illustrate the difficulty in making aetiological inferences from time trend analysis. First we may ask: do the trends in mortality accurately reflect underlying trends in incidence? Sullivan *et al.* (1972) compared incidence and mortality trends in Connecticut over a 30-year period; they were not parallel for either the breast or the large bowel. For cancer of the large bowel, particularly, mortality showed much greater evidence of a fall (as shown in Fig. 2) than did incidence. Incidence measurement, however, is subject to error and apparent incidence rates may show an increase over time because of improved ascertainment of cases of cancer. In a careful consideration of incidence (cancer registration) and mortality data as indicators of time trends, Doll and Peto (1981) concluded that 'mortality data seem generally more trustworthy'.

Secondly there is the problem of 'lag time'. How soon after a change in

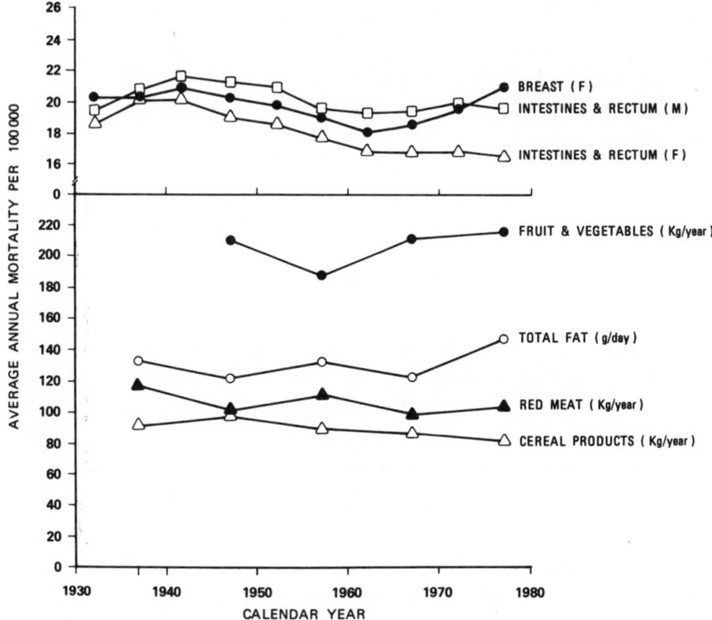

Fig. 3. Trends in mortality from cancer of the breast, intestines, and rectum in Australia in relation to trends in apparent intake of fat, meat, cereals, and fruit and vegetables. Data from Australian Bureau of Statistics (1981) and Holman and Armstrong (1982).

food intake should cancer rates change? The descriptions given above of the trends in Figs 2 and 3 have assumed no lag; that is likely to be an incorrect assumption but what lag period should be assumed? Any assumption will depend on speculation as to, or evidence of, the stage of carcinogenesis at which a particular food or nutrient is operating. For fat and breast cancer at least, late-stage effects are possible (Armstrong 1983).

Thirdly, it may be, for example, in countries such as the U.S. and Australia, that fat intake is now so high that fluctuations around the prevailing level have no further effect on rates of breast or colorectal cancer, i.e., a plateau has been reached on the dose-effect curve. Recent experience in Japan provides some support for this explanation. Fat intake in that country more than doubled between 1955 and 1973 from an initially very low level, and breast cancer mortality increased substantially, particularly in young and middle-aged women, over the same period (Hirayama 1979).

Ideally, trends in mortality and dietary intake by cohort of birth would be compared. This has provided strong descriptive evidence, for example, of the relationship between cigarette smoking and bladder cancer

(Armstrong and Doll 1974). Diet, like smoking, is presumably a matter of habit fixed fairly early in life and retained thereafter to a substantial degree. Unfortunately such analyses of diet are not possible because of the lack of any description of dietary intake specified by age (and sex) over long periods of time.

Correlation across strata defined by personal characteristics

One of the best illustrations of this approach is provided by studies of diet and cancer risk across ethnic groups (Caucasian, Japanese, Hawaiian, Filipino, Chinese) and sex in the population of Hawaii (Kolonel *et al.* 1981). Cancer incidence data for the period 1973–1977 came from the Hawaii Tumour Registry and dietary data were collected annually from a 2 per cent random sample of the population beginning in 1977. In this study, as in the geographical correlation studies described above, there was a very high correlation between fat and particularly saturated fat intake ($r = 0.95$) and incidence of breast cancer; this association is shown graphically in Fig. 4. In contrast, incidence of cancers of the colon and rectum showed no important association with any of the dietary variables examined – total fat and its components, total protein and its components, carbohydrates, and vitamins A and C.

Religion has also been used to subdivide populations for ecological studies. Seventh-day Adventists in California, some 50 per cent of whom are lacto-ovo-vegetarians, have lower mortality rates from cancers of the breast and colon, among other cancers, than other Californians. These differences have been attributed to the vegetarian diet – they appear to be independent of educational level and smoking habits (Phillips 1980). Some doubt that the vegetarian diet is the explanation, however, comes from studies showing that non-vegetarian Mormons, another conservative protestant sect, have rates of colon cancer similar to those in Seventh-day Adventists (Lyon *et al.* 1980) and that vegetarian nuns have rates of colorectal and breast cancer similar to those of the general population (Kinlen 1982).

Metabolic epidemiology

The measurement of metabolic variables which may bear on the mechanisms of environmental carcinogenesis, or may reflect exposure to environmental carcinogens, has been attempted both in the study of geographical variation in cancer risk and variation between subgroups of a single population. The former approach will be illustrated here with reference to metabolic studies in Scandinavian populations the latter by

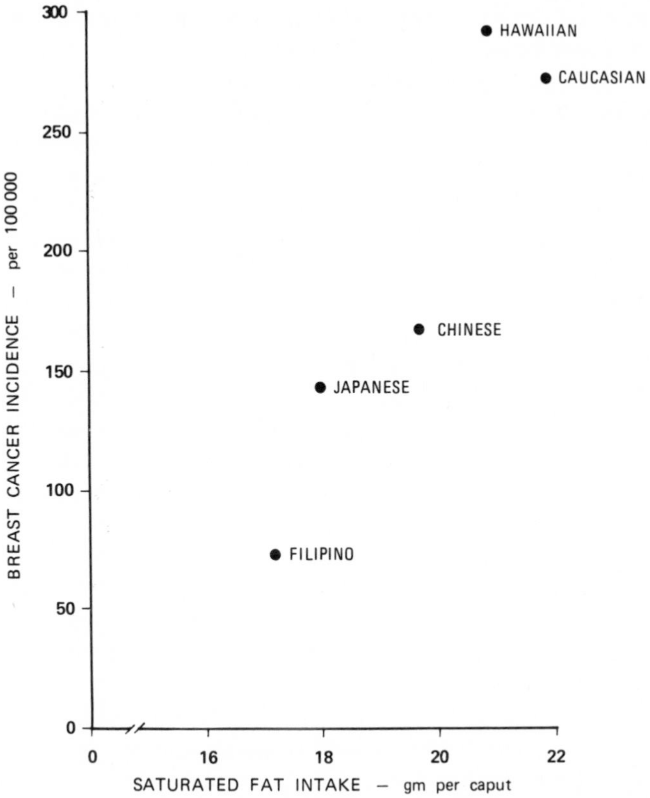

Fig. 4. Correlation of age-standardized annual average breast cancer incidence (45+ years of age) in five ethnic groups in Hawaii with estimated average daily fat intake. Data from Kolonel *et al.* (1981) and Rellahan (1982).

hormonal studies in vegetarian women as they may bear on the influence of diet on risk of breast cancer.

In the study of colorectal cancer, interest has concentrated on several diet-related metabolic variables: faecal bulk and stool transit time, faecal steroids, faecal enzymes, faecal bacteria, particularly anaerobes, and faecal mutagens. Jensen *et al.* (1982) observed a negative association of risk of colorectal cancer with faecal bulk and a positive association with concentration of acid steroids (bile acids) across four populations in Finland and Denmark. These observations were concordant with their observed negative association of fibre intake with colorectal cancer; fibre presumably increased faecal bulk and, in consequence, diluted the acid steroids in faeces. There was no significant variation in total acid steroid output between the regions studied, consistent with absence of significant variation in fat intake. There was no apparently relevant variation in content or concentration of faecal bacteria.

These results have been interpreted as suggesting that the main dietary influence in colon carcinogenesis is the effect of dietary fibre to dilute carcinogenic faecal constituents. Similar results were obtained in a comparison of males in rural Finland (low risk for colorectal cancer) and metropolitan New York (high risk for colorectal cancer: Reddy *et al.* 1978). In an extension of this study, however, faecal mutagen activity was found to be higher in New Yorkers than Finns and absent from the faeces of vegetarian Seventh-day Adventists in New York (Reddy *et al.* 1980). The Finns had a similar total fat intake to that of the New Yorkers but relatively less fat from meat and correspondingly more from dairy products. Dietary fibre may lead to dilution of faecal mutagens but the extent to which mutagens are produced in faeces, or are present in the diet, may be determined by other dietary constituents (e.g. meat).

Several studies have sought to explain, by hormonal measurements, the lower recorded mortality from breast cancer in vegetarian than non-vegetarian women (Phillips 1980). Hill and Wynder (1979), in a follow-up of studies showing that dietary fat influences prolactin production in rodents, showed evidence of suppression of prolactin production by a vegetarian diet. Subsequently Armstrong *et al.* (1981) found lower mean plasma prolactin levels in vegetarian than non-vegetarian postmenopausal women. They also found lower urinary excretion of oestrogens, particularly of oestriol, in vegetarian women, and higher plasma sex hormone binding globulin in vegetarian than non-vegetarian women. An increase in plasma sex hormone binding globulin would be expected to reduce plasma free oestrogen concentrations and cellular clearance of oestrogens (Siiteri 1981). Schultz and Leklem (1980) reported lower plasma oestrone and oestradiol concentrations in vegetarians than non-vegetarians, further reinforcing the impression that a vegetarian diet is associated with reduced oestrogen activity.

More recently Goldin *et al.* (1982) confirmed the reduced plasma and urinary oestrogen concentrations in vegetarian women and found them to be almost completely explained by increased faecal excretion of oestrogens. The latter correlated with faecal bulk and could be due to the high fibre content of a vegetarian diet. Alternatively, as it was shown that vegetarians had low faecal ß-glucuronidase activity, it may be that reduced deconjugation of conjugated oestrogens decreases the enterohepatic circulation of oestrogens. Intake of beef and fat has been shown to increase faecal ß-glucuronidase activity (Goldin and Gorbach 1976).

These studies suggest that a vegetarian diet could reduce breast cancer risk either through effects on prolactin activity, oestrogen activity, or both. On present evidence, however, it is not possible to attribute its action or actions to a specific nutrient. Dietary fibre or fat, or some other component of meat remain as candidate agents.

Discussion

Ecological studies of the type described above share a number of weaknesses which limit their usefulness, particularly in making causal inferences. In all except special surveys, for example, of the type conducted in Scandinavia in relation to colorectal cancer (Jensen *et al.* 1982), the quality of data on diet and disease is not under the investigators' control. The larger the population units under study, the cruder the data are likely to be. Thus at the level of whole countries the only dietary data are those from apparent consumption, i.e. food balance or 'disappearance' statistics and the only disease data may be mortality statistics. Both are subject to error (Greaves and Hollingsworth 1966; Percy *et al.* 1981).

This error may have several consequences. First, it will affect the strength of any true correlations that exist, and generally, move the measure of association such as the correlation coefficient towards the null value. If the degree of error varies, as is likely, from one food or nutrient to another, the relative strengths of disease correlations with highly inter-correlated dietary variables will vary somewhat arbitrarily. In consequence the results of a multiple variable (multiple regression, partial correlation) analysis aimed at selecting variables which are independently correlated with the disease may be misleading in selecting, perhaps, the most error-free variables rather than the true causal variables. Secondly, it may create spurious correlations. For example if the quality of disease recording varies with economic development, spurious correlations may appear between a disease and dietary variables which also vary with economic development both geographically and over time. Certainly, measures of economic activity are commonly highly correlated with cancer rates (Armstrong and Doll 1975) but the extent, if any, to which this contributes to correlations with food intake is unknown.

Problems of error and spurious correlation are probably less in correlation studies across geographical units in a single country than across many countries. In a single country, uniform methods of data collection may be expected and more valid methods may be used. For example, the household survey method of collection of dietary data commonly used within a country (see Bingham *et al.* 1979) is almost certainly better than the apparent-consumption method. Even in a single country, however, the quality of data may vary over time and thus influence time trend analysis.

Restriction of analysis to routinely collected data may also mean that measurements of the most relevant dietary variables are not available. Thus, for example, in international correlation studies and time trend analyses, cereal intake or fruit and vegetable intake have been used as surrogates for the components of fibre most relevant to large-bowel function. While they may include these components they are imprecise and inaccurate measures of them and their use will probably weaken the strength of any real associations, if not be quite misleading.

In ecological studies it is virtually never possible to exclude with confidence the possibility that the observed association between food and disease is explained by a relationship between some other variable (which is correlated with intake of the food) and the disease. Table 3 shows the five variables, among those studied, which were correlated most highly with incidence of cancer of the breast and corpus uteri in 23 countries (Armstrong and Doll 1975). Note the very high correlations with gross national product, a measure of economic activity. Although the dietary correlations have logical appeal, it is not possible on these data to select which, if any, of the dietary variables is the most relevant or to exclude the possibility that some unmeasured agent, highly correlated with economic development, is the explanatory variable.

The same problem arises in interpreting, for example, the differences in disease frequency between vegetarian Seventh-day Adventists and the general population. Seventh-day Adventists differ from the general population in a variety of ways (Phillips 1975), some measurable (e.g. alcohol and tobacco consumption) and some not (e.g. religious belief and commitment). In the absence of more discriminating studies, any of these other characteristics of Seventh-day Adventist behaviour should be considered as potential explanations for observed differences in disease frequency.

Measures of association between disease frequency and a dietary or other variable derived from ecological studies may not reflect at all well the true strength of association in individuals even when an association exists

Table 3. Most highly correlated variables in a correlation study of food intake and economic variables and incidence of cancer of the breast and corpus uteri in 23 countries (Armstrong and Doll 1975)

Breast cancer		Cancer of corpus uteri	
Correlated variable	Correlation coefficient	Correlated variable	Correlation coefficient
Gross national product	0.83	Total fat	0.85
Total fat	0.79	Gross national product	0.82
Meat	0.78	Meat	0.78
Animal protein	0.77	Fats and oils	0.76
Eggs	0.71	Animal protein	0.74

and is causal. This 'cross-level' bias (Morgenstern 1982), a manifestation of the so-called 'ecological fallacy', may be due both to confounding effects which would be observed in studies of individuals and an 'aggregation bias' due to the grouping of individuals in the ecological study. Its effects are unpredictable but generally exaggerate the strength of the true association.

Most of the problems described above lead to claims of positive associations between food and disease when the truth is otherwise. The opposite may also occur either because of gross error in measurement or lack of heterogeneity in a dietary variable over the units studied. For example, in relation to dietary fat and breast cancer, Enstrom (1981) has argued against an association because of apparent lack of correlation across the United States of America. It might reasonably be questioned, however, whether the degree of variation in fat intake across the United States, in relation to measurement error and other variables which also influence breast cancer frequency, is sufficient to produce an association. This negative result, therefore, is not persuasive. Similarly the absence of association between total fat intake and frequency of colorectal cancer across Scandinavia (Jensen *et al.* 1982) cannot exonerate fat from a role in the aetiology of this disease because there was little heterogeneity in fat intake. It may mean only that in this study situation some other variable, perhaps dietary fibre, explained the observed variation in disease frequency.

The above considerations indicate the limits of the usefulness of ecological studies in establishing cause-effect relationships. The main value of these studies is in providing hypotheses which can be studied by other means. Indeed they have served as the starting-point for much recent research in diet and cancer. In addition they can add valuable evidence to data on causation from other sources, adding, or perhaps removing in some instances, the element of coherence necessary in the establishment of cause-effect relationships (Hill 1977). Thus, for example, the increasing breast cancer rates now being observed in Japan in parallel with increasing fat intake contribute to the coherence of the evidence that dietary fat influences breast cancer risk. Conversely evidence that saccharin might be a cause of bladder cancer was reasonably held in question when it was observed that substantial increases in saccharin intake over time in England and Wales has not been followed, within the limits of the time elapsed since saccharin intake began to rise, by an increase in bladder cancer mortality (Armstrong and Doll 1974).

Analytical epidemiology

Analytical epidemiological studies are usually set up to examine hypotheses suggested by descriptive studies. They differ from descriptive studies primarily in that data are collected for individuals rather than groups or populations and they may be specifically designed to control as far as possible for confounding variables. There are three principal analytical approaches: case-control studies, cohort studies, and intervention studies. In case-control studies dietary information and data relating to possible confounding variables are collected for cases with a specific type of cancer and compared with similar exposure data for an appropriate non-cancer control group. In cohort studies exposure data are collected for disease-free people amongst whom it is possible to observe cancer incidence over a prolonged period of time. Occurrence rates are then examined in relation to dietary and other characteristics recorded before the onset of the disease (or diseases) under consideration. Intervention studies have usually been undertaken to assess the effectiveness of a new treatment but although they are only occasionally appropriate to the question of diet and cancer, they do offer a unique opportunity for establishing true causal relationships. In intervention studies, volunteers are randomized into two or more groups which are exposed (or not exposed) to various levels of the substance being tested. Disease incidence may then be related to the level of exposure without some of the biases inherent in the case-control and cohort methods.

Case-control studies

A major difficulty in setting up and interpreting case-control studies of diet and cancer concerns the method by which dietary data are collected. For accurate assessment of nutrient intake, *dietary* and *food records* are usually regarded as the most satisfactory method. Subjects record as accurately as possible (by weighing or estimating quantity) all food eaten during a specified time interval, usually a week; recording food eaten away from home as well as in the home. There are several problems with this technique: recording and weighing may result in the modification of eating habits; it can be extremely difficult (and sometimes impossible) to obtain recipes of dishes eaten away from home; the method is time consuming and only motivated people are likely to cooperate, introducing the possibility of participant selection bias. In addition the method does not take into account seasonal variation of food intake and is not suitable for large studies since instructing participants and coding the dietary diaries are time consuming.

Recent recall is probably the most commonly used approach: participants are asked what food they ate over a recent specified time interval, usually 1–7 days before the interview is carried out, or a questionnaire is completed. Intake of food varies considerably from day to day and it is usually necessary to collect information for at least three days. This technique is particularly useful for assessing nutrients or food constituents that are derived from a limited number of sources (such as dietary fibre).

A disadvantage of both these methods in case-control studies of cancer is that the symptoms of the condition may result in a change of dietary habit so that current diet bears little resemblance to that before the onset of the disease. The *dietary history* technique has therefore been used to collect food consumption data relating to the period before the onset of symptoms, or even an earlier period if this is thought to be aetiologically relevant. Problems of recall limit the reliability of this method and information is usually limited to frequency of consumption of various foods. Careful training of interviewers, or the subjects themselves if questionnaires are to be used, is essential. However, several investigators have developed detailed dietary history methods (involving the recall of large numbers of foods) from which nutrients can be quantified, which appear to correlate well with other methods (e.g. dietary records).

Problems with dietary methods can be so great that some have concluded that the case-control approach is suitable only for conditions with acute onset and not conditions wih an insidious onset such as most cancers. Another difficulty which besets all nutritional studies is the fact that several nutritional variables are so closely related that it may be difficult to disentangle separate effects even when detailed dietary data are available. However, despite these serious limitations, some useful information has been derived from the case-control approach.

Dietary fat and breast cancer Phillips (1975) studied 77 breast cancer cases discharged from Seventh-Day Adventist hospitals during 1969–1972. Three types of age, sex, and race matched Adventists were selected as controls to test the hypothesis that a high fat intake, a low fibre intake or both are associated with an increased risk of breast cancer. Details of the diet history method were not provided. Of the large number of foods about which enquiry was made only five were related in any way to breast cancer. Fried foods (heavy and medium intake versus light intake), fried potatoes (any versus none), dairy products except milk (heavy and medium versus light), and white bread 'most of the time' (yes versus no) were associated with relative risks ranging from 1.6 to 2.6, the highest being for fried potatoes.

Lubin *et al.* (1981) have reported data relating to 577 breast cancer patients, representing 95 per cent of all cases aged 30–80 years reported to the Alberta Cancer Registry during the years 1976–1977: 826 disease-free women selected from the general population formed the control group. They represented only 72 per cent of the age-stratified sample originally drawn, but energetic attempts to study at least a proportion of non-responders showed no major differences between them and those responding to the initial invitation. The study questionnaire concerned mainly demographic, reproductive, and medical histories but it also covered the frequency with which eight food items (beef and other red meat, pork, chicken and other fowl, fish, eggs, cheese, creams, and sweet desserts) were usually eaten. Questions were also asked about the amount and type of milk consumed and the use of butter. Relative risk increased significantly with increasing intake of beef, pork, and sweet desserts. Elevated risks were also noted for the use of butter at the table and for frying with butter or margarine as opposed to vegetable oils. The associations were not appreciably altered by controlling for any of the other factors known to be associated with breast cancer. Recall bias is unlikely to explain these associations as there seems to be no good reason why breast cancer patients should selectively remember certain dietary items as compared with controls. However, apart from the crudeness of the dietary methods, one further potentially important factor needs to be borne in mind: the interviews for the cases were conducted at a referral clinic by nurses during 1976–77, whereas professional interviewers questioned controls in their homes during 1978. The authors attempted to evaluate the possibility that interviewer or temporal bias might account for their findings by comparing the responses to eight foods between 45 cases, who did not attend the clinic and were interviewed in their homes by the professional interviewers and the 526 cases interviewed by the nurses. No major differences were apparent. In fact the only difference was a slightly higher frequency of pork consumption for the nurse-interviewed cases. Given the limitations of the study, the results are consistent with an association beween breast cancer and animal fat and protein.

Graham *et al.* (1982) reported results of a similar study based on limited food frequency data collected from patients at the Roswell Park Memorial Institute between 1958 and 1965. There was no apparent association between estimated monthly intake of 'animal fats' and breast cancer risk. No measure of total fat intake was provided.

Miller *et al.* (1978) reported the results of a case-control study of diet and breast cancer carried out between 1973 and 1976 in four Canadian provinces. A total of 400 cases and 400 individually matched neighbourhood controls were interviewed for the study. Information on diet was collected in three ways: a 24-hour recall in which subjects were asked what they had eaten in the previous 24 hours; a four-day record which involved subjects writing down everything they ate during a four-day period; and a diet history in which the amount and frequency with which more than 150 different foods were consumed, were ascertained. The diet-history method addressed both the time immediately preceding the interview and a time period six months before the interview (i.e. before the diagnosis and treatment of the breast cancer cases). Estimates of daily nutrient intake in terms of calories, total fat, saturated fat, oleic and linoleic acids, and cholesterol were calculated separately for the various dietary methods. The initial analysis considered nutrient intake based on the diet history for a period of six months before the interview and it was concluded that there was some evidence for a weak association between fat intake and risk of breast cancer though small numbers led to a rather wide confidence interval around the relative risk.

A recent re-analysis of these data (Howe 1983) has used nutrient intake estimates based on both the 24-hour recall and the diet history relating to six months before interview. (The diet histories at the time of interview were so highly correlated with the earlier diet history that they were not included in the analysis, nor was the four-day record, since the response rate was only 87 per cent.) Table 4 shows the relative risk estimates and trend based on the mean daily intake of the six nutrients using both the 24-hour recall and the diet history, compared with the earlier analysis which used only the diet history. The estimates were made using a linear logistc regression model. Saturated fat was the only nutrient which showed a statistically significant trend, with increasing risk being apparent with increasing daily intake. When oleic and linoleic acids and cholesterol were included in the model (in order to examine for possible confounding since the different fat components are highly correlated) the relative risk estimates for saturated fat were increased. When the data were analysed separately for premenopausal and postmenopausal women the effects were restricted to premenopausal women in whom the relative risk was appreciably larger than in the whole group (Table 5).

Table 4. Relative risk estimates and trend tests for breast cancer in relation to various nutrients based on diet history alone and diet history together with 24-hour recall (from Howe 1983)

Nutrient	Estimated dietary intake							
	Diet history alone				Diet history and 24-hour recall			
	Low	Medium	High	Trend test *p* value	Low	Medium	High	Trend test *p* value
Total calories	1.0	1.1	1.0	0.88	1.0	1.1	1.3	0.16
Total fat	1.0	0.9	1.1	0.54	1.0	1.1	1.3	0.13
Saturated fat	1.0	1.4	1.3	0.18	1.0	1.3	1.5	0.03
Oleic acid	1.0	1.1	1.2	0.35	1.0	1.0	1.1	0.47
Linoleic acid	1.0	1.2	1.1	0.84	1.0	1.2	1.2	0.42
Cholesterol	1.0	1.1	1.1	0.52	1.0	1.2	1.2	0.28

Table 5. Relative risk estimates and trend tests for breast cancer in relation to saturated fat and oleic acid considered separately for pre- and post-menopausal women (from Howe 1983)

Status	Nutrient	Estimated daily intake			Trend test
		Low	Medium	High	p value
Premenopausal	Saturated fat	1.0	3.1	5.9	0.006
	Oleic acid	1.0	0.4	0.2	0.012
Postmenopausal	Saturated fat	1.0	1.2	1.5	0.358
	Oleic acid	1.0	0.8	1.0	0.894

Dietary fibre and colorectal cancer The frequency with which certain food items were eaten by patients with cancer of the colon or rectum and hospital or neighbourhood controls has been considered by many investigators (reviewed briefly by Haines 1983). For the purpose of illustration we have detailed below those studies which have provided a specific measure of dietary fibre intake.

Modan *et al.* (1975) studied 198 patients with colon cancer and 77 with rectal cancer identified during a three-year period in surgical wards of six hospitals in Tel Aviv, Israel. Neighbourhood and hospital controls were selected for each case and matched according to sex, age, country of origin, and length of residence in Israel. Interviewers of the hospitalized patients did not know whether patients were cases or controls. Information was requested for 243 different foods and overall response rate was 98 per cent. Subjects were asked to score a frequency of consumption category for each food. Fourteen food groups were identified and scores for each patient obtained from the sum of the consumption frequencies of items in each food group. Of the major food groups studied only dietary fibre differed significantly between patients with colon cancer and both hospital and neighbourhood controls. Differences were apparent for a wide range of fibre-containing foods. No such differences were seen for patients with rectal cancer and their controls. Bjelke (1980) in Norway and Minnesota and Dales *et al.* (1978) in a study of colorectal cancer among blacks in the U.S. found a similar reduction in the frequency of consumption of fibre-containing foods among cancer patients as compared with controls. Dales *et al.* also found a consistent dose-response effect of fibre and an association with food high in saturated fat.

Two recent case-control studies have adopted more sophisticated dietary methods. A Canadian study identified 348 cases of colon cancer and 194 cases of cancer of the rectum (Jain *et al.* 1980): 542 age- and sex-matched neighbourhood controls and 535 hospital controls (who had undergone abdominal surgery) formed the comparison groups. All were interviewed in their homes. The detailed dietary questionnaire concerned the usual amounts and frequency of a large number of food items comprising those found in the majority of diets. Food models were used to ascertain quantity and other questions were aimed at determining the types of food used in food preparation (e.g. the types of fats used for cooking, frying, etc). It was thus possible to quantify the intake of various nutrients in the two dietary periods to which the interview related: the two-month period immediately before interview and the two-month period at the end of six months before the interview date. The latter period, which usually antedated diagnosis and surgery (for both cases and hospital controls), was used for the major analysis.

A higher energy intake, and increased intakes of total protein, saturated fat, oleic acid, and cholesterol characterized patients with both colonic and rectal cancer as compared with controls. No association was seen with intakes of crude fibre, vitamin C, and linoleic acid. The nutrients associated with an increased risk were highly correlated with one other, but multivariate analysis suggested that the strongest association was with intake of saturated fat with evidence of dose-response relationship. Findings were essentially similar for both control groups. The most important potential source of bias in this study is the possibility that cases, having lost weight, were attempting to counteract the effect by eating more. The authors regard this as unlikely for the following reasons: the questionnaire was directed towards a period before weight loss; the effect of the disease (and the treatment) tends to reduce the food intake of cases compared with controls; and the association with saturated fat intake was far greater than for total energy intake.

The South Australian Cancer Registry was used to identify 368 consecutive cases of large bowel cancer who were studied with 732 controls selected from the general population via the electoral role (Potter *et al.* 1982). Once again a detailed food-frequency questionnaire which could be converted to nutrient intake was used. Highly significant associations were found with intake of total energy, protein, saturated fat, and alcohol. Dietary fibre intake (measured as total dietary fibre, rather than crude fibre as measured by Jain *et al.* (1980)) was identical in the cases and controls, although there is a suggestion that amongst men a high fat-low fibre diet is associated with a higher relative risk (2.4) than a high intake of saturated fat alone (1.7). This was not apparent in women.

Comment The case-control studies of dietary fat and fibre in relation to cancers of the breast and colon and rectum illustrate well the evolution that has occurred in dietary methods. In early studies, the approach was crude, with enquiries relating to a small number of foods. More recent investigators have developed questionnaires concerning many hundreds of foods (including all those likely to form part of the local diet) and food preparation, in a way which enables quantification of nutrients. The studies of Miller *et al.* (1978) in relation to breast cancer and Jain *et al.* (1980) and Potter *et al.* (1982) in relation to colorectal cancer are good examples. Unfortunately, questionnaires developed by these groups cannot be applied universally since they must always be related to local eating habits. It is therefore necessary before using such a questionnaire in a new environment to revalidate it in terms of repeatability as well as in relation to some other standardized dietary method (usually a dietary record). It is still not possible, however, to be totally confident that symptoms have not influenced recall. Howe's (1983) re-analysis of the breast cancer data published earlier by Miller *et al.* (1978) emphasizes the potential value in analysing data collected by more than one method.

The studies also underline the difficulty of identifying a single dietary variable when nutrients are so closely related. The danger of studying only one or two dietary factors is now fully appreciated. Dietary methods which permit translation into nutrient intake are amenable to sophisticated statistical analysis to examine for possible confounding but it needs to be stressed that even advanced statistical techniques should be interpreted with caution when identifying one of a number of interrelated nutritional variables as being independently associated with a particular cancer.

Cohort studies

In theory a cohort study can overcome some of the potential biases associated with case-control studies. In particular, dietary data are collected before the onset of symptoms and there is therefore no possibility that the condition may in some way influence dietary habits or recollection of them. Furthermore, it is possible to study the relationship between dietary factors and cancer at all sites. However, there are several problems associated with this approach. Most cancers are relatively uncommon and it is therefore usually necessary to study a large number of people for a very long period of time in order to obtain a sufficient number of 'events' to examine the relationship with dietary factors. The need for detailed dietary data, as well as information about other potentially confounding variables, remains and the work involved in setting up such a study is considerable. Identifying cohorts on whom it will be possible to maintain long-term follow-up presents particular problems and often results in the criticism that the cohorts studied are not representative of the population at large.

One of the most important cohort studies relating diet to cancer is that conducted by Hirayama on 265 118 adults aged 40 years and over who comprised 91–99 per cent of the census population in 29 health centre districts in Japan. The subjects were interviewed in 1965 and followed for 10 years with observation of 27 993 deaths, 7377 of them from cancer (Hirayama 1979). Diet was also documented to a limited extent in the prospective Adult Health Survey in Hiroshima (Hirayama 1978).

The limited data on diet and breast cancer reported from these two studies are summarized in Table 6. Both studies showed an association between meat intake and breast cancer and there is an association also with intake of diary produce in the Hiroshima study. The question of confounding by variables other than age, however, was not dealt with in the analysis and the causal significance of these associations is uncertain. There is also a very strong social-class gradient for breast cancer in Japan (Hirayama 1978) and one may assume that breast cancer is, in general, associated with 'Westernization' of the population. Associations with specific nutrients have also not been addressed in these analyses and it is probable that the dietary data collected were insufficient for quantitation of nutrient intake.

Probably because of limitations in his dietary data, Hirayama has not reported on fibre intake and colorectal cancer. He found no consistent association between meat intake and risk of colorectal cancer (Hirayama 1979).

Table 6. Relative risks of breast cancer associated with intakes of foods of animal origin in two cohort studies in Japan (from Hirayama 1978)

1 Study in 29 health centre districts

Age group and food	Frequency of intake	
	Less than daily	Daily
Age 40–54 years; meat	1.00	1.26
Age 55+ years; meat	1.00	2.38

2 Adult health study, Hiroshima

Food	Frequency of intake		
	Less than once a week	2–4 times a week	Almost daily
Meat	1.00	2.55	3.83
Eggs	1.00	1.91	2.86
Butter or cheese	1.00	3.23	2.10
Fish	1.00	0.76	0.94
Ham or sausage	1.00	0.75	0.73

A novel approach to analysis of data from the Japan-Hawaii Cancer Study, a cohort study of 6860 men of Japanese origin in Hawaii, has provided some confirmation of the results obtained by Hirayama in Japan (Nomura *et al.* 1978). Breast cancer was found in 86 wives of men in the study and the dietary data obtained from their husbands compared with that obtained from the rest of the men in the study. Dietary data had been collected both by food-frequency questionnaire and dietary recall. The husbands of the breast cancer cases were more frequent consumers of butter, margarine, cheese, and meat, and less frequent consumers of green tea and seaweeds (characteristic of the Japanese diet) than the husbands of non-cases. There was, however, only a small difference in total fat intake (in the expected direction) which was not statistically significant. Similar results were obtained from a comparison of the dietary recalls.

These various studies strongly suggest a correlation, at the individual level, between Westernization of diet and increasing risk of breast cancer in Japanese women. The Hawaii study, of course, assumes a close correlation between the dietary habits of husband and wife; to the extent that this assumption is not true the associations between breast cancer and dietary variables would probably have been weakened. It is not possible, however, from these studies to draw firm conclusions about specific nutrients and breast cancer although they are consistent with an association between fat intake and the disease.

The question of fibre intake and colorectal cancer has been addressed to only a very limited extent in cohort studies. Kromhout *et al.* (1982) related 10 years' mortality from all causes to fibre intake in 871 middle-aged men from Zutphen in the Netherlands. Nutrient intake estimates were based on formal dietary histories taken at the beginning of the study. Mortality from all causes, and mortality from all cancers increased as fibre intake decreased. There were, however, only five deaths from colon cancer. The inverse relationship between fibre intake and cancer mortality appeared to be mainly with death from lung cancer.

Although it contributes few relevant data itself, this study points to potential sources of additional data in the other populations from the Seven Countries Study of coronary disease and other cohort studies of coronary disease in which diet has been documented. Some of these studies have been analysed with respect to the relationship of death from cancer to blood cholesterol and also intake of ß-carotene/vitamin A (Kark *et al.* 1981; Shekelle *et al.* 1981; Feinleib 1981). Fibre and other potentially confounding nutrients merit some attention.

The cohort studies in Japanese and Japanese migrant populations illustrate the value of studying populations which can provide substantial dietary heterogeneity, particularly on variables of interest in current hypotheses. The need for heterogeneity has led to some carefully planned cohort studies of vegetarian populations. Phillips (1975, 1980) and his colleagues at Loma Linda University have collected dietary and other lifestyle data from some 100 000 Seventh-day Adventists in California. About 50 per cent of Adventists are vegetarian. This study should eliminate the problem of confounding inherent in simple comparisons of disease frequency between Adventists and the general population.

Similarly, a study has begun in Oxford into which some 6000 vegetarians, mainly members of the Vegetarian Society of the U.K., have been recruited. A comparison cohort, non-vegetarian friends of the vegetarians, has also been recruited and is similar in most relevant respects, except diet (e.g. smoking habits, parity, social class, alcohol intake), to the vegetarians. All participants are completing a four-day diet record and answering supplementary questions on diet (e.g. concerning food preparation, foods not eaten during the recorded period, seasonal variation) which will permit calculation of average daily nutrient intakes. The participants have been 'flagged' in the National Health Service Control Registry so that all deaths and cancer registrations are notified to the investigators. The dietary heterogeneity provided by the vegetarian and comparison cohorts and the accurate estimation of nutrient intake provided by the four-day diaries should contribute substantially to knowledge of the association between diet and the more common cancers.

Intervention studies

Intervention studies provide the best evidence in human populations of a causal association. Such studies are rarely feasible in the study of diet and cancer. One such study has, however, been started in the U.S. in which ß-carotene or placebo is being given in a randomized controlled clinical trial. Reduced intake of vitamin A has been implicated in the aetiology of several cancers on the basis of descriptive studies and cohort studies and this approach offers the possibility of conclusive confirmation.

The application of this approach to the prevention of relatively common lesions which are believed to be precursors of cancer, at least in a proportion of cases, may also be rewarding. Thus, for example, studies are under way aimed at preventing recurrent adenomatous polyps of the large bowel by use of a high-fibre diet and recurrent benign mammary dysplasia by use of a low-fat diet. It will be difficult to decide, however, whether a change in frequency of a benign condition will necessarily translate into a change in frequency of the corresponding cancer.

Discussion

The principal limitation in most of the analytical studies of diet and cancer which have been conducted so far lies in the dietary methods. Methods in case-control studies have improved substantially but uncertainty remains about the validity of recall of diets in the somewhat distant past. Cohort studies which have been reported have, in general, used rudimentary dietary methods and have not provided data on intake of specific nutrients.

In spite of these problems, there is some consistency at least in the association between dietary fat and breast cancer. It was suggested by descriptive studies, has been shown by several recent case-control studies, and is consistent with the results of the cohort studies we have reviewed. Such an association has substantial biological plausibility (Armstrong 1979).

The situation for large bowel cancer is much less clear. Dietary factors seem to be involved, particularly from the evidence of the descriptive data, but the analytical studies have shown no consistent pattern. Whether, therefore, diet really is important and, if so, whether fat, meat, fibre, all three, or some other dietary constituent is the most important remains to be resolved. Analytical studies of colorectal cancer would benefit from refinements in dietary methods, accurate estimation of nutrient intake, and the adequate documentation and control of confounding variables.

That we have limited our detailed discussion of the facts to these two themes, fat and breast cancer and fibre and colorectal cancer, should not be taken to mean that they have been the most thoroughly elucidated. There are substantial data on other relationships to which we will refer, at least briefly, below.

Diet and cancer prevention

For the mainly methodological reasons which we have treated in some detail above, there are few indisputable facts about the role of diet in the aetiology of human cancer. Nonetheless, because we believe that preventive action should be taken early rather than late in the course of investigation of disease aetiology, we will summarize the state of knowledge as we now understand it and consider its implications for cancer prevention.

Table 7 summarizes and classifies food-derived variables thought or known to be related to risk of human cancer. As suggested above, there are few firmly established facts: alcoholic drinks, dietary fat, obesity, and arsenic (not certainly a nutrient and not certainly associated with cancer at usual dietary levels of intake) as causes and vegetables and vitamin A, ß-carotene, or both as protective (and not necessarily independently of each other); some of these are disputed.

Palmer (1983) reviewed in detail the health-related dietary policies adopted by various organizations, both in the U.S. and elsewhere. There was a remarkable degree of consensus between them: 'ideal' body weight

Table 7. Dietary components that may either cause of protect against the development of cancer in humans; disputed, speculative, and less well-established effects are indicated by a question mark (?); modified from Armstrong *et al.* (1982)

Classes of food	
Causative:	Alcoholic drinks, meat (?), coffee (?), bracken fern (?)
Protective:	Vegetables, fruit (?), milk (?)
Nutrients	
Major nutrients	
Causative:	Total energy (obesity), fat, alcohol (?)
Protective:	Fibre (?)
Minor nutrients	
Causative:	Arsenic, cadmium (?)
Protective:	Vitamin A and/or ß-carotene, riboflavin (?), vitamin C (?), vitamin E (?), folate (?), iodine (?), iron (?), selenium (?)
Non-nutrients	
Natural components of food	
Causative:	Cycasin (?)
Protective:	Certain indoles and other chemicals in cruciferous vegetables (?)
Food additives	
Causative:	Nitrates and nitrites (?), AF2 (?)
Protective:	BHA and BHT (? – animal experimental evidence only)
Food contaminants	
Causative:	Aflatoxins, *N*-nitroso compounds (?), polycyclic aromatic hydrocarbons (?)
Protective:	No example

should be maintained, total fat intake reduced, saturated fat intake reduced disproportionately, intake of simple sugars reduced, complex carbohydrate intake increased, fibre intake increased, sodium intake decreased, and moderation in alcohol advised. There was less agreement on reduction in cholesterol intake and an absolute increase in polyunsaturated fat intake.

A comparison of these recommendations, not based specifically on considerations of cancer control, with the summary given in Table 7 suggests that they are fairly well targeted to cancer control. On considering the evidence in detail, the Committee on Diet, Nutrition and Cancer (1982) of the National Academy of Sciences recommended a reduction in total fat intake, increased consumption of whole grains, fruits, and vegetables (without a specific recommendation regarding fibre), a reduction in intake of salt-cured, pickled, and smoked foods and moderation in alcohol intake. Maintenance of ideal body weight might reasonably have been recommended by the National Academy of Sciences Committee (almost certainly prophylactic against endometrial cancer and gallbladder cancer and possibly breast cancer) and increased use of whole grains, fruits, and vegetables, while not specified by other groups, is implicit in limitation of intake of simple sugars and increased intake of complex carbohydrates (although the micronutrients and fibre in grains, fruits and vegetables are probably the most relevant to cancer prevention. It appears, therefore, considerations of carcinogen contamination of food and some naturally occurring carcinogens apart, that a diet which is both 'ideal' nutritionally and for the prevention of other chronic diseases may also be that which minimizes the risk of cancer.

References

Ahlbom, H.E. (1936). Simple achlorhydric anaemia, Plummer-Vinson syndrome, and carcinoma of the mouth, pharynx, and oesophagus in women. *Brit. med. J.* **ii**, 331–3.

Armstrong, B.K. (1979). Diet and hormones in the epidemiology of breast and endometrial cancers. *Nutr. Cancer* **1**, 90–5.

Armstrong, B. (1976). Recent trends in breast-cancer incidence and mortality in relation to changes in possible risk factors. *Int. J. Cancer* **17**, 204–11.

Armstrong, B. (1982). Endocrine factors in human carcinogenesis. In *Host factors in human carcinogenesis* (ed. H. Bartsch and B. Armstrong), pp. 193–221. International Agency for Research on Cancer, Lyon. (IARC Scientific Publications No. 39.)

Armstrong, B. and Doll, R. (1974). Bladder cancer mortality in England and Wales in relation to cigarette smoking and saccharin consumption. *Brit. J. prev. soc. Med.* **28**, 233–40.

Armstrong, B. and Doll, R. (1975). Environmental factors and cancer incidence and mortality in different countries, with special reference to dietary practices. *Int. J. Cancer* **15**, 617–31.

Armstrong, B.K., Brown, J.B., Clark, H.T., Crooke, D.K., Hahnel, R., Masarei, J.R., and Ratajczak, T. (1981). Diet and reproductive hormones: A study of vegetarian and non-vegetarian postmenopausal women. *J. nat. Cancer Inst.* **67**, 761–7.

Armstrong, B.K., McMichael, A.J., and MacLennan, R. (1982). Diet. In *Cancer epidemiology and prevention* (ed. D. Schottenfeld and J. Fraumeni, Jr.), pp. 419–33. Saunders, Philadelphia.

Australian Bureau of Statistics (1981). *Apparent consumption of foodstuffs and nutrients: Australia 1970–80*. Australian Bureau of Statistics, Canberra (Catalogue No. 4306.0).

Bingham, S., Williams, D.R.R., Cole, T.J., and James, W.P.T. (1979). Dietary fibre and regional large-bowel cancer mortality in Britain. *Brit. J. Cancer* **40**, 456–63.

Bjelke, E. (1980). Epidemiology of colorectal cancer with emphasis on diet. In *Human cancer: its characterisation and treatment* (ed. W. Davis, K.R. Harrap and G. Stathopoulos), pp. 158–74. Proceedings of the Eighth International Symposium on the Biological Characterization of Human Tumours, Athens, 8–11 May, 1979. Excerpta Medica, Amsterdam. (International Congress Series No. 484.)

Carroll, K.K., Gammal, E.B., and Plunkett, E.R. (1968). Dietary fat and mammary cancer. *Can. med. Ass. J.* **98**, 590–4.

Committee on Diet, Nutrition and Cancer (1982). *Diet, nutrition and cancer.* National Academy Press, Washington D.C.

Cummings, J.H. (1981). Dietary fibre and large bowel cancer. *Proc. nutr. Soc.* **40**, 7–14.

Cummings, J.H., Branch, W.J., Jenkins, D.J.A., Southgate, D.A.T., Houston, H., and James, W.P.T. (1978). Colonic response to dietary fibre from carrot, cabbage, apple, bran and guar gum. *Lancet* **i**, 5–9.

Dales, L.G., Friedman, G.D., Ury, H.K., Grossman, S., and Williams, S.R. (1978). A case-control study of relationships of diet and other traits to colorectal cancer in American blacks. *Amer. J. Epidemiol.* **109**, 132–44.

Devesa, S.S. and Silverman, D.T. (1978). Cancer incidence and mortality trends in the United States: 1935–74. *J. nat. Cancer Inst.* **60**, 545–71.

Doll, R. (1979). Nutrition and cancer: a review. *Nutr. Cancer* **1**, 35–45.

Doll, R. and Peto, R. (1981). The causes of cancer: quantitative estimates of avoidable risks of cancer in the United States today. *J. nat. Cancer Inst.* **66**, 1194–1308.

Doll, R. and Smith, P.G. (1982). Comparison between registries: age-standardized rates. In *Cancer incidence in five continents* (ed. J. Waterhouse, C. Muir, K. Shanmugaratnam, and J. Powell), Vol. 4, pp. 671–3. International Agency for Research on Cancer, Lyon. (IARC Scientific Publications No. 42.)

Drasar, B.S. and Irving, D. (1973). Environmental factors and cancer of the colon and breast. *Brit. J. Cancer* **27**, 167–72.

Enstrom, J.E. (1981). Reassessment of the role of dietary fat in cancer etiology. *Cancer Res.* **41**, 3722–3.

Feinleib, M. (1981). On a possible inverse relationship between serum cholesterol and cancer mortality. *Amer. J. Epidemiol.* **114**, 5–10.

Fleming, N.T., Armstrong, B.K., Sheiner, H.J., and James, I.R. (1981). Occurrence of breast cancer in Australian women. *Med. J. Aust.* **1**, 290–3.

Food and Agriculture Organization (1971). *Food balance sheets. Average, 1964–66.* Food and Agriculture Organization, Rome.

Friend, B. (1967). Nutrients in United States food supply: A review of trends, 1909–1913 to 1965. *Amer. J. clin. Nutr.* **20**, 907–14.

Gaskill, S.P., McGuire, W.L., Osborne, C.K., and Stern, M.P. (1979). Breast cancer mortality and diet in the United States. *Cancer Res.* **39**, 3628–37.

Goldin, B.R. and Gorbach, S.L. (1976). The relationship between diet and rat fecal bacterial enzymes implicated in colon cancer. *J. nat. Cancer Inst.* **57**, 371–5.

Goldin, B.R., Adlercreutz, H., Gorbach, S.L., Warram, J.R., Dwyer, J.T., Swenson, L., and Woods, M.N. (1982). Estrogen excretion patterns and plasma levels in vegetarian and omnivorous women. *New Engl. J. Med.* **307**, 1542–7.

Gortner, W.A. (1975). Nutrition in the United States, 1900 to 1974. *Cancer Res.* **35**, 3246–53.

Graham, S., Marshall, J., Mettlin, C., Rzepka, T., Nemoto, T., and Byers, T. (1982). Diet in the epidemiology of breast cancer. *Amer. J. Epidemiol.* **116**, 68–75.

Gray, G.E., Pike, M.C., and Henderson, B.E. (1979). Breast-cancer incidence and mortality rates in different countries in relation to known risk factors and dietary practices. *Brit. J. Cancer* **39**, 1–7.

Greaves, J.P. and Hollingsworth, D.F. (1966). Trends in food consumption in the United Kingdom. *World Rev. Nutr. Diet.* **6**, 34–89.

Haines, A.P. (1983). Dietary fat intake and the causation of cancer: The epidemiological perspective. *Biochem. Soc. Trans.* **11**, 254–6.

Hems, G. (1970). Epidemiological characteristics of breast cancer in middle and late age. *Brit. J. Cancer* **24**, 226–7.

Hems, G. (1978). The contributions of diet and childbearing to breast-cancer rates. *Brit. J. Cancer* **37**, 974–82.

Hill, A.B. (1977). *A short textbook of medical statistics*, p. 293, Hodder and Stoughton, London.

Hill, P.B. and Wynder, E.L. (1979). Effect of a vegetarian diet and dexamethasone on plasma prolactin, testosterone and dehydroepiandrosterone in men and women. *Cancer Letters* **7**, 273–82.

Hirayama, T. (1978). Epidemiology of breast cancer with special reference to the role of diet. *Prev. Med.* **7**, 173–95.

Hirayama, T. (1979). Diet and cancer. *Nutr. Cancer* **1**, 67–81.

Holman, D. and Armstrong, B. (1982). *Cancer mortality trends in Australia 1910–1979*, Parts 1 and 2. Cancer Council of Western Australia, Perth.

Howe, G.R. (1983). The use of polytomous response data to increase power in case-control studies: an application to the association between dietary fat and breast cancer. Invited paper. Annual Meeting of the American Statistics Association, Toronto, August 1983.

Howell, M.A. (1975). Diet as an etiological factor in the development of cancers of the colon and rectum. *J. chron. Dis.* **28**, 67–80.

Hutchinson, J. (1982). On cancer and malignant processes in general. *Arch. Surg.* **3**, 47–59.

Irving, D. and Drasar, B.S. (1973). Fibre and cancer of the colon. *Brit. J. Cancer* **28,** 462–3.

Jain, M., Cook, G.M., Davis, F.G., Grace, M.G., Howe, G.R., and Miller, A.B. (1980). A case-control study of diet and colo-rectal cancer. *Int. J. Cancer* **26**, 757–68.

Jensen, O.M., MacLennan, R., and Wahrendorf, J. (1982). Diet, bowel function, fecal characteristics, and large bowel cancer in Denmark and Finland. *Nutr. Cancer* **4**, 5–19.

Kark, J.D., Smith, A.H., Switzer, B.R., and Hames, C.G. (1981). Serum vitamin A (retinol) and cancer incidence in Evans County, Georgia. *J. nat. Cancer Inst.* **66**, 7–16.

Kinlen, L.J. (1982). Meat and fat consumption and cancer mortality: a study of strict religious orders in Britain. *Lancet* **i**, 946–9.

Knox, E.G. (1977). Foods and diseases. *Brit. J. prev. soc. Med.* **31**, 71–80.

Kolonel, L.N., Hankin, J.H., Lee, J., Chu, S.Y., Nomura, A.M.Y., and Hinds, M.W. (1981). Nutrient intakes in relation to cancer incidence in Hawaii. *Brit. J. Cancer* **44**, 332–9.

Kromhout, D., Bosschieter, E.B., and DeLezenne Coulander, C. (1982). Dietary fibre and 10-year mortality from coronary heart disease, cancer, and all causes: the Zutphen Study. *Lancet* **ii**, 518–22.

Lea, A.J. (1967). Neoplasms and environmental factors. *Ann. roy. Coll. Surg. Engl.* **41**, 432–8.

Li, J-Y. (1982). Epidemiology of esophageal cancer in China. *Nat. Cancer Inst. Mono.* **62**, 113–20.

Lubin, J.H., Burns, P.E., Blot, W.J., Ziegler, R.G., and Fraumeni, J.F., Jr (1981). Dietary factors and breast cancer risk. *Int. J. Cancer* **28**, 685–9.

Liu, K., Stamler, J., Moss, D., Garside, D., Persky, V., and Soltero, I. (1979). Dietary cholesterol, fat, and fibre and colon-cancer mortality: an analysis of international data. *Lancet* **ii**. 782–5.

Lyon, J.L., Gardner, J.W., and West, D.W. (1980). Cancer incidence in Mormons and non-Mormons in Utah during 1967–75. *J. nat. Cancer Inst.* **65**, 1055–61.

McCoy, T.A. (1959). Neoplasia and nutrition. *World Rev. Nutr. Diet.* **1**, 177–203.

MacLennan, R., Jensen, O.M., Mosbech, J., and Vuori, H. (1978). Diet, transit time, stool weight, and colon cancer in two Scandinavian populations. *Amer. J. clin. Nutr.* **31**, s239–s242.

McMichael, A.J. (1979). Alimentary tract cancer in Australia in relation to diet and alcohol. *Nutr. Cancer* **1**, 82–9.

Maruchi, N., Aoki, S., Tsuda, K., Tanaka, Y., and Toyokawa, H. (1977). Relation of food consumption to cancer mortality in Japan, with special reference to international figures. *Gann* **68**, 1–13.

Miller, A.B., Kelly, A., Choi, N.W., Matthew, V., Morgan, R.W., Munan, L., Burch, J.D., Feather, J., Howe, G.R., and Jain, M. (1978). A study of diet and breast cancer. *Amer. J. Epidemiol.* **107**, 499–509.

Modan, B., Barell, V., Lubin, F., Modan, M., Greenberg, R.A., and Graham, S. (1975). Low-fiber intake as an etiologic factor in cancer of the colon. *J. nat. Cancer Inst.* **55**, 15–18.

Morgenstern, H. (1982). Uses of ecologic analysis in epidemiologic research. *Amer. J. publ. Hlth* **72**, 1336–44.

Nomura, A., Henderson, B.E., and Lee, J. (1978). Breast cancer and diet among the Japanese in Hawaii. *Amer. J. clin. Nutr.* **31**, 2020–25.

Palmer, S. (1983). Diet, nutrition, and cancer: The future of dietary policy. *Cancer Res.* (Suppl.) **43**, 2509–14.

Percy, C., Stanek, E., and Gloekler, L. (1981). Accuracy of cancer death certificates and its effect on cancer mortality statistics. *Amer. J. publ. Hlth* **71**, 242–50.

Phillips, R.L. (1975). Role of life-style and dietary habits in risk of cancer among Seventh-day Adventists. *Cancer Res.* **35**, 3513–22.

Phillips, R.L. (1980). Cancer among Seventh-day Adventists. *J. environ. Pathol. Toxicol.* **3**, 157–69.

Potter, J.D., McMichael, A.J., and Bonett, A.Z. (1982). Diet, alcohol and large bowel cancer: a case-control study. *Proc. Nutr. Soc. Aust.* **7**, 123–6.

Reddy, B.S., Hedges, A., Laakso, K., and Wynder, E.L. (1978). Fecal constituents of a high-risk North American and a low-risk Finnish population for the development of large bowel cancer. *Cancer Letters* **4**, 217–22.

Reddy, B.S., Sharma, C., Darby, L., Laakso, K., and Wynder, E.L. (1980). Metabolic epidemiology of large bowel cancer. Fecal mutagens in high- and low-risk populations for colon cancer: A preliminary report. *Nutr. Res.* **72**, 511–22.

Rellahan, W. (1982). U.S.A. Hawaii. In *Cancer incidence in five continents*, Vol. 4 (ed. J. Waterhouse, C. Muir, K. Shanmugaratnam, and J. Powell), pp. 616–20. International Agency for Research on Cancer, Lyon (IARC Scientific Publications No. 42.)

Schrauzer, G.N. (1976). Cancer mortality correlation studies. II. Regional associations of mortalities with the consumption of food and other commodities. *Med. Hypoth.* **2**, 39–49.

Shekelle, R.B., Liu, S., Raynor, W.J., Jr, Lepper, M., Maliza, C., and Rossof, A.H. (1981). Dietary vitamin A and risk of cancer in the Western Electric Study. *Lancet* **ii**, 1185–90.

Schultz, T.D. and Leklem, J.E. (1980). Dietary fat intake and plasma estrogen levels in pre-menopausal vegetarian and non-vegetarian women. *Fed. Proc.* **39**, 432.

Siiteri, P.K. (1981). Extraglandular oestrogen formation and serum binding of oestradiol: Relationship to cancer. *J. Endocrinol.* **89**, 119–29P.

Stocks, P. (1916/17). Cancer and goitre. *Biometrika* **16**, 364–401.

Stocks, P. (1947). *Regional and local differences in cancer death rates*. His Majesty's Stationary Office, London (Studies on Medical and Population Subjects No. 1).

Stocks, P. (1970). Breast cancer anomalies. *Brit. J. Cancer* **24**, 633–43.

Stocks, P. and Kay, M.N. (1933). A co-operative study of the habits, home life, dietary and family histories of 450 cancer patients and of an equal number of control patients. *Ann. Eugen.* **5**, 277–80.

Sullivan, P.D., Christine, B., Connelly, R., and Barrett, H. (1972). Analysis of trends in age-adjusted incidence rates for 10 major sites of cancer. *Amer. J. publ. Hlth* **62**, 1065–71.

Tannenbaum, A. (1940). Relationship of body weight to cancer incidence. *Arch. Pathol.* **30**, 509–17.

5 Occupation

Rodolfo Saracci

Occupational cancer has, for about two centuries, provided a continuous flow of observations, clinical and epidemiological, leading to the identification of individual carcinogens, opening the way to the understanding of carcinogenesis by chemicals and providing support for the now commonly accepted view that exogenous agents play a major role in cancer causation. Publications on the history of occupational cancer have appeared in the literature on numerous occasions (Hueper 1942; Hunter 1975). Notwithstanding this long history and its central importance in cancer research, occupational cancer remains from a public-health viewpoint a somewhat elusive entity in most countries, both with respect to its present impact and future evolution.

A key feature of occupational cancer is that it is preventable by avoidance of exposures in the workplace, but what the law regards as cancer due to occupation varies markedly even within industrialized countries (Montesano and Tomatis 1972), as does its medical recognition. Also, in developed countries there are trends at work acting in opposite directions on the occurrence of cancers due to workplace exposures: on the one hand large numbers of new chemicals are continuously being synthesized and put into use, while, on the other, control of exposure to hazardous materials is becoming more rigorous and smaller numbers of workers are exposed to them. Some modern technology is now beginning to be transferred to developing countries, where it runs side by side with earlier technologies and conditions of exposure similar to those prevalent several decades ago in industrialized countries. One hopes that the net balance of these trends is a decreasing incidence, worldwide, of occupational cancers, but this cannot come about without sustained effort in research and action on prevention. The level of interest is reflected by discussions and developments which have taken place during the last decade within both the scientific and lay communities. Rather than attempting to review these developments comprehensively I will touch on a few aspects, mostly drawing from collaborative work in which I have a direct involvement at the International Agency for Research on Cancer (IARC).

Proportion of cancer attributable to occupation

A major and recurring theme in discussion has been the magnitude of the present-day impact of occupational factors in the causation of cancer, the question often being formulated as: 'What proportion of all cancers in industrialized countries is attributable to occupation?'. Framed in this way, the question addresses the impact of occupation in relative rather than in absolute terms. If other things are equal, the proportion of cancers attributable to occupation *must* be higher in populations experiencing a comparatively low overall cancer rate: for example, in non-smoking communities. Also, the impact is viewed in the aggregate, lumping together not only all cancers but, more importantly, a spectrum of exposures heterogeneous in type and intensity, variably distributed within a population. Finally, the question does not address the fact that when interactions occur between different agents (for example, an occupational exposure and smoking) a cancer is simultaneously attributable to more than one agent. Questions of this kind, soliciting a single figure as an answer to a complex question, are not uncommon, particularly on socially sensitive issues: another well-known example is: 'What proportion of intelligence is due to heredity?'. To the extent that the detailed data necessary to dissect a complex problem and reduce it to a simple form are inadequate or non-existent, any single-figure answer to such questions will inevitably embody a variety of assumptions and will thus be subject to much uncertainty, difficult for the uninitiated reader to appreciate. As J. Bernal (1969) once wrote: 'Figures are as flexible as words, and more deceptive because they convey with them the air of neutral facts.' Not suprisingly, for the proportion of all cancers attributable to occupation, figures ranging from 1 per cent (or even less) to 20 per cent (or even more) have been quoted (Wynder and Gori 1977; Bridbord *et al.* 1981). This state of affairs reflects the incomplete (particularly from the quantitative angle) information at present available on the risk associated with given exposures and the mostly indirect nature of the information on how many workers are in fact exposed, compounded by variations between countries.

In 1981 Doll and Peto reviewed, mostly from an epidemiological angle, what is known about the causes of cancer: they discussed critically the main limitations involved in attributing cancer to specific causes and expressed explicitly the uncertainty in their own estimates. They put the proportion of all cancers attributable to occupation within the U.S. at 4 per cent, with an 'acceptable range' from 2 per cent to 8 per cent. These are overall figures, averaged over the whole population. They carry the implication that in the 20 per cent or so of the population in which the occupation-related cancers are almost exclusively concentrated (manual workers aged 20 and over in mining, agriculture, and industry, broadly defined, numbering 31 million out of a total U.S. population aged 20 and over of 158 million (International Labour Office 1982)), as much as one cancer out of every five may be attributable to exposures in the workplace.

Occupations carrying an increased risk of cancer

The first question that can be asked, relevant for research purposes as much as for prevention, is: which occupations have been shown to carry an increased risk of cancer? An accurate answer would require an evaluation of all the data available from the observation of occupationally exposed human groups. The task is made considerably lighter by the existence of classifications, mostly of chemicals and mixtures of chemicals, according to the degree of evidence of carcinogenicity. A well-known classification, internationally used as a term of reference, is that provided by the IARC Programme on the Evaluation of the Carcinogenic Risk of Chemicals to Humans (International Agency for Research on Cancer 1972–82). Within this programme, Working Groups develop evaluations of carcinogenic risk to humans in the form of overall judgments, combining initially separate assessments of evidence for carcinogenicity from studies in humans and in experimental animals (supplemented by data on short-term tests). By 1981, the ongoing programme (initiated in 1971) had produced 29 volumes, containing evaluations or re-evaluations of 585 chemicals, groups of chemicals, industrial processes, and occupational exposures; a synthesis of the programme (Volumes 1–29) has been published as IARC Monographs Supplement No. 4 (International Agency for Research on Cancer 1982). Of the 155 agents and exposures reviewed in this supplement for which some data (often scanty) pertinent to carcinogenicity evaluations in humans were available, 30 were classified as causally associated with cancer and 61 were probably carcinogenic to humans. (Sixty-four could not be classified as to their carcinogenicity in humans due to inadequate data.)

Using the Monographs as a source, supplemented by whatever additional epidemiological information was available, Table 1 has been prepared in an attempt to portray those industries and occupations showing an increased risk of cancer. Table 1, which appears in the third (1983) edition of the International Labour Office *Encyclopaedia of occupational health and safety* (Simonato and Saracci 1983), is reproduced here in its entirety for easy consultation. In part (a) of Table 1 occupations are included for which an increase in risk of cancer at a given site, causally related to the occupation, can be regarded as well established. In part (b) occupations are listed which have been reported in published studies as presenting an increased cancer risk at some site(s), but for which a definitive statement about the causal relation with occupation is not possible. This category encompasses, at one extreme, occupations reported as associated with an increased risk in a single study and, at the other, occupations reported in several studies each of which is, however, affected by limitations that prevent the drawing of firm inferences. Some occupations appear in parts (a) and (b), but for different cancer sites. The occupational groups in Table 1 are *only* those quoted in the studies contributing the evidence of an increased cancer risk: they are not the groups, most likely larger in size, in which the relevant carcinogenic exposure(s) may occur. Excluded from the studies contributing evidence of an increased risk of cancer were case reports, ecological studies, and investigations reporting ill-defined occupations. Also excluded were occupations of historical interest which are non-existent today. More generally, a consideration of time is essential in qualifying the content of Table 1; what appears in it is strictly related to those occupations which have up to now attracted enough attention to be investigated epidemiologically and that, under past conditions of exposure, have showed an increased risk of cancer at some site(s). Thus, occupations not included in Table 1 cannot be considered not to present an excess risk (they may simply not have been investigated well enough or not at all), whereas occupations included in Table 1 do not necessarily still carry the hazard if conditions of exposure have changed with time.

Interacting carcinogens: asbestos and smoking

Varying conditions of exposure and changes in risk with time also affect the investigation of an emerging aspect of occupational carcinogenesis of potential general relevance, namely the interaction of different occupational agents between themselves and with other non-occupational agents such as those deriving from personal habits. The example of the interaction of asbestos and smoking on lung cancer is one on which results from several studies exist, and which is generally instructive. The development of knowledge on this topic can be highlighted through a few key references:

1. In 1955, Doll first showed, among asbestos-exposed workers in a British textile factory, a lung cancer mortality about 14 times higher than in the general population. This observation placed on firm epidemiological grounds the evidence for the carcinogenic action of occupational exposure to asbestos, which up to that time had been based only on scattered clinical and pathological reports.

2. In 1968, Selikoff *et al.* confirmed this finding in a U.S. group of 370 insulation workers and first showed that the excess in workers who smoked was much greater than one would expect from a simple additive effect of asbestos and smoking on lung cancer rates. In fact, while lung cancer mortality appeared to be increased about nine times when workers were

Table 1. Occupations carrying an increased risk of cancer

Industry	Occupation	Site	Reported or suspected causative agent
(a) *Occupations recognized to present an increased risk of cancer, causally related to the occupation.*			
Agriculture, forestry, and fishing	Vineyard workers using arsenical insecticides	Lung, skin	Arsenic
Extractive	Arsenic mining	Lung, skin	Arsenic
	Iron-ore mining	Lung	Causative agent not identified
	Asbestos mining	Lung, pleural and peritoneal mesothelioma	Asbestos
	Uranium mining	Lung	Radon
Asbestos production industry	Insulated material production (pipes, sheeting, textile, clothes, masks, asbestos cement manufacts)	Lung, pleural and peritoneal mesothelioma	Asbestos
Petroleum industry	Wax pressmen	Scrotum	Polycyclic hydrocarbons
Metal industry	Copper smelting	Lung	Arsenic
	Chromate producing	Lung	Chromium
	Chromium plating	Lung	Chromium
	Ferrochromium producing	Lung	Chromium
	Steel production	Lung	Benzo(a)pyrene
	Nickel refining	Nasal sinuses, lung	Nickel
Shipbuilding, motor vehicles and transport	Shipyard and dock-yard workers	Lung, pleural and peritoneal mesothelioma	Asbestos
Chemical industry	BCME and CMME products and users	Lung (oat cell carcinoma)	BCME, CMME
	Vinyl chloride producers	Liver angiosarcoma	Vinyl chloride monomer
	Isopropyl alcohol manufacturing (strong acid process) workers	Paranasal sinuses	Causative agent not identified
	Pigment chromate producing	Lung	Chromium
	Dye manufacturers and users	Bladder	Benzidine, 2-naphthy-lamine, 4-aminodi-phenyl
	Auramine manufacture	Bladder	Auramine (together with the other aromatic amines used in the process)
Pesticides and herbicides production industry	Arsenical insecticides production and packaging	Lung	Arsenic
Gas industry	Coke plant workers	Lung	Benzo(a)pyrene

Industry	Occupation	Site	Reported or suspected causative agent
	Gas workers	Lung, bladder, scrotum	Coal carbonization products, ß-naphthylamine
	Gas-retort house workers	Bladder	α/ß-naphthylamine
Rubber industry	Rubber manufacture	Lymphatic and haematopoietic system (leukaemia)	Benzene
		Bladder	Aromatic amines
	Calendering, tyre curing, tyre building	Lymphatic and haematopoietic system (leukaemia)	Benzene
	Millers, mixers	Bladder	Aromatic amines
	Synthetic latex producers, tyre curing, calender operatives, reclaim, cable makers	Bladder	Aromatic amines
Construction industry	Insulators and pipe coverers	Lung, pleural and peritoneal mesothelioma	Asbestos
Leather industry	Boot and shoe manufacturers, repairers	Nose, marrow (leukaemia)	Leather dust, benzene
Wood pulp and paper industry	Furniture and cabinet makers	Nose (adenocarcinoma)	Wood dust
Other	Roofers, asphalt workers	Lung	BAP

(b) *Occupations reported to present an increased risk of cancer, but for which the assessment of the causal relation with the occupation is not definitive*

Industry	Occupation	Site	Reported or suspected causative agent
Agriculture, forestry and fishing	Fishermen	Skin, lip	Pitch, ultraviolet radiation
	Farmers	Lymphatic and haematopoietic system (leukaemia, lymphoma)	Undefined
	Basal bark spraying	Lymphatic and haematopoietic system (lymphoma), soft tissue sarcomas	Phenoxyacetic acids, chlorophenols (presumably contaminated with PCDF, PCDD, and polychlorinated benzodioxins)
	Railway embankment spraying	Lymphatic and haematopoietic system (lymphoma), lung cancer	Phenoxyacetic acids, amitrol, monuron, durion
	Pesticide-appliers	Lung	Hexachlorocyclohexane combined and other pesticides

Industry	Occupation	Site	Reported or suspected causative agent
Extractive	Zinc–lead mining	Lung	Radiations
	Coal	Stomach	Coal dust
	Talc	Lung, pleura	Talc (contaminated with asbestos?)
	Asbestos mining	Gastrointestinal tract	Asbestos
Asbestos production industry	Insulation material production pipes, sheeting, textiles, clothes, masks, asbestos cement manufacts)	Larynx, gastro-intestinal tract	Asbestos
Petroleum industry	Oil refining	Oesophagus, stomach, lung	Polycyclic hydrocarbons
	Boilermakers, painters, welders, oilfield workers	Lung	Polycyclic hydrocarbons
	Petrochemical plant workers	Brain, stomach	Polycyclic hydrocarbons
	Petroleum refining	Marrow (leukaemia)	Benzene
Metal industry	Aluminium production	Lung	Benzo(a)pyrene
	Beryllium refining	Lung	Beryllium
	Smelters	Respiratory and digestive system	Lead
	Nickel refining	Larynx	Nickel
	Battery plant workers, cadmium alloy producers, electro-plating workers	Prostate, kidney	Cadmium
	Cadmium smelters	Prostate, lung	Cadmium
Shipbuilding, motor vehicles and transport	Filling station, bus and truck drivers, operators of excavating machines	Marrow (leukaemia)	Petroleum products and combustion residues containing benzene
	Hauliers	Lung	Polycyclic aromatic hydrocarbons
	Shipyard and dock-yard workers	Larynx, digestive system	Asbestos
Chemical industry	Acrylonitrile production	Lung, colon	Acrylonitrile
	Vinylidene chloride producers	Lung	Vinylidene chloride (mixed exposure to VC and acrylonitrile)
	Isopropyl alcohol manufacturing (strong acid process) workers	Larynx	Undefined
	Polychloroprene producers	Lung	Chloroprene
	Dimethylsulphate producers	Lung	Dimethylsulphate
	Epichlorohydrin producers	Lung, lymphatic and haemato-poietic system (leukaemia)	Epichlorohydrin

Industry	Occupation	Site	Reported or suspected causative agent
	Ethylene oxide producers	Lymphatic and haematopoietic system (leukaemia), stomach	Ethylene oxide
	Ethylene dibromide producers	Digestive system	Ethylene dibromide
	Flame retardant and plasticiser users	Skin (melanoma)	Polychlorinated biphenyls
	Styrene and polystyrene producers	Lymphatic and haematopoietic system (leukaemia)	Styrene
	Ortho- and *para-*toluidine producers	Bladder	*Ortho/para*-toluidine
	Benzoylchloride producers	Lung	Benzoylchloride
	Magenta producers	Bladder	Aniline, *o*-toluidine
Pesticides and herbicides production industry	Tetrachlorodibenzodioxin producers and those exposed after accidents	Lung, stomach	DCDD and TCDD dichlorodibenzodioxin, trichlorodibenzodioxin
Rubber industry	Rubber manufacturing	Lymphopoietic system, stomach, brain, pancreas	Undefined
	Processors, composers, cementing synthetic plant	Stomach	Undefined
	General service	Lymphatic and haematopoietic system (leukaemia), lymphatic and haemopoietic tissue	Undefined
	Synthetic latex producers and tyre curing	Lung	Undefined
	Calender operatives and reclaim	Prostate, lung	Undefined
	Compounding, mixing and calendering	Prostate	Undefined
	Styrene butadione rubber producers	Lymphatic and haematopoietic system (lymphomas)	Styrene
	Pliofilm producers	Lymphatic and haematopoietic system (leukaemia)	Benzene
	Rubber compounding, extruding, milling	Stomach	Undefined
	Tyre assembly	Skin Brain	Mineral extender oil Undefined
Construction industry	Insulators and pipe coverers	Larynx, gastro-intestinal tract	Asbestos

Industry	Occupation	Site	Reported or suspected causative agent
Printing industry	Rotogravure workers, binders	Marrow (leukaemia)	Benzene
	Printing pressmen	Buccal cavity, rectum, pancreas, lung, prostate, kidney	Oil mist, solvents, dyes, cadmium, lead
	Newspaper pressmen	Buccal cavity	Oil mist, solvents, dyes, cadmium, lead
	Commercial pressmen	Pancreas, rectum	Oil mist, solvents, dyes, cadmium, lead
	Compositors	Multiple myeloma	Solvents
	Machine room workers	Lung	Oil mist
Leather industry	Tanners and processors	Bladder, nasal, lung	Leather dust, other chemicals, chromium
	Leather workers, unspecified	Nose, larynx, lung, bladder, lymphatic and haemato-poietic system (lymphomas)	Undefined
	Boot and shoe manu-facturers and repairers	Buccal cavity	Undefined
	Other leather goods manufacturers	Marrow (leukaemia)	Benzene
Textile industry	Cotton and wool workers	Mouth, pharynx	Cotton and wool dust
Wood pulp and paper industry	Lumbermen and saw-mill workers	Nose, Hodgkin's lymphoma	Wood dust, chloro-phenols
	Pulp and papermill workers	Lymphopoietic tissue	Undefined
	Carpenters, joiners	Nose, Hodgkin's	Wood dust, solvents
	Wood workers, un-specified	Lymphomas	Undefined
Other	Radium dial workers	Breast	Radon
	Laundry and dry cleaners	Lung, skin, cervix uteri	Tritetrachloroethylene and carbon tetra-chloride
	Roofers, asphalt workers	Mouth, pharynx, larynx, oesophagus, stomach	Benzo(a)pyrene, other pitch volatile agents

From Simonato, L. and Saracci, R. (1983) (slightly modified)

compared with a population of similar sex, age, and smoking habits, the increase was more than 90 times when the comparison was made with a population of non-smokers, indicating the great rise in effect deriving from joint exposure to asbestos and smoking. Also, a feature common to this study and several subsequent ones was that the excess lung cancer could be discerned only in smokers. For non-smoking workers, however, the number of person-years of observation was usually small and so was the corresponding number of expected lung cancer deaths (say 0.1–0.5), so that an observed number of 0 lung cancer deaths could easily come about by chance. Such a result might, however, also mean that the excess was confined only to smokers and this interpretation, namely that asbestos could not increase the lung cancer risk in the absence of smoking, was often put forward as the one most consistent with the available observations. The practical implication was that, at least as far as lung cancer went, asbestos was not a risk factor unless the exposed subject was a smoker.

3. An analysis by Doll in 1971 of the data from the previously mentioned study of Selikoff *et al.*, as well as an analysis by Berry *et al.* (1972), of a new set of data from a British textile factory, suggested that the observed excess of lung cancer might be adequately represented by a multiplicative model predicting that the relative risk due to the combined exposure to asbestos and smoking would equal the product of the relative risks due to each agent separately. Having reviewed in some detail all published studies up to 1977 providing enough information on occupational asbestos exposure, smoking habits, and lung cancer risk, I concluded (Saracci 1977) that in the absence of new evidence to the contrary, the multiplicative model appeared the most plausible interpretation of the asbestos–smoking interaction on human lung cancer production.

A set of data which fits this model was reported in 1979 by Hammond *et al.* and Frank as a result of their follow-up of a cohort of 17 800 U.S. and Canadian insulation workers (Table 2). It can be seen in column 2 that the relative risk in workers who also smoked very closely approximates the product of the relative risk among non-smoking asbestos workers multiplied by the relative risk among smokers not exposed to asbestos (respectively 53.24 and (5.17 × 10.85) = 56.09).

Table 2. Lung cancer and all causes mortality rates (per 100 000 person-years) occurring 20 years or more after onset of exposure to asbestos

Exposure group	Lung cancer			All causes	
	Mortality rate (1)	Relative rate (2)	Excess rate (3)	Mortality rate (4)	Excess rate (5)
Asbestos − Smoking −	11.3	1.00	–	980.9	–
Asbestos + Smoking −	58.4	5.17	47.1	1430.9	450.0
Asbestos − Smoking +	122.6	10.85	111.3	1580.7	599.8
Asbestos + Smoking +	601.6	53.24	590.3	2659.0	1678.1

Clearly, the interpretation of the data as an expression of a multiplicative interaction is basically different from the interpretation previously mentioned (point 2) in which asbestos could increase the risk of lung cancer only in the presence of smoking: in the multiplicative model, instead, both agents are capable of increasing the risk of lung cancer by themselves and, moreover, their effect is reciprocally amplified when exposure to the two agents occurs simultaneously. A multiplicative interaction may often (depending on the relative risk for the individual agents involved) be a strong one, implying that the joint effect is quantitatively dominant in comparison with the separate effects of each agent. This is illustrated for lung cancer in column 3 of Table 2, from which the size of the excess lung cancer risk which would be eliminated by avoiding exposure to asbestos or to smoking can immediately be obtained. Eliminating smoking would cause the excess among people exposed to both agents to be reduced by 543.2 (590.3 − 47.1) or 92 per cent of the excess, while completely removing asbestos would reduce the excess rate by 479.0 (590.3 − 111.3) or 81 per cent of the excess. Elimination of smoking thus appears somewhat more effective (1.13 times = 543.2/479.0) than elimination of asbestos; also the bulk of the excess ((92 + 81) − 100 = 73 per cent) may be eliminated by removing either smoking or asbestos, as it derives from their joint action.

From a preventive viewpoint, therefore, attack on *either* agent (and *a fortiori* on both) would offer a substantial benefit. In the same practical perspective it may be more relevant to look at all causes of mortality in the groups with different exposures (columns 4 and 5 of Table 2) rather than focusing only on lung cancer, which constitutes just one pathological effect of asbestos as well as of smoking. Simple calculations similar to those made for lung cancer (using the figures from column 5) show that removal of smoking would eliminate 73 per cent of the excess in all causes rate and removal of asbestos 64 per cent, implying that a sizeable fraction (37 per cent) could be avoided by eliminating one or the other agent. Therefore, whether one looks at lung cancer rates, which appear to conform to a multiplicative interaction, or to all causes rates, the conclusion holds that acting on *either* agent removes an important fraction of the excess rate.

4. As further results have accumulated, it begins to appear that the interaction of asbestos and smoking on lung cancer may be smaller, perhaps considerably so, than the one implied by a multiplicative model. While a key feature of the latter is that the relative risk due to asbestos is the same in smokers and non-smokers, Berry *et al.* (1984) quote six studies (involving a total of 37 observed lung cancer deaths in non-smokers), three of which (involving 32 of the 37 lung cancer deaths) show relative risks due to asbestos *higher* (1.8–5.3 times) in non-smokers than in smokers, a

feature that points towards a simple additive effect of asbestos and smoking. The preventive implication of this would be that, to the extent that the total effect derives from addition of separate effects with no important fraction coming from the joint action of the two agents, the option of acting through removal of *either* agent becomes inadequate and one has instead to act on *both* agents.

It is still unclear whether the quantitatively variable forms of the interaction of asbestos and smoking on lung cancer derive from (a) variable conditions of exposure in the different study populations; (b) the fact that as time passes more cases of lung cancer are observed in a given study population and a better representation of the 'true' situation can emerge; (c) a changing form of the interaction as time from first exposure goes by; (d) a combination of the previous conditions.

Whatever the final picture turns out to be, the points just outlined using the asbestos–smoking example throw light on the joint action between any interacting agents which also carries implications for the preventive options open for their control.

Investigating substitutes for an occupational carcinogen: a study of man-made vitreous fibres.

Among the available methods of preventing further exposure of workers to recognized occupational carcinogens, replacement of a non-carcinogenic substitute may seem attractive, but may, however, turn out to be of doubtful value if the health effects of the substitute, which may be a newer type of material, are still poorly known. A case in point is that of asbestos, the carcinogenic effect of which is well established. As substitutes for some of the asbestos fibre applications, man-made vitreous fibres (MMVF) appear to be satisfactory. These fibres, also designated as man-made mineral fibres (MMMF), include different inorganic wool products (slag-wool, rockwool, glasswool) widely used as thermal and acoustic insulation material and as filament products (continuous filament) employed for textile manufacturing and for the reinforcing of plastic materials. Production of MMVF reached an estimated world annual total of 4.5 million tons in 1973, thus being close to that of asbestos (WHO-Euro 1983). Considering Western Europe alone, it can be estimated that the workforce in the production industry numbered about 30 000 by the end of the 1970s, and an even larger number of workers were involved in handling the products in user trades like the building industry. Biologically, some experiments in animal systems have indicated that MMVF may have pathogenic effects (Kuschner and Wright 1976; Stanton and Wrench 1972; Pott and Friederichs 1972) (fibrogenic and carcinogenic) but until recently there was a dearth of pertinent epidemiological observations on pulmonary fibrosis (or, more generally, chronic respiratory diseases) and on respiratory cancer in exposed subjects (Saracci 1980).

For these reasons a large international research programme on the health effects of MMVF was launched in the mid 1970s with the support of the Joint European Medical Research Board (a registered charity founded by industry). One major component of the programme was an epidemiological study coordinated by the IARC, the structure and currently available results of which (Saracci *et al.* 1984) I will comment on in some detail. The study took the form of an international historical cohort investigation of mortality and cancer incidence among workers in the MMVF production industry carried out at 13 plants in seven Western European countries (Denmark, Finland, Federal Republic of Germany, Italy, Norway, Sweden, U.K.). In each country a collaborating national research team took responsibility for the local conduct of the investigation. The 13 plants were selected out of the 72 included in early 1976 in the list of companies belonging to the European Insulation Manufacturers' Association (EURIMA) and to the Comité International de la Rayonne et des Fibres Synthetiques (CIRFS), located in 15 countries. The 13 plants represent 18 per cent of the total on the list, and 20 per cent of the workforce in 1976. Criteria for selection were: (a) no loss of or destruction of personnel records, i.e. total cohort identifiable; (b) MMVF production process operating for at least 20 years; (c) facilities for follow-up available with regard to mortality and, whenever possible, cancer incidence; (d) plants with a history of processing asbestos materials excluded. This last requirement proved in the end not to be fulfilled at one factory, at which also it was not possible to perform an environmental survey (the plant having been closed).

An environmental study was conducted at the other 12 plants by a team from the Institute of Occupational Medicine, Edinburgh, to measure present concentrations of fibres in air samples collected through personal samplers used during an eight-hour shift by workers operating in different jobs and plant areas. These data, together with a personal work history, enabled the construction for an individual worker of a cumulative index of exposure in fibres × years/ml air inspired.

Follow-up of workers was carried out at least to 31 December 1977 and national rates (mortality and, when applicable, cancer incidence) were used for each of the seven countries for comparison with the mortality and cancer incidence experience of the exposed cohort. The total number of workers in the cohort was 25 146 (20 766 males and 4 380 females) contributing a total of 309 353 person-years of observation (248 438 in males and 60 915 for females) and a total of 1659 deaths (1505 in males, 154 in females). The overall mean duration of employment was 5.1 years (plant averages varying from 2.3 to 11.3) and the median duration 2.2 years (plant medians varying from 0.5 to 4.6 years); 745 workers (3.9 per cent of the total) were lost to follow-up. A number of findings emerged from the analysis.

1. Of the three types of production process 'rockwool' (six plants) showed an average concentration of (respirable) fibres of 0.04/ml, 'glasswool' (four plants) 0.02/ml, and 'continuous filament' of 0.006/ml. Workers' cumulative levels of exposure as derived from these measurements of airborne concentrations of MMVF (under present production conditions) are low, generally in the range of 0.1 fibres × years/ml to 1–2 fibres × years/ml. However, environmental fibre concentrations *may* have been higher in the past, perhaps by an order of magnitude. It may be recalled that in investigations of asbestos workers cumulative exposures in the range of 10 to several hundred fibres × years/ml have commonly been reported.

2. A single mesothelioma death was reported out of the total 309 353 person-years at risk.

3. There were no consistent across-factories departures of the observed numbers from those expected on the basis of the experience of the general population for individual causes of death or for individual cancer sites with the exception of lung cancer.

4. There was a tendency for the risk of lung cancer to increase with time from first employment. The results for males are presented in Table 3. When the data for the three production processes (all plants) were pooled a statistically significantly increased standardized mortality ratio of 192 (95

Table 3. Lung cancer mortality by production process and by time since first employment (men)

Factory	Time since first employment (years)											
	0–19			20–29			30+			Total		
	O	E	SMR	O	E	SMR	O	E	SMR	O	E	SMR
Rockwool (7 factories)	27	29.8	91	12	9.7	124	11	5.7	195	50	45.1	111
Rockwool (6 factories only)†	21	23.4	90	8	5.4	148	5	3.1	163	34	31.9	107
Glasswool (4 factories)	30	31.2	96	10	13.2	76	4	2.6	157	44	46.9	94
Continuous filament (2 factories)‡	11	7.9	139	2	1.9	104	2	0.6	333	15	10.5	143
Total (13 factories)	68	69.0	98	24	24.8	97	17	8.9	192	109	102.6	106

† Excluding the factory in which asbestos use was reported.
‡ Glasswool predominant at one factory until 1962, when discontinued; observed and expected figures at this factory for the three time periods were: 6, 4.0; 2, 1.5; 2, 0.5.
O = observed deaths; E = expected deaths; SMR = standardized mortality ratio.

per cent confidence limits 117–307) appeared in the group in which 30 years or more had passed since first employment.

5. No relation was found when the risk of lung cancer was related to cumulative exposure to MMVF.

The outstanding question that these results raise is whether the increased risk of lung cancer observed 30 or more years from first employment is due to exposure to MMVF, an interpretation which would indict these fibres as carcinogenic in man. The increase occurs at a site – the lung – and at a time – several decades after first employment – at which an effect if present could be expected to appear. On the other hand, the increase is not related to cumulative exposure to MMVF nor is it related to type of production process: although the trend is more obvious with the rockwool production process (i.e. the one with comparatively higher average environmental concentrations of fibres), it is not absent with the two other production processes. Also, no consistent excess was found in the incidence of lung cancer, but this may be due to the very small amount of data available on incidence (in contrast to mortality). Finally, the possible role in the observed increase of occupational and non-occupational confounding factors, such as previous occupational history or (of great importance) smoking, cannot be assessed or ruled out. Among all the factors which point against an aetiological role for MMVF, the lack of a relation with cumulative exposure must be regarded with particular caution. This is because the relatively small number of subjects followed for 30 or more years for whom it was possible to construct an exposure index (yielding 11 lung cancer deaths) prevents a reliable evaluation of an exposure–response relationship within the one period in which an increase in risk was observed. In this respect it is also worth mentioning a point of general importance for epidemiological studies: the full potential of this study was curtailed by legal restrictions denying access to individual death certificates in some countries. In fact, two countries – France and the Federal Republic of Germany – which included as many as one-third of the plants in the initial list of 72, ended up by being represented by only one factory suitable for the historical cohort study. In both countries, follow-up of workers was assessed as impossible or highly problematical. As a consequence of this type of impediment alone, five factories which would otherwise have been included in the study had to be left out and it can be estimated that their inclusion would have increased the study population by some 30 per cent.

In conclusion, the question of the meaning of the observed increase in lung cancer risk remains open, even when placed within the framework of all other experimental and epidemiological results, notably those of the large multicentre study conducted within the U.S. by Enterline and Marsh (1984), which have recently been reviewed (Saracci *et al.* 1984; Saracci and Simonato 1982). More generally, what still remains open to further investigation is the question: 'Are man-made vitreous fibres carcinogenic when inhaled by Man?'. An extension of the follow-up of workers included in the study co-ordinated by the IARC is in progress and should help to answer this question.

Detecting occupational carcinogens

The example of MMVF, assessing the safety of a partial substitute for a well-known carcinogen (asbestos), points both to the desirability and to the feasibility of carrying out international multicentre cohort studies as a way of investigating possible carcinogenic exposures in the workplace. In fact, in occupational epidemiology, as in epidemiology in general, repeatability or (more generally) consistency of results obtained through the observation of different working populations is crucial in establishing a causal association between an exposure occurring in the working environment and a disease. This is all the more critical in that often the size of a single working population (i.e. the workforce of a factory) is small, and results derived from observing its members may be affected by large sampling errors. As a consequence a strong case exists both for extending the study of a possible occupational carcinogen to several different working populations and for doing this in a planned and organized way, rather than just waiting for replicate studies (which may never occur) to be performed by different research workers. An obvious means to this end is by way of a multicentre cohort study carried out nationally or (and often this may be the only option of an adequately large size) internationally. Not only cancers, but also other possible health effects from an occupational exposure may be investigated through this type of study. Simultaneous replication, reducing the chances of both false-positive and false-negative results, can be cited (Saracci 1983) as the first among the advantages of the multicentre cohort study, which stands as a valuable and relatively recent development in occupational epidemiology.

Other lines of epidemiological research include: company- or industry-wide prospective morbidity and/or mortality surveillance (Schottenfeld *et al.* 1981; Austin 1981), ongoing and systematic case-control monitoring of cancer at several sites (Siemiatycki *et al.* 1981) (special attention being given to conversion of job titles into exposure to specific chemicals) (MRC Environmental Epidemiology Unit 1983), geographical correlation (Blot and Fraumeni 1976), cross-examination of current occupational mortality (or morbidity) statistics across countries to pinpoint 'suspect' occupations (Lynge, personal communication), use of biological markers of exposure to carcinogens (especially those damaging DNA) (Berlin *et al.* 1984), and utilization of statistical models for data analysis (e.g. Day and Brown 1980). Apart from prospective surveillance systems and the utilization of statistical models (which facilitate the extraction of whatever information is embodied in a set of data on such important issues as exposure-response relationship, reversibility of effects, and interactions of several agents) the other approaches mentioned appear at present to be exploratory. I for one find them more encouraging as a sign of awareness of the occupational cancer problem than enlightening as to whether a problem may materialize.

Also, one has to reckon with the limitations of the epidemiological approach. An occupational carcinogen may have caused in the past, and may cause *a fortiori* in the future if trends towards cleaner workplaces continue, only a 'small' increase in the risk of cancer at a given site (say 50 per cent or less). Such increases are difficult to detect not only because they require the study of large samples if they are to be distinguished from pure chance fluctuations, but also because they can barely (if at all) be discriminated from variations, often of the same order of magnitude, produced by biasing factors intrinsic to observational studies. But a 'small' 50 per cent increase in, say, lung cancer implies that for the persons exposed one out of three lung cancers will develop because of the exposure. Also, the epidemiological method is sharper at investigating mixtures of (chemical) agents as they naturally occur in the workplace than at pinpointing a specific pathogenic chemical. Certainly, both on account of the latter consideration and for practical reasons it is quite impossible to investigate epidemiologically, now or in the future, all compounds (70 000 or so) in commercial use! As far as new substances (synthetic molecules) are concerned, which could be revealed as carcinogenic in man in 20 or 30 years, reliance should be placed on controlling their use now rather than on late *a posteriori* observations of cancers in humans.

To overcome the limitations of direct observation in Man it is natural to turn to observation in other living systems: epidemiology naturally directs attention to the experimental approach. This provides not only reproducible and clear demonstrations of the carcinogenic effects of a variety of physical, chemical, and biological agents in laboratory animals, but also extensive information of a basic nature on the mechanisms of carcinogenesis. For the more restricted purpose of detecting carcinogens, both short-term tests, using as classes of end-points DNA damage, mutagenicity, and chromosome damage, and long-term (often lifetime) carcinogencity tests in whole animals (usually rodents), are in current experimental use. Consistent positive results in short-term tests with different end-point classes is usually regarded as indicating the *potential* carcinogenicity of the tested agent (through direct action on the DNA), but only clear positive results in adequate long-term animal tests is regarded as demonstration of the carcinogenicity of an agent independently of mechanism.

The crucial issue is, of course, what this tells us about carcinogenicity in Man. Although presently available animal tests fall short of the ideal of enabling one to extrapolate from animals to Man (and a search for better testing approaches is warranted) there is certainly a good empirical basis for their utilization as predictors of carcinogenicity in humans. In fact, of the 23 chemical compounds classified as carcinogenic to humans in the IARC Monographs Programme, only one (arsenic) is not positive in animal tests. This points towards a high sensitivity of long-term animal tests in detecting human carcinogens, although it would be going too far to attach a precise figure to 'sensitivity' in the formal sense (the relation between animal test results and human study results being affected, for instance, by different intensities of investigation and testing for different compounds). Even more, the 'specificity' of these animal tests cannot be quantified as there are simply no reliable figures for the frequencies with which compounds well investigated and clearly shown to be negative for carcinogenicity in humans are positive or negative in animal experiments.

What can be said, on the basis of these considerations, about compounds which have sufficient evidence of carcinogenicity for animals and for which no human epidemiological data are available? Of the 585 compounds in the first 29 volumes of the IARC Monographs Programme there were 103 such compounds, a major fraction (63/103) of them entailing human exposure in the workplace. Based on a prudent interpretation of the sensitivity of animal tests in respect of carcinogens for humans, the following statement is made about those compounds in the Monographs series (International Agency for Research on Cancer 1983): 'In the absence of adequate data on humans it is reasonable, *for practical purposes*, to regard the chemical as if it presented a carcinogenic risk to humans.' Of course, when moving to the realm of the practical, as opposed to the realm of the purely scientific, other considerations come into play as well, like the technical and economic feasibility of avoiding exposure to these carcinogens. Without going in any detail into the area of prevention and risk management, I would simply like to point out that technical and economic considerations cannot change or obscure the fundamental public health principle, that the benefit of doubt should first go to the people exposed to a hazard, particuarly when this is of an involuntary nature, as is the case with a potential occupational carcinogen.

References

Austin, S.G. (1981). An industry-sponsored mortality surveillance program. In *Quantification of occupational cancer* (ed. R. Peto and M. Schneiderman), pp. 347–55. Banbury Report No. 9. Cold Spring Harbor Laboratory.

Berlin, A., Draper, M., Hemminki, K., and Vainio, H. (eds) (1984). *Monitoring human exposure to carcinogenic and mutagenic agents*. Proceedings of a Seminar organized by the Institute of Occupational Health, Helsinki, the IARC, the

International Programme on Chemical Safety and the Commission of the European Communities, 12–15 December 1983. International Agency for Research on Cancer, Lyon. (IARC Scientific Publication No. 59.)

Bernal, J.D. (1969). *Science in history*, Vol. 4, p. 1143. Penguin Books, Harmondsworth.

Berry, G., Newhouse, M.L., and Turok, M. (1972). Combined effects of asbestos exposure and smoking on mortality from lung cancer in factory workers. *Lancet* **ii**, 476–9.

Berry, G., Newhouse, M.L., and Antonis, P. (1985). Combined effect of asbestos and smoking on mortality from lung cancer and mesothelioma in factory workers. *Brit. J. indust. Med.* **42**, 12–8.

Blot, W.J. and Fraumeni, J.F. (1976). Geographic pattern of lung cancer: industrial correlations. *Amer. J. Epidemiol.* **103**, 539–50.

Bridbord, K., Decoufle, P., Faumeni, J.F., Hoel, D.G., Hoover, R.N., Rall, D.P., Saffiotti, U., Schneiderman, M.A., Upton, A.C., and Day, N. (1981). Estimates of the fraction of cancer in the United States related to occupational factors. In *Quantification of occupational cancer* (ed. R. Peto and M. Schneiderman), pp. 701–26. Banbury Report No. 9, Cold Spring Harbor Laboratory.

Day, N.E. and Brown, C.C. (1980). Multistage models and primary prevention of cancer. *J. nat. Cancer Inst.* **64**, 977–89.

Doll, R. (1955). Mortality from lung cancer in asbestos workers. *Brit. J. indust. Med.* **12**, 81–6.

Doll, R. (1971). The age distribution of cancer: implications for models of carcinogenesis. *Roy. stat. Soc. J.* Series A, **134**, 133–5.

Doll, R. and Peto, R. (1981). *The causes of cancer*. Oxford University Press.

Enterline, P.E. and Marsh, G.M. (1984). Mortality of workers in the MMMF industry. In *Biological effects of man-made mineral fibres*, pp. 311–39. Proceedings of a WHO/IARC Conference, WHO, Copenhagen.

Frank, A.L. (1979). Public health significance of smoking–asbestos interactions. *Ann. N.Y. Acad. Sci.* **330**, 791–4.

Hammond, E.C., Selikoff, I.J., and Seidman, H. (1979). Asbestos exposure, cigarette smoking and death rates. *Ann. N.Y. Acad. Sci.* **330**, 473–90.

Hueper, W.C. (1942). *Occupational tumors and allied diseases*. L.C. Thomas, Springfield, Illinois.

Hunter, D. (1975). *The diseases of occupation* 5th ed. Little Brown, Boston.

International Agency for Research on Cancer (1972–82). *IARC Monographs on the evaluation of the carcinogenic risk of chemicals to humans*, Vols 1–29. IARC, Lyon.

International Agency for Research on Cancer (1982). *Chemicals, industrial processes and industries associated with cancer in humans*. Supplement No. 4 to the IARC Monographs, Volumes 1–29. IARC, Lyon.

International Agency for Research on Cancer (1983). *Miscellaneous pesticides*, p. 18. IARC Monographs on the Evaluation of the Carcinogenic Risk of Chemicals to Humans. IARC, Lyon.

International Labour Office (1982). *Yearbook of labour statistics*. ILO Geneva.

Kuschner, M. and Wright, G.W. (1976). The effects of intratracheal instillation of glass fiber of varying size in guinea-pigs. In *Occupational exposure to fibrous glass*, pp. 151–68. US Department of Health, Education and Welfare Publication No. NIOSH, 76–151. National Institute for Occupational Safety and Health, Washington, DC.

Montesano, R. and Tomatis, L. (1972). Legislation concerning chemical carcinogens in several industrialized countries. *Cancer Res.* **37**, 310.

MRC Environmental Epidemiology Unit (1983). *Job exposure matrices.* Scientific Report No. 2, Medical Research Council.

Pott, F. and Friederichs, K.H. (1972). Tumoren der Ratte nach i.p.Injektion faserförmiger Stäube. *Naturwissenschaften* **59**, 318.

Saracci, R. (1977). Asbestos and lung cancer: an analysis of the epidemiological evidence on the asbestos–smoking interaction. *Int. J. Cancer* **20**, 323–31.

Saracci, R. (1980). Epidemiology of groups exposed to other mineral fibres. In *Biological effects of mineral fibres*, Vol. 2 (ed. J.C. Wagner), pp. 951–63. IARC Scientific Publication No. 30. IARC, Lyon.

Saracci, R. (1983). Studies in occupational epidemiology: the case for international collaboration. *J. Univ. occup. environ. Hlth* **5**, Suppl., 207–14.

Saracci, R. and Simonato, L. (1982). Man-made vitreous fibers and workers' health: an overview of the epidemiological evidence. *Scand. J. Work environ. Hlth* **8**, 234–42.

Saracci, R., Simonato, L., Acheson, E.D., Andersen, A., Bertazzi, P.A., Claude, J., Charnay, N., Estève, J., Frentzel-Beyme, R.R., Gardner, M.J., Jensen, O.M., Maasing, R., Olsen, J.H., Teppo, L., Westerholm, P., and Zocchetti, C. (1984). Mortality and cancer incidence of workers in the man-made vitreous fibres producing industry: an international investigation at thirteen European plants. *Brit. J. indust. Med.* **41**, 425.

Schottenfeld, D., Worshauer, M.E., Zauber, A.G., Meikle, J.G., and Hart, B.R. (1981). A prospective study of morbidity and mortality in petroleum industry employees in the United States. A preliminary report. In *Quantification of occupational cancer* (ed. R. Peto and M. Schneiderman), pp. 247–60. Banbury Report No. 9. Cold Spring Harbor Laboratory.

Selikoff, I.J., Hammond, E.C., and Chung, J. (1968). Asbestos exposure, smoking and neoplasia. *J. Am. med. Ass.* **204**, 106–10.

Siemiatycki, J., Gerin, M., and Hubert, J. (1981). Exposure-based case-control approach to discovering occupational carcinogens: preliminary findings. In *Quantification of occupational cancer* (ed. R. Peto and M. Schneiderman), pp. 471–81. Banbury Report No. 9. Cold Spring Harbor Laboratory.

Simonato, L. and Saracci, R. (1983). Cancer: occupational. In *Encyclopaedia of occupational health and safety* (ed. L. Parmeggiani), pp. 369–75. International Labour Office, Geneva.

Stanton, M.F. and Wrench, C. (1972). Mechanisms of mesothelioma induction with asbestos and fibrous glass. *J. nat. Cancer Inst.* **48**, 797–821.

WHO-Euro (1983). *Biological effects of man-made mineral fibres.* pp. 10–11. Euro Reports and Studies 81. WHO, Copenhagen.

Wynder, E.L. and Gori, G.B. (1977). Contribution of the environment to cancer incidence: an epidemiological exercise. *J. nat. Cancer Inst.* **58**, 825–32.

6 Radiation

P.G. Smith

Introduction

Ionizing radiations are carcinogens to which human exposure is ubiquitous. Current estimates of the risks associated with exposure, however, suggest that such radiations are responsible for only a relatively small proportion of all cancers. About two-thirds of the radiation dose received by the U.K. population is from natural sources, i.e. from cosmic radiation, from rocks and soil, and from within the body. Most of the remaining one-third is contributed by radiation used in medical procedures, both diagnostic and therapeutic. The amount contributed by nuclear fallout, occupational exposure, and the disposal of radioactive wastes is about 1 per cent of the total population exposure. Taylor and Webb (1978) have estimated the average per caput dose from all sources to be of the order of 0.15 rem per year. In the United Nations report on the effects of radiation (UNSCEAR 1977) it is estimated that exposure of one million persons to one rad of ionizing radiation will induce about 20 leukaemias, and 100 fatal cancers of other sites. On this basis we might attribute to radiation exposure about 150 (5 per cent) of the 3000 leukaemia deaths a year in England and Wales and 750 (0.6 per cent) of the 120 000 deaths from other malignant disease. Jablon and Bailar (1980) conducted a detailed analysis of this kind for the U.S. and concluded that less than 3 per cent of cancers may be attributed to radiation.

Although it seems that radiation is not a very powerful human carcinogen, it is among those that have been most extensively studied and it is certainly one about which there is much public concern. The reasons for the latter may be at least threefold. First, because of the association of radiation exposure with nuclear weapons (though the immediate catastrophic effects of the use of such weapons are of a higher order of concern than the long-term carcinogenic effects). Secondly, because it seems likely that increasing numbers of people will be at risk of exposure to radiation with the development of nuclear power as other energy sources are depleted. Thirdly, because the assumptions underlying the current estimates of the carcinogenic effects of low doses of radiation have been questioned by some workers.

In this review a summary is made of some of the main epidemiological investigations upon which current estimates of radiation effects and risks are based and some of the difficulties of interpretation are discussed. More extensive discussions of these and other studies have been published by UNSCEAR (1977) and BEIR (1980). For the most part, attention is focused in this chapter on studies of persons exposed to radiation as a consequence of medical investigations or treatment. Not only have such studies been among the most important sources of information, but also it is primarily, though not exclusively, in the conduct of such investigations that Richard Doll, mostly in collaboration with the late Michael Court Brown, has made major contributions to knowledge of the long-term effects of radiation exposure.

Studies of exposed populations

Apart from the consequences of nuclear welfare, most public-health interest in the long-term effects of exposure to ionizing radiations is concentrated on the consequences for those exposed to low doses. In the normal course of events, high doses are likely to be received only by rare accident or in the treatment of malignant disease, for which the long-term hazards of radiotherapy are usually far outweighed by the immediate therapeutic benefits. Very large populations, however, are exposed to low doses of radiation, in addition to that derived from natural sources, as a consequence of their employment (e.g. in nuclear installations) or through diagnostic radiology.

If the carcinogenic effects of radiation were such as to produce cancers of a type that were clearly distinguishable from those due to other causes, it would be relatively easy to identify small effects in populations exposed to very low doses. Unfortunately, this is not the case as tumours induced by radiation are presently indistinguishable from those due to other causes. It is necessary to search, therefore, for radiation effects superimposed on the background level of cancers due to all other causes. In such circumstances, even if very large populations (of size perhaps a million or more) exposed to low doses are studied, the chance of detecting carcinogenic effects of the size of current risk estimates may be small (Land 1980). For this reason many of the epidemiological investigations on radiation effects have been conducted on groups of persons exposed to doses of radiation larger than those that are of most public-health concern. By study of such groups it was hoped, first, that it would be easier to identify radiation effects, because of their anticipated greater magnitude, and, secondly, that it would be possible to predict the effect of low doses based upon observations at higher doses. Such backwards extrapolation requires that assumptions are made about the form of dose-response relationships and it is this problem that has proved perhaps more complicated than was initially anticipated.

Background radiation

To detect the carcinogenic effects of exposure to very low doses of radiation it is necessary to examine the disease experience of very large populations, if radiation risks are as low as have been estimated by international bodies (Land 1980). An apparently attractive way of doing this is to study populations with different exposures to natural background radiation. Such exposures vary with altitude, with the geological composition of the earth, and according to the materials from which dwellings are constructed. Studies which have tried to associate cancer mortality with variations in background radiation have not, however, demonstrated clear effects. Court Brown *et al.* (1960a) conducted a study of this kind by examining mortality from leukaemia over an 18-year period in different parts of Scotland, including some areas in which measurements of background radiation were also made. Although it was found that inhabitants of the 'granite city' of Aberdeen received a background radiation dose that was 20 per cent higher than that of persons living in Edinburgh and also that the rate of leukaemia was higher in the former city, the authors considered that the overall variation in leukaemia risk between areas could not be attributed to background radiation. They concluded that in studying geographical variations in leukaemia rates it was insufficient to consider only variation in the background levels of radiation and it would be necessary to take into account social and economic factors that might relate to the risk of leukaemia or to the probability of its diagnosis.

It is perhaps for these reasons that similar studies of this kind, seeking to relate background radiation to an increased risk of cancer, have been unrewarding. The contribution of other factors, beside radiation, to cancer induction is so large that it is very difficult to rule out their confounding effects in relating geographic variations in mortality to background radiation exposures.

In utero exposures

Evidence that *in utero* exposure to diagnostic radiation might lead to the development of childhood leukaemia and other cancers was first reported by Stewart and her colleagues in Oxford on the basis of a national case-control study of childhood cancers (Stewart *et al.* 1956; Stewart *et al.* 1958). These workers attempted to interview the parents of all children who had died of leukaemia or cancer before their tenth birthday in England and Wales during the years 1953–1955. By comparing the responses of the parents to questions about *in utero* radiation with those of the parents of selected control children they showed that *in utero* exposure to diagnostic

X-rays appeared to increase the risk of childhood leukaemia and other cancers about two fold. The findings of this study created considerable controversy and the causative nature of the association was questioned. Criticisms were directed especially at the retrospective method of enquiry used in the survey, as biased recall of radiation exposure by the parents of children who had died of cancers, relative to that of the parents of the control children, could not be excluded.

In an attempt to overcome this problem Court Brown *et al.* (1960b) adopted a different approach. From the radiological records in four London and four Edinburgh hospitals they compiled a list of about 40 000 women who had received a diagnostic X-ray examination to the pelvis or abdomen during pregnancy in the period 1945–1956. By linking the names of the children in this cohort to a national leukaemia registry they were able to identify 9 who had died of leukaemia, against an expected number of 10.5 based upon national mortality rates. Thus the findings from this study appeared to offer no support to the observations of Stewart and her colleagues.

A study was conducted by MacMahon (1962) in the U.S. of over 700 000 children born between 1947 and 1954 in 37 maternity hospitals. Deaths from cancer among all the children in the period 1947–1960 were traced (by searching State death records). The frequency of prenatal exposure to radiation among those who had died of cancer was contrasted with that of a 1 per cent sample of all children who had been born in the same 37 hospitals. It was found that irradiated children had a mortality rate from both leukaemia and other cancers that was about 45 per cent higher than that of non-irradiated children. This study was later extended to include a further 5 hospitals and also to include all deaths from cancer between 1947 and 1967 among children born in the 42 hospitals between 1947 and 1960 (Monson and MacMahon 1984). No excess risk of leukaemia or other cancers was apparent among *in-utero*-irradiated children after the age of 10 years. Before this age irradiated children had a 50 per cent increased risk of death from leukaemia compared with non-irradiated children, similar to the finding in the initial study. The risk of death from a cancer other than leukaemia was only 30 per cent higher in the irradiated group; lower than the 50 per cent excess observed in the initial study. The findings with respect to leukaemia and solid tumours were not significantly different, however, and Monson and MacMahon (1984) attributed the apparent discrepancy to chance.

A number of other studies of this issue have been reported (UNSCEAR 1977) and most, including that of Court Brown *et al.* (1960b), are consistent with an increased risk of leukaemia and other cancers among irradiated children of about 40 per cent. A possible bias, which is hard to rule out in all of these studies, is that the increased cancer risk is related to the reason the women were irradiated rather than due to the X-ray exposure. Some evidence against this interpretation was provided by Stewart and her co-workers (Stewart and Kneale 1968, 1970; Bithell and Stewart 1975), who reported updated data from the Oxford Survey of Childhood Cancers. Analysing data on 8513 childhood cancer deaths in the period 1953–1967 and an equal number of matched control children, they showed, overall, irradiated children had a 50 per cent higher risk of cancer than those who had not been exposed to *in utero* radiation. Furthermore, the cancer risk was directly related to the number of times that X-ray exposure had occurred in the pregnancy. A steadily declining risk was found with year of birth and it was suggested that this was due, at least in part, to a reduction in both the number of exposures and the radiation dose for each exposure over the period of the study (Bithell and Stewart 1975).

Further evidence favouring a causative interpretation of the association was given by Mole (1974), who noted that in the Oxford survey, 55 per cent of twin pregnancies were investigated radiologically compared with only 10 per cent of singletons. He found, however, that the risk of a subsequent tumour was similar in an irradiated twin and an irradiated singleton. He argued that such a finding was unlikely unless the cancers were attributable to the radiation exposure.

Studies of the survivors of the atomic bomb (A-bomb) explosions, which have contributed much to our knowledge of the carcinogenic effects of radiation, have given results with respect to *in utero* radiation which appear to conflict with other epidemiological studies. Jablon and Kato (1970) found only one cancer death among children who had been *in utero* at the time of the atomic bomb explosions against about 0.4 expected on Japanese national rates. Assuming a linear dose-response relationship between radiation dose and cancer induction they argued that the small excess they observed was incompatible with the effect expected based on the estimates given by Stewart and Kneale (1970) from the Oxford survey. A possible explanation of this apparent discrepancy was offered by Mole (1974) who questioned the assumption of a linear dose-response relationship and showed that if a 'cell-killing' effect of radiation was taken into account the findings from the A-bomb survivors appear to be not so discrepant from those of other studies. The argument that he advanced has relevance to studies among adults also and will be discussed later in this chapter (p. 136).

Relative risks of the order of 1.5 in epidemiological studies often pose problems with respect to causal interpretations. While there is still room for some doubt that *in utero* radiation exposure does increase the risk of childhood cancers, the weight of the evidence would seem to favour a cause-effect interpretation. Furthermore, the available data suggest that the foetus may be especially sensitive to the carcinogenic effect of small doses of radiation. This was taken into account by UNSCEAR (1977) who estimated that the risk of a fatal malignancy might be in the region of 200–250 per million exposures of 1 rad, about twice as high as the risk estimated for adults.

Radiologists

Radiologists have been studied for longer than any other defined population to assess the late effects of exposure to ionizing radiations received as a consequence of their occupation.

In the mid-1950s there were reports that the average age at death of American radiologists was about five years less than that of American physicians who were not routinely exposed to radiation. It was suggested that radiation was having a non-specific life-shortening effect causing the radiologists to 'age' at an increased rate due to the accumulation of genetic damage in the somatic tissues. Comparisons of average ages at death usually have to be regarded with some caution, especially in situations in which persons may enter the compared groups at different ages and also leave for reasons other than death. Nevertheless, there was clear evidence that the deaths of some pioneer radiologists were directly attributable to their exposure to radiation sources (for example, due to cancers of the skin of the hand) and in 1956 Court Brown and Doll (1958) initiated a study of the mortality experience of those who had been members of the two major British radiological societies between 1897 and 1954. About 1300 radiologists were identified and reports have been published on their mortality experience up until 1957 (Court Brown and Doll 1958) and, later, up until 1977 (Smith and Doll 1981).

In the early days of radiology the potential hazards of radiation exposure were not appreciated and precautions against exposure were either minimal or non-existent. It was only around 1920, following recommendations from the X-ray and Radium Protection Committee, that protective measures became widespread in the U.K. Thus many of those who practised radiology before 1921 are likely to have accumulated exposure to very high radiation doses. In this group there was evidence of a substantial excess of cancer (75 per cent higher than that expected from rates for men in social class 1 and about 50 per cent higher than that of other doctors). The sites for which the excesses were most apparent were for leukaemia (four deaths against 0.65 expected) and cancers of the skin (six deaths against 0.77 expected) and there were also significant excesses of cancers of the lung and pancreas. Among those who joined the societies after 1920 there was no overall excess of cancer deaths but there was a statistically significant increase in the ratio of observed to expected deaths with increasing length of follow-up. Thus it appears that a cancer risk may be emerging as the follow-up time of this group increases.

Unfortunately, it has proved impossible to make good estimates of the doses which the men in this study are likely to have received. Some of those who joined the societies before 1921 may have accumulated, over a period of years, whole-body doses of over 1000 rad and even many of those who joined later may have accumulated whole-body doses of the order of 100–500 rad (Smith and Doll 1981). The uncertainties about individual radiation doses limit the usefulness of this population in quantifying the effects of repeated exposure to low doses of radiation.

To obtain a rough idea of how the findings in the radiologists compare with the risk estimates upon which current radiation protection standards are based, consider the group of about 1000 men who entered radiology after 1920. All of these were followed for at least 20 years. If we assume that the average dose of radiation accumulated was 100 rad per person (and this may be too low an estimate), and apply the UNSCEAR (1977) estimate of the leukaemogenic effect of low doses of radiation (1 case induced/million persons/rad/year for the first 20 years after exposure) we would expect about 2 induced leukaemias in this group. In fact 4 cases were observed against 2.6 expected, an excess of 1.4 cases. Thus, given the assumptions that have been made, the excess is compatible with the leukaemia induction rate suggested by UNSCEAR (1977) but is not, for example, compatible with a risk of, say, 10 times this amount (under which assumption we would have expected 20 cases of leukaemia in the radiologists). It should be stressed, however, that because the true doses received by the radiologists are not known, these computations are rather speculative.

Studies of U.S. radiologists have also shown excess cancer mortality rates compared to physicians in other specialties (Seltzer and Sartwell 1959: 1965; Matanoski *et al.* 1975a, b: 1981) but for this group also it has not been possible to relate the excess mortality to radiation dose other than through the presumed reductions in doses to which radiologists have been exposed in more recent years.

A contrasting finding in the U.S. studies has been an apparent increased risk of death from causes other than cancer. This has been interpreted as being consistent with a non-specific ageing effect of radiation, as originally postulated on the basis of the age-of-death comparisons. There is, however, little support for this theory of radiation action from other studies on human populations. British radiologists, even those who entered the profession before 1921, had a mortality rate from all causes other than cancer which was less than that of other doctors or other men in social class 1. Furthermore, no life-shortening effect, other than through the induction of cancer, has been found among survivors of the atomic bomb explosions (Beebe *et al.* 1978a; Kato *et al.* 1982). Nor is such an effect apparent among patients irradiated for ankylosing spondylitis (Radford *et al.* 1977; Smith *et al*. 1977) or for the induction of an artifical menopause (Smith and Doll 1976).

Atomic bomb survivors

One of the most important sources of information on the long-term effects of exposure to ionizing radiation has been provided by the experience of the survivors of the atomic bomb explosions in Hiroshima and Nagasaki. In 1950 a Japanese National census enumerated 283 500 persons who claimed exposure to the bombs in August 1945. A sample of 82 000 of the survivors was selected (the 'lifespan' study group) and members of this group have been carefully followed until the present time, through the family registration system of Japan, to measure the long-term effects of the exposure on mortality.

This chapter is concerned with the long-term effects of radiation and especially with the effects of low-dose exposures. It is perhaps important, however, when considering the A-bomb survivors, to put the short and long-term effects of nuclear explosions into some perspective. At the time the bombs were exploded it has been estimated that the non-military population of the two cities was about 429 000. Within a day of the explosions about 67 000 people had died as a direct effect of blast or burns and over the next few months another 36 000 died, including those dying of acute radiation sickness. Thus after four months only 75 per cent of the population of the cities was surviving (Ohkita 1975). The long-term carcinogenic effects are lower by two orders of magnitude.

Between 1950 and 1978 it has been estimated that there were about 67 000 deaths from all causes among the 283 000 survivors alive in 1950. Of these deaths only about 530 (0.8 per cent) are likely to be attributable to the radiation exposure; 190 of the 530 were due to leukaemia (49 per cent of all leukaemia deaths) and 340 were due to other cancers (3 per cent of other cancer deaths) (Kato and Schull 1982). One reason for the small proportion of deaths due to radiation is the low value (16 rad) of the mean radiation dose received by the survivors. The 'lifespan' sample was deliberately selected in such a way that persons estimated to have received low radiation doses were under-represented but, even so, the average radiation dose of persons in the sample was only about 27 rad.

One of the main problems in interpreting the data from this study has been because of uncertainties with respect to individual dose estimates. Whereas details of the type and quantity of radiation have been, in general, well documented for patients who were treated with radiotherapy (see p. 127), much cruder methods of dose estimation have had to be used for the atomic bomb survivors. Shortly after the sample of survivors was defined they were carefully questioned as to their exact location at the time the bombs exploded. Using this information and data on the likely shielding provided by buildings between each individual and the hypocentre of the explosion, estimates of exposure doses were calculated for each individual. Tentative dose estimates made in 1965 ('T65' doses) have been used in the examination of radiation effects in the two cities (Milton and Shohoji 1968). Recently, however, the basis of those estimates has been questioned and it is believed that the estimates of the neutron dose from the Hiroshima bomb were too high (Loewe and Mendelsohn 1981). Until revised estimates have been calculated it will not be clear how this will effect the interpretation of the A-bomb survivor data. It seems likely, however, that the main effect will be on the interpretation of apparent differences in the effects of Hiroshima and Nagasaki bombs. Previously some of these differences have been ascribed to variations in the neutron dose but this explanation may now be less tenable.

Two basic methods of analysis have been adopted in relating mortality rates to radiation doses among those exposed to the A-bombs. First the mortality rates of persons estimated to have received different doses have been compared with the mortality rates of the entire Japanese population (for example, Jablon and Kato 1972). A second approach has been used to make 'internal' comparisons of the mortality of persons exposed to different doses within the study cohort (Beebe *et al.* 1971; Beebe *et al.* 1978b; Kato and Schull 1982).

This brief summary hardly does justice to the very extensive programme of studies that originated under the Atomic Bomb Casualty Commission (ABCC) and are being continued by the Radiation Effects Research Foundation (RERF). A more extensive summary is given in BEIR (1980) and, of course, in reports from the RERF. The results of some of these studies will be discussed in pp. 131–42.

Patients treated with radiation

Before the long-term hazards of radiation exposure were appreciated the use of relatively high doses of radiation in the treatment of benign disease was not uncommon. X-ray therapy was used, for example, to reduce enlarged thymus glands (Hempelmann *et al.* 1975) and for the treatment of ringworm of the scalp (Ron and Modan 1980) and in both of these series excesses of thyroid cancers were reported. There were also small excesses of leukaemias, though this was not significant in the latter series. Radioactive isotopes have also been widely used in the investigation and treatment of benign conditions (see Boice and Land (1982) for a recent brief review of the results of studies on these groups).

Below we discuss three studies on patients treated with radiotherapy that have, in some respects, produced apparently conflicting results.

Radiation-induced menopause From the 1930s onwards X-irradiation of the ovaries was a commonly used method used to induce an artificial menopause among women with benign menopausal bleeding. Court Brown suggested that it would be of considerable interest to study the mortality experience of women so treated. It was possible to identify about 2000 women who had had a radiation-induced menopause at three Scottish radiotherapy centres between 1940 and 1960 and their subsequent mortality experience was contrasted with that of the general population of Scotland (Doll and Smith 1968; Smith and Doll 1976). By the early 1970s 25 per cent of the women had died and there had been seven deaths from leukaemia (against 2.7 expected on the basis of general population rates, $p < 0.03$). Deaths from cancers other than leukaemia were divided into those originating in sites that would have been directly in the radiation treatment beams (mainly intestines, rectum, uterus, ovary, and bladder) and those in other sites. There was a statistically significant excess of deaths from cancers of the pelvic sites combined but no excess of other cancers. The excess of cancers in the irradiated sites first became apparent five to nine years after treatment and an excess cancer risk persisted beyond 20 years after treatment. These findings were in line with other studies on similar groups of women in the U.K. and in the U.S. (Smith 1977). No 'control' series treated by means other than radiation has been studied and it has not been possible to exclude the possibility that any increased risk of malignancy is associated with the presenting condition and not the radiation exposure. Evidence against this interpretation is provided by the finding that excess risk was confined to those sites in the radiation fields and that the increased risk was not confined to genital sites. It was estimated that the excess risk of leukaemia (per rad) was very similar to that observed among the atomic bomb survivors and among patients with ankylosing spondylitis treated with radiotherapy (Smith and Doll 1976).

Radiation treatment of cervix cancer Apparently contradictory findings have come from studies of women irradiated in the treatment of cancer of the cervix. Cervix cancer is usually treated by the insertion of radium or by high doses of X-rays directed at the cancer, or by both of these methods. Survival following treatment is relatively good and it seemed that a population of such women would be well suited to study the leukaemogenic effects of radiation exposure. There was some surprise therefore when no excess of leukaemia cases was found in a study of over 70 000 women treated in this way (16 observed against about 16 expected) (Simon *et al*. 1960). It was thought, at first, that inadequate follow-up of patients in this study may have been responsible for the failure to find the expected excess of leukaemia deaths, but other studies of similar groups of women treated for cervix cancer, including a large international collaborative study (Hutchinson 1968; Boice and Hutchinson 1980) also reported no excess of leukaemia deaths (Smith 1977). The results have recently been reported of a collaborative study of the follow-up of over 80 000 women treated with radiotherapy for cancer of the cervix in one or other of eight countries (Boice *et al.* 1984). Altogether there were 77 cases of leukaemia arising in these women against about 66 cases expected on the basis of national leukaemia incidence rates.

It has been estimated that the average dose to the active bone marrow in patients treated with radiotherapy for cervix cancer was probably several hundred rads and, in some patients, would have been several thousand rads. Using the radiation risk estimates given by UNSCEAR (1977) it would be predicted that in the study of Boice *et al.* (1984) there would have been several hundred leukaemias induced as a result of the radiation doses received, yet the actual leukaemia excess was only 11 cases. This, perhaps more than any other epidemiological finding, has led to the conclusion that the assumption of a linear relationship between the induction of leukaemia and radiation dose is invalid, at least in so far as very high radiation doses are concerned. Discussion as to the possible reasons for this finding among the cervix cancer patients will be deferred until p. 136.

X-ray treatment of ankylosing spondylitis The study initiated by Court Brown and Doll of the mortality experience of patients given radiotherapy for ankylosing spondylitis was one of the first to be set up to assess the carcinogenic hazards of radiation exposure and it has also been among the most informative. There are several reasons for this. First, the group of patients followed was large, over 14 000. Secondly, there has been a long period of follow-up of the irradiated population. Thirdly, reasonably high radiation doses were used in the treatment of this benign condition so that the radiation effects have been correspondingly large.

In the period 1930–1955 the recorded leukaemia mortality rate in England and Wales nearly tripled (Hewitt 1955). Although it was thought that some of the recorded increase might be due to improved diagnostic procedures there was concern that some of the rise might have been due to the increasing exposure of the population to ionizing radiations through diagnostic and therapeutic radiology and fallout from nuclear tests. Around the same time the first reports were appearing of an excess leukaemia rate among the atomic bomb survivors (Folley *et al.* 1952). Court Brown and Abatt (1955) had also identified patients with ankylosing spondylitis treated with X-irradiation as possibly being at increased risk of leukaemia.

With this background the Medical Research Council, which was being pressed by Parliament to report on the hazards to Man of radiation exposure, asked Court Brown and Doll to investigate the leukaemogenic effect of exposure to ionizing radiations among patients with ankylosing spondylitis who had been treated with X-rays.

Starting in August 1955 an attempt was made to identify all the patients who had been treated with X-rays for this condition between 1935 and 1954 in 81 radiotherapy centres distributed throughout the U.K. Over 13 000 such patients were identified by the team working under the direction of Court Brown and Doll. Patients who had died of leukaemia subsequent to the radiation treatment were identified either through follow-up information available at the original treatment centre or by checking the names against a national registry of leukaemia deaths that had been set up especially for this study. With remarkable speed, the basic data were assembled, the preliminary results were analysed, and the findings were summarized for inclusion in a Parliamentary White Paper in June 1956, and within a year the detailed report on the findings with respect to leukaemia was available (Court Brown and Doll 1957).

The initial report dealt with the mortality from leukaemia up until 1956 (Court Brown and Doll 1957). The follow-up was later extended to 1960 and the numbers of deaths from leukaemia and other specific causes were compared with the numbers that would have been expected had the patients died at the same rate as the general population of England and Wales (Court Brown and Doll 1965).

From these first two reports it was clear that the patients had suffered a substantially increased risk of leukaemia and aplastic anaemia (67 deaths against 6.0 expected) and of cancer (285 deaths against 194.5 expected). Furthermore, the excess cancer mortality rate was largely confined to those sites that were likely to have been directly in the radiation beams. Other sites, designated 'lightly irradiated' as they might have received some radiation exposure due to scatter from the main beams, showed only a slight and non-significant excess (60 deaths against 52.4 expected). It was also found that the patients suffered an excess mortality from causes other than cancer. About 10 per cent of the deaths were attributed to spondylitis itself or to a closely allied condition, but in addition there was substantial excess mortality from a variety of other conditions not all of which had previously been thought to be associated with the presenting condition (Court Brown and Doll 1965).

In a study of this kind, in which the mortality experience of a diseased group receiving some specific treatment is compared with that of the general population, there is concern that any differences observed may not be attributable to the treatment but rather to a different disease susceptibility associated with the condition for which treatment was given. Thus, for the study of the spondylitic patients, at least two possibilities had to be considered. First that the excess cancer rate was either unrelated or only partially related to the radiation treatment and, secondly, that the excess of deaths from causes other than cancer may have been related to the radiation treatment, a finding which would have been consistent with the suggestion that radiation exposure has a non-specific ageing effect.

Court Brown and Doll (1965) advanced arguments to support their interpretation that the excess cancer risk was attributable to the radiation exposure but that the increased mortality from other causes was associated with the underlying condition. Support for this conclusion was provided later by a follow-up study of about 1000 patients with ankylosing spondylitis who had been identified at the time of the original survey but who, for various reasons, had not received radiation therapy. There was no evidence of an excess risk of leukaemia (0 deaths against 0.44 expected) or of other cancers (18 deaths against 17.21 expected) (Smith *et al.* 1977). The size of this non-irradiated group was small and only 80 per cent were completely traced. It is not possible to rule out completely the possibility that these patients were at increased risk of cancer but the findings for leukaemia, at least, were significantly different from those for irradiated patients. For causes of death other than cancer the experience of this group of patients was very similar to that of the irradiated patients. It thus seems that patients with ankylosing spondylitis were at substantially increased risk of death from a variety of different causes, compared to the general population, but that except for cancer and aplastic anaemia, this risk was unrelated to the radiation treatment (Radford *et al.* 1977).

Many of the patients who were included in the studies of leukaemia (Court Brown and Doll 1957) and other cancers (Court Brown and Doll 1965) had been treated with X-rays for their spondylitis on more than one occasion. This introduced a complication into the interpretation of the late effects of the radiation treatment on mortality as it was not clear to what extent the second and subsequent treatment courses were responsible for the excess of deaths that persisted many years after the first radiation treatment. To overcome this problem in recent analyses, patients who received more than one course of treatment have been excluded from consideration shortly after receiving their second course. By thus confining the analysis to the mortality of patients following a single treatment course it has been possible to examine how the excess of leukaemia and other cancer deaths varies with time since exposure, age at exposure, and, for leukaemia, with radiation dose (Smith and Doll 1982). The results of these analyses will be discussed in the following section.

Radiation carcinogenesis

There is abundant evidence that exposure to ionizing radiations increases the risk of leukaemia and other cancers and this relationship is beyond serious dispute. Certain important aspects of the association, however, are less clear. These include: the evolution and duration of risk following exposure, the magnitude of the risk following exposure to different types and doses of radiation, and the way in which radiation interacts with other causes of cancer to affect risk. Some of these issues are discussed in the following sections.

Distribution of induction periods

The way in which the risk of a radiation-induced cancer varies with the time since exposure is easiest to look at in populations in which only one exposure of short duration has occurred. Two of the groups best suited in this respect are the atomic bomb survivors and patients with ankylosing spondylitis following a single treatment course. Both of these groups are large and substantial numbers of radiation-induced cancers have occurred. Neither group, unfortunately, is well suited to examine the risk in the period immediately following exposure. The A-bomb cohort was not defined until 1950 and thus does not include deaths from cancers other than leukaemia occurring in the first five years after the explosion of the bombs. (Surveillance for cases of leukaemia was started in 1946.) Patients treated for ankylosing spondylitis may include some persons who, at the time of the first treatment, had a cancer that was causing symptoms that were incorrectly ascribed to spondylitis and which therefore provoked the radiation treatment. This, for example, seems the likely explanation for the five deaths from pancreas cancer that occurred within two years of first treatment whereas only one such death would have been expected based on national rates (Smith and Doll 1982). In both the spondylitic population and the A-bomb survivors the induced leukaemias appeared, on average, considerably before other cancers. Fig. 1 shows the change in the risk of a radiation-induced leukaemia with time since exposure. For the spondylitics 'expected' numbers of leukaemia deaths have been calculated on the basis of general population death rates (Smith and Doll 1982) whereas, in the most recent publication of data on the A-bomb survivors, the leukaemia induction rates have been derived by fitting linear dose-response relationships to those estimated to have received different doses of radiation (Kato and Schull 1982). These differences limit the comparisons that may be made between the two sets of curves but the way in which the leukaemia risk changes with time since exposure may be compared for the two groups. Graphs are shown for both relative risk and excess risk. In the spondylitics the leukaemia risk is greatest three to five years after exposure and subsequently declines such that by 20 years there is no evidence of an excess risk. It should be noted, however, that the total number of leukaemia deaths is small and the follow-up of the population beyond 20 years is not extensive (Smith and Doll 1982). The apparent secondary peak

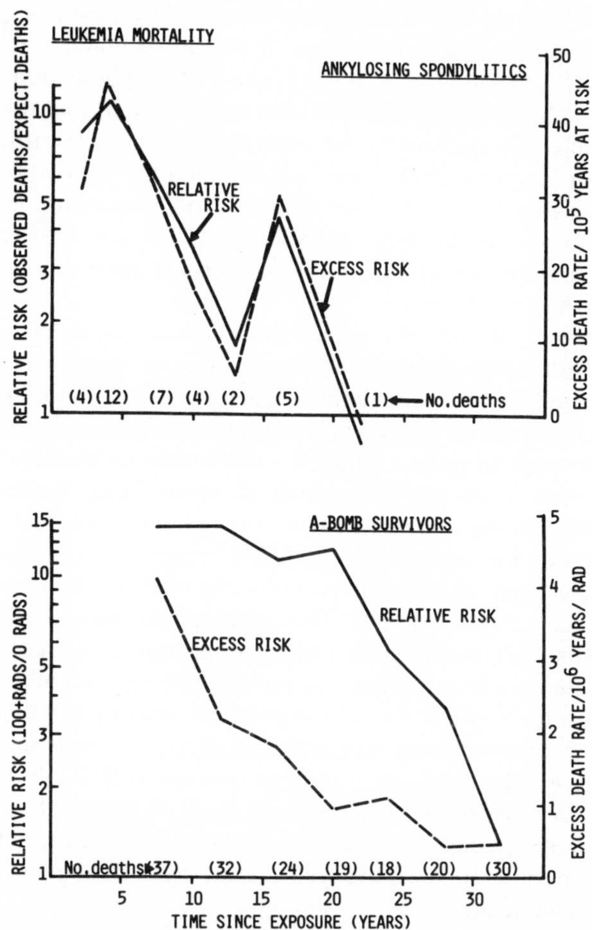

Fig. 1. Risk of radiation-induced leukaemia deaths at different times after exposure in ankylosing spondylitics and A-bomb survivors. Derived from Smith and Doll (1982), and Kato and Schull (1982).

of leukaemias 15–17 years after exposure is based on only five cases and is probably an artifact.

No data are given by Kato and Schull (1982) for the first five years after exposure among the A-bomb survivors but the greatest measured risk is in the period immediately following this, five to nine years after exposure. Subsequently the excess risk declines in a fairly regular manner and there is only a small excess mortality 25 or more years after exposure. Thus it seems reasonable to conclude from these results, first, that most radiation-induced leukaemias occur by 10–15 years after exposure and, secondly, that beyond 20 or 25 years the risk associated with radiation may be near zero. The veracity of this latter conclusion should become apparent with further follow-up of both populations. It should be noted that the curves shown include leukaemia of all types but in neither population is there an excess risk of chronic lymphatic leukaemia and it seems that this disease is less susceptible to induction by radiation than other forms of leukaemia.

It has been suggested that in the A-bomb data the interval between the radiation exposure and the development of leukaemia increases in proportion to age at the time of exposure (Ichimaru *et al.* 1978). The evidence in support of such an effect is not strong and it is not apparent in the data on the spondylitics.

The evolution of the risk of radiation-induced cancers, other than leukaemia, following exposure shows a different pattern from that of leukaemia, both among the ankylosing spondylitics and the A-bomb survivors. This is shown in Fig. 2. The numbers of induced cancers are, in general, too small to permit detailed examination of the changes in risk with time since exposure for individual sites. Thus for the A-bomb survivors the graphs shown are for all cancers combined (excluding leukaemia). For the spondylitics, data for cancers of all sites that were likely to have been directly in the radiation beams ('heavily irradiated' sites) have been combined. The excess risk among the spondylitics in the first few years after treatment is difficult to interpret, for reasons already discussed, and may be an artifact. A notable increase in both relative and excess risk occurs between 9 and 11 years after exposure and the excess risk remains at an approximately constant level thereafter until about 20 years after exposure. The subsequent decline, though graphically dramatic, is based on a comparison of only small numbers of observed and expected cases and is not statistically significant. The apparent decline in the relative risk in the period 10 or more years after first treatment is also not statistically significant.

Among the A-bomb survivors the excess risk 5–9 years after exposure is just significant ($p = 0.02$) but there is no risk apparent in the following five years and only 15 or more years after exposure is the increased risk highly significant. Subsequently the relative risk remains approximately constant with a tendency to increase in the most recent data collected 30 years after exposure. This disturbing trend is even more striking for the excess risk, the highest risk of an induced cancer being 30 or more years after exposure. This last point shown on this graph is based on reasonable numbers of deaths and may indicate a true increase in the risk at very long intervals after exposure (the lower 90 per cent confidence limit on the excess risk 30 more more years after exposure is 6.5 cancers per million person years per rad) (Kato and Schull 1982).

Consideration of changes in the risk of radiation-induced cancers with time since exposure must be examined in conjunction with the ages at

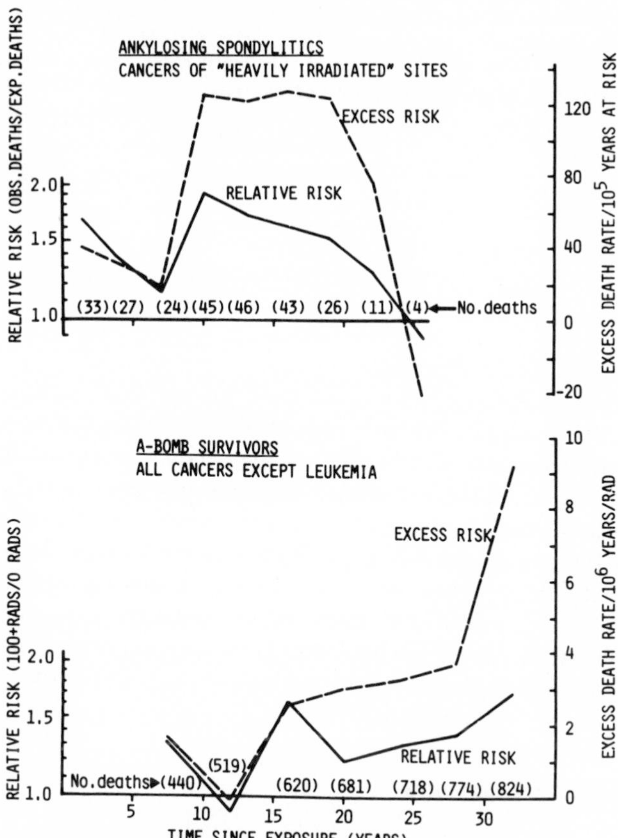

Fig. 2. Risk of radiation-induced cancer deaths (other than leukaemia) at different times after exposure in ankylosing spondylitics and A-bomb survivors. Derived from Smith and Doll (1982), and Kato and Schull (1982).

which the exposures occurred. In interpreting the data on the A-bomb survivors it is important to take into account the observation that those irradiated under the age of 10 years have a higher *relative* risk of a radiation-induced cancer than those exposed at a later age. This is illustrated in Table 1 which is taken from Kato and Schull (1982) and also in Fig. 4. The increase in the excess risk of cancer among the A-bomb survivors, shown in Fig. 2, is due, at least in part, to those who appear to be at high relative risk of a radiation-induced cancer reaching ages at which the 'natural' rate of cancer is becoming high.

It may be concluded that the risk of a radiation-induced cancer, other than leukaemia, may be small in the first 10 years following exposure but, subsequently, the risk remains elevated until at least 20 years after

Table 1. Relative risk of death from a cancer, other than leukaemia, among atomic bomb survivors by age at irradiation and age at death. The numbers shown in the body of the table are the ratios of the death rates among those exposed to more than 100 rad compared to those not exposed (Kato and Schull 1982)

Age at exposure (y) (in 1945)	Age at death (y)					
	<30	30–39	40–49	50–59	60–69	70+
< 10	15.1	5.0	6.8	–	–	–
10–19	1.0	2.5	2.4	8.2	–	–
20–24	–	1.8	1.9	2.0	1.6	–
35–49	–	–	1.2	1.1	1.3	1.4
50+	–	–	–	2.2	1.0	1.4

exposure and possibly for the rest of life. Further follow-up will be necessary to determine whether or not the excess cancer rate increases at very long periods after exposure. This has not been observed in the spondylitics (in fact at present the reverse appears to be the case) but, currently, the person-years of experience beyond 20 years is small in this series. It should perhaps be noted also that among women given a radiation-induced menopause there is no evidence that the risk of a radiation-induced cancer declines 20 years after exposure, though again this observation is based on small numbers of deaths (13 observed against 9.8 expected; Smith and Doll 1976).

Dose–response relationships

Most public-health interest centres on the likely effect of low doses of radiation as it is to these which a substantial proportion of the population may be exposed. The spondylitics were, in general, exposed to large doses of radiation as were many of the A-bomb survivors, though most of the latter group received doses of less than 10 rad. There are clear advantages in studying a group in which exposure has been high as effects of a larger magnitude are to be expected. The problems become manifest when attempts are made to extrapolate from the observations to estimate the effects of exposure to very low doses. The simplest assumption to make is that effects are linearly related to dose and to extrapolate backwards on this basis. This has been the general approach adopted for many of the analyses of data from studies of the A-bomb survivors. For leukaemia, the cause of death for which the radiation-induced excess is most apparent, this form of dose–response relationship fits the data quite well though it is a better fit for the Hiroshima data than for the Nagasaki data and also the leukaemia risk, for a specified dose, seems to be higher in Hiroshima than Nagasaki. In part this difference may be due to the different relative contributions of neutron and gamma radiation in the two cities, but this will have to be reassessed when the revised dosimetry on the A-bomb survivors is available.

If the data from the two cities are combined and linear dose–response curves are fitted to the leukaemia excess mortality the estimate of the induction rate is 1.9 leukaemia deaths per million person years at risk per rad and for other cancers the rate is 2.2 per million person years at risk per rad (Beebe *et al.* 1978b). These authors also give estimates of the induction rates for cancers of individual sites.

For the spondylitics, detailed organ dose estimates are not yet available, except for the bone marrow, though some approximate estimates are given in BEIR (1980). Estimates of the mean bone marrow dose of radiation have been made for patients dying of leukaemia and for a random sample of all patients and these have been used to relate the excess leukaemia risk to radiation dose. Details of the procedures used are given in Smith and Doll (1982) and Fig. 3 is taken from that paper.

The greatest risk of leukaemia induction is in those patients with a mean marrow dose of 100–200 rad. At high doses the risk appears to be reduced. The data are not well fitted by a linear dose–response curve passing through the origin (line 1 in Fig. 3) and, indeed, the assumption that the excess risk is unrelated to dose fits the data better (line 0 in Fig. 3). This surprising finding was not apparent in the original analyses (Court Brown and Doll 1957) when patients receiving multiple courses of X-ray treatment were included and marrow dose estimates from the different courses were simply added. In that analysis a linear dose–response relationship, passing through the origin, appeared reasonable. The reasons for these differences are not clear but it is possible that the effect of two or more courses of radiation may be greater than the same amount of radiation given in a single course.

Evidence that a simple linear dose–response relationship for the induction of leukaemia may be incorrect was provided by the finding of little or no excess risk of leukaemia among women irradiated for the treatment of cervix cancer. Women given a radiation-induced menopause received a substantially smaller dose to the bone marrow and yet showed a statistically significant excess mortality for leukaemia. It was suggested that patients irradiated for cervix cancer may not be at greatly increased risk of leukaemia because the radiation treatment is given in such a way that some of the bone marrow received a very high dose or radiation, sufficient to sterilize the marrow cells in the vicinity of the cervix, and that the dose to the marrow falls off rapidly with distance from the cervix such that the mean dose to surviving cells may be quite small. Thus the 'effective' dose for leukaemia induction is small (Hutchison 1968; Mole 1973; Boice *et al.* 1984).

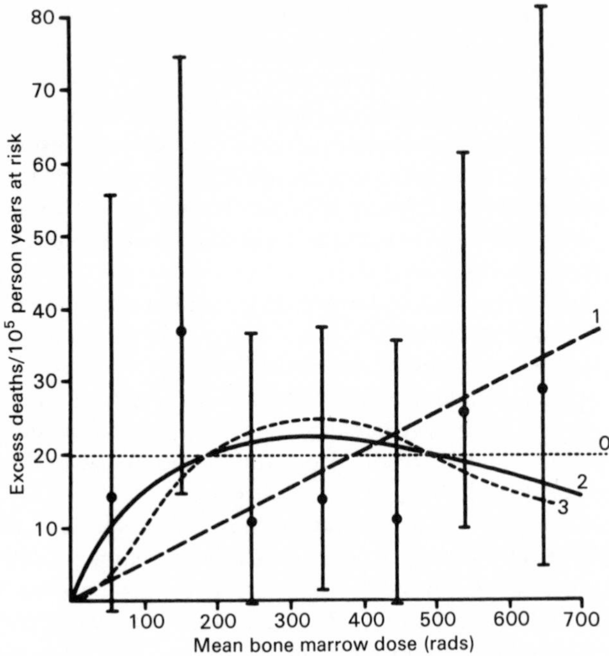

Fig. 3. Excess death rate from leukaemia among ankylosing spondylitics according to mean bone marrow radiation dose. Curves are based on maximum likelihood fit of the following models: (0) E.R. = b; $b = 19.6 \times 10^{-5}$; (1) E.R. = bD; $b = 0.52 \times 10^{-6}$; (2) E.R. = $bDe^{-\lambda D}$; $b = 2.02 \times 10^{-6}$, $\lambda = 0.33 \times 10^{-2}$; (3) E.R. = $bD^2e^{\lambda D}$ $b = 0.018 \times 10^{-6}$, $\lambda = 0.63 \times 10^{-2}$, where E.R. is the excess leukaemia death rate, D is the mean bone marrow dose and b and λ are constants estimated by the method of maximum likelihood (from Smith and Doll (1982) reproduced by kind permission of the editor of the *British Medical Journal*).

In the treatment of ankylosing spondylitis, usually only the spine and sacroiliac joints were irradiated but the doses shown in Fig. 3 relate to the mean marrow dose. The dose to cells directly in the radiation field may have been higher than the mean dose by a factor of two or more (as the spinal marrow constitutes about 40 per cent of the total bone marrow). Thus at the higher doses many of the cells directly in the line of radiation may have received a dose large enough to sterilize them and thus render them incapable of becoming leukaemic.

Dose–response curves for cancer induction that take account of the cell-sterilizing effect of radiation have been discussed by Gray (1965), Mole (1975), and others. Mole and his colleagues have also developed a mouse system for the induction of leukaemia by X-rays in CBA mice in which the leukaemia-induction data is well fitted by a mathematical model assuming an exponential cell-sterilization effect, and a leukaemia-induction rate among non-sterilized cells proportional to the square of the radiation dose (Major and Mole 1978; Mole *et al.* 1983). We have fitted models of this general form to the data shown in Fig. 3. Line 2 shows the best fit of a curve predicting the excess death rates as aDe^{-bD}, where D is the mean marrow dose and a and b are constants which are estimated. Line 3 fits a model of the form aD^2e^{-bD}, which does not fit quite as well. Unfortunately the confidence bands on the leukaemia excess risk at each dose point are sufficiently large that a wide range of different possible models would fit the data. It should be noted also that it is not strictly appropriate to fit models of this form for this data set. As only part of the marrow is irradiated, and the fraction varies from patient to patient, different portions of the marrow will receive different doses and this should be taken into account in the model-fitting procedure. The necessary data relating to the dose to different parts of the marrow for each patient are not yet available, however.

A further complication in interpreting these data derives from the fact that a radiation treatment course for ankylosing spondylitis may have been spread over a month or more. In calculating the marrow dose we simply added together the contributions from the different fractions. It is well established that the cell-killing effect of radiation is modified by fractionation of the radiation dose and it has been suggested that the same may be true for leukaemia induction. Using the same mouse model as discussed above, Mole and Major (1983) have demonstrated recently that with fractionated exposure a dose–response curve is obtained remarkably similar to that which has been observed for the spondylitics. The relevance of the mouse model for human data is unclear but, at least, it suggests that extrapolating from the effects of high radiation doses given at high dose rates to predict the effects of low doses at low dose rates may be a more complicated procedure than was perhaps initially anticipated!

Age at exposure

Several workers have advanced the hypothesis that individuals may vary in their susceptibility to a radiation-induced cancer. Bross and Natarajan (1972) in particular, have suggested, with respect to *in utero* radiation exposure, that some fetuses may be many times more susceptible than others to radiation carcinogenesis. Whilst this is a plausible theory the evidence advanced to support the argument has been unconvincing. There is, however, good evidence that age at exposure is related to radiation risk. We have mentioned earlier that the fetus seems to be more sensitive to radiation than are adults (UNSCEAR 1977) and in Figs 4 and 5 the induction rates of leukaemia and other cancers are compared among

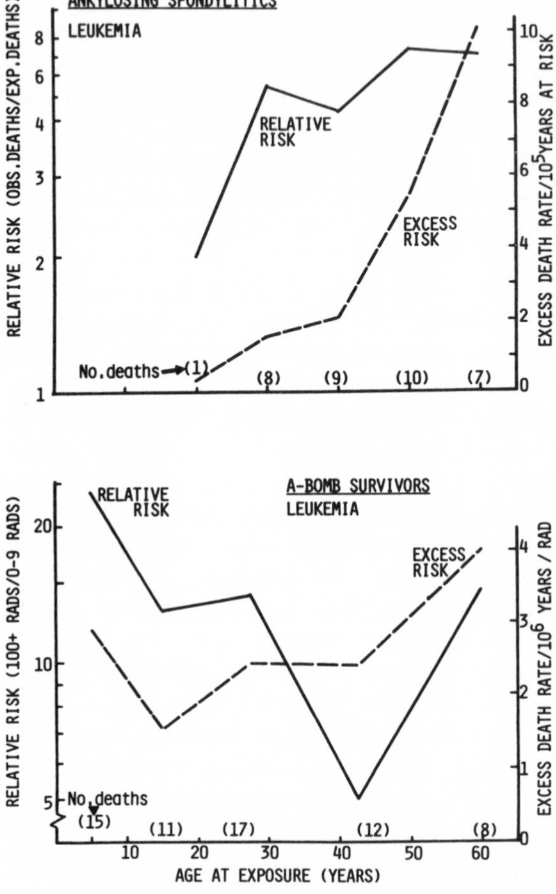

Fig. 4. Risk of radiation-induced leukaemia deaths at different ages at exposure in ankylosing spondylitics and A-bomb survivors. Derived from Smith and Doll (1982) and Beebe *et al.* (1977).

patients with ankylosing spondylitis and the A-bomb survivors according to their ages at the time of the radiation exposure.

Among the spondylitics, there is no evidence that the *relative* risk of leukaemia varies significantly with age at exposure (note that the point for patients aged less than 25 years is based on only one case) but the excess risks show a steep and, statistically, highly significant increase as the age at exposure increases.

There were no young children among the spondylitics but among the A-bomb survivors there is evidence that children may be especially susceptible to leukaemia induction (at least as measured by the relative

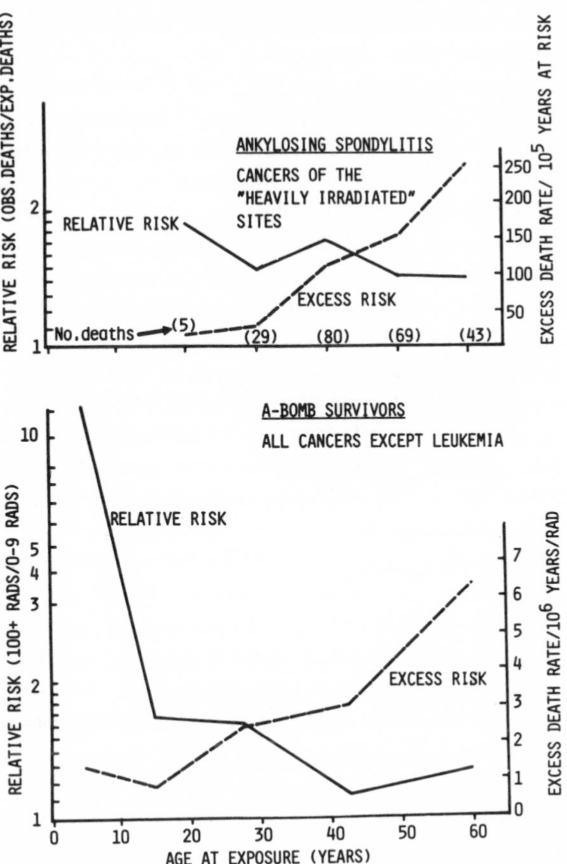

Fig. 5. Risk of radiation-induced cancer deaths (other than leukaemia) at different ages at exposure in ankylosing spondylitics and A-bomb survivors. Derived from Smith and Doll (1982) and Beebe *et al.* (1977).

risk). The excess risk among children is similar to that among adults up to the age of 50 years and it rises slightly after this. The increase in the excess risk with age is much steeper among the spondylitics than in the A-bomb survivors. Doll (1970) noted that the incidence of leukaemia among non-irradiated persons also increased much more steeply with age in Britain than in Japan. This suggests that, among adults at least, radiation may be interacting in a multiplicative way with other factors which induce leukaemia.

For cancers other than leukaemia the situation appears to be similar (Fig. 5 and Table 1). In both population groups shown the excess risk increases regularly with age at exposure among adults. The relative risk among those who were children at the time of the A-bomb explosions is especially high. In the spondylitics the relative risk of a radiation-induced cancer shows no significant variation with age but the excess risk for those irradiated at age 55 years or more is over 10 times higher than that for persons irradiated at ages under 35 years. These observations also suggest, as for leukaemia, that radiation interacts in a way that may be approximately multiplicative with other factors which induce cancer. Of relevance in this respect also is the observation that for most individual cancers the radiation risk is approximately proportional to the expected death rate from the cancer in the absence of radiation (Smith and Doll 1972; Kato and Schull 1982). These conclusions must be tentative, however, as it remains to be seen how the risk of radiation-induced cancers will evolve in later life among persons irradiated at a young age. There is some evidence also that the effect of age at irradiation is not the same for all cancers. For example, among the A-bomb survivors, McGregor *et al.* (1977) found that the risk of radiation-induced breast cancer was highest among those exposed at ages 10–19 years and showed a significant decrease associated with exposure at older ages. More recent observations on the A-bomb survivors indicate that those exposed under the age of 10 years are also at increased risk of breast cancer. At present the radiation-associated *excess* risk of breast cancer among those irradiated as young children is lower than that of those aged 10–19 years at the time of the explosions. The *relative* risk of breast cancer is higher, however, among those irradiated in the first decade of life (Tokunaga *et al.* 1984). Thus it is possible, with further follow-up of the population, that those irradiated at the youngest ages may be at greatest absolute risk of a radiation-induced breast cancer.

Future work

Ionizing radiations are one of the most well studied of carcinogens yet there is still considerable controversy regarding the magnitude of their effect in the induction of cancer at low doses. This is perhaps not surprising as they are a relatively weak carcinogen and it seems likely that they are responsible for only a small proportion of all human cancers. Thus to separate out their effects from those of other, and often more powerful, carcinogenic agents poses considerable difficulties. This is especially likely to be the case when populations whose members have been exposed to very low levels of radiation are studied. It is perhaps for these reasons that studies of cancer mortality in geographical areas with different levels of background radiation have been unrewarding. Most public-health interest in the carcinogenic effects of radiation is with respect to populations who might have a low, but higher than average, exposure as a consequence of their occupation or through exposure to the products of nuclear industries or to diagnostic radiation. The risk estimates on which existing international exposure standards are based would suggest that exposure at the limit of recommended levels are likely to produce only a small increase in an individual's cancer risk – of a magnitude that would be very difficult to detect even in large epidemiological studies (Land 1980). Nevertheless, we have seen above that there are still several important areas of uncertainty that should encourage caution in deducing the effects of low-level exposure from effects seen in special population groups exposed to high radiation doses.

There are theoretical and experimental grounds for believing that the dose–response curve for X-ray induction of cancer is not simply linear but should include a quadratic component and take account of cell sterilization. If this is the case, it has been assumed that fitting linear dose–response curves may lead to overestimates of the effects of low-level exposure (ICRP 1977). Whilst it seems unlikely that the carcinogenic effects of low levels of radiation have been seriously underestimated this possibility cannot be completely excluded and, therefore, it will be important to monitor carefully the experience of those whose employment involves radiation exposure. Fortunately many of those in this position have worn film badges which enable reasonable estimates to be made of the magnitude of exposure and it should thus be possible to relate cancer risk to dose. Studies of this kind have been conducted on U.S. atomic energy workers and studies of similar U.K. populations are under way. The confidence intervals on any estimates of risk obtained from these studies will be wide but they should, at least, provide information on whether or not the current estimates of risk (based on extrapolation from populations exposed to high doses) are out by an order of magnitude.

The choice of an appropriate dose–response curve for extrapolation is still a matter of considerable controversy and uncertainty (BEIR 1980) and this is an area where more work is needed. Unfortunately the way forward is not entirely clear. It is likely that the revised dose estimates for the A-bomb survivors that are now being derived will lead to changes in the risk estimates based on this population. They may also lead to a reassessment of the relative carcinogenic effects of gamma and neutron radiation. The basic methods by which dose estimates for this population are derived are, however, necessarily crude and this may frustrate attempts to elucidate the detailed shape of dose–response relationships. The estimation of the radiation dose to the spondylitic patients is, in principle, easier as reasonably good data are available on the treatment schedules employed for a sample of patients. Interpretation is complicated, however, as organs, including the bone marrow, were not uniformly irradiated and, furthermore, the radiation exposure may have been given over a period of a month or more. Mole and his colleagues have suggested, and also shown in their mouse model, that it may be important to take account of both of these factors in constructing dose–response relationships, although the way in which this should be done, especially with respect to fractionation, is unclear. By taking account of the dose-distribution to different parts of the marrow it should be possible to fit more appropriate models, incorporating cell-sterilization effects, of the form illustated in Fig. 3.

At present efforts are being made to extend the follow-up of spondylitis patients who received more than one course of radiotherapy. It is likely that comparison of the cancer risks to such patients with the risks to patients following a single treatment course will enable the effects of exposures separated in time to be estimated. This is of interest as, for example, in situations of occupational exposure, radiation doses to workers are likely to be accumulated in this way, though at lower doses. There may be considerable difficulties, however, in extrapolating the effects seen at the high doses received by patients with spondylitis to predict effects at much lower dose levels.

Studies of the way in which radiation interacts with other carcinogens are of considerable scientific and public-health interest. The finding that the excess risk of leukaemia and other cancers following radiation exposure varies according to the age at exposure strongly suggests that the effects of radiation are not independent of other carcinogenic factors. Unfortunately in few of the published studies of population groups exposed to moderate doses of radiation is there any information on exposure to other potential carcinogens. For example, among the spondylitics, deaths from lung cancer are a high proportion of all deaths from cancers of 'heavily irradiated' sites. There are, however, no data available on the smoking habits of the patients in this series so that it is possible neither to assess how much of the excess risk of lung cancer is due to differences in smoking habits from those of the general population nor to determine how rates of radiation-induced lung cancer vary with smoking habits. Whittlemore and McMillan (1983) analysed data on the mortality of uranium miners from lung cancer in relation to both their smoking habits and estimated radiation exposure. They found that a model in which the risk associated with exposure to both factors was estimted by a multiplication of the risks associated with each factor alone gave a satisfactory fit to the data whereas an additive model did not. Prentice *et al.* (1983) could not distinguish between the two types of model in their analysis of data on lung cancer mortality and smoking habits among survivors of the atomic bomb explosions. For smoking-related cancers of other sites, however, these authors found that the joint effects of smoking and radiation exposure were not only less than multiplicative but, for some cancer sites, there was some evidence that the joint effects were less than additive.

Although the risk of a radiation-induced leukaemia appears to decline by 10 years after exposure, and may be near zero more than 20 years after exposure, the risk of other radiation-induced cancers remains relatively high in this period. In order to estimate the total numbers of cancers induced by a given radiation exposure it will be necessary to follow the members of exposed populations for many decades and probably throughout life. It is possible that the induced cancer risk will persist throughout life or it may even increase in later years. Among the A-bomb survivors the relative risk of a cancer other than leukaemia among those estimated to have received more than 100 rad, compared with those not irradiated, is greatest among those irradiated at the youngest ages. If these relative risks remain constant throughout life, the absolute risk of a radiation-associated cancer will increase as the follow-up time increases. There is a disturbing suggestion of such a trend in recent data from the A-bomb survivors (Fig. 2 and Kato and Schull 1982). It is especially important to continue to follow population groups that have already been under study for several decades (e.g. the A-bomb survivors and patients with ankylosing spondylitis) as there is presently little information on radiation effects 30 or more years after exposure.

Acknowledgements

I am grateful to Gilbert Beebe and John Boice for their comments on an earlier version of this chapter.

References

Beebe, G.W., Kato, H., and Land, C.E. (1971). Studies of the mortality of A-bomb survivors. 4. Mortality and radiation dose 1950–1966. *Radiat. Res.* **48**, 613–49.

Beebe, G.W., Kato, H., and Land C.E. (1977). *Mortality experience of atomic bomb survivors 1950–74.* Radiation Effects Research Foundation Lifespan Study Report 8. Technical report RERF TR 1–77.

Beebe, G.W., Land, C.E., and Kato, H. (1978a). The hypothesis of radiation-accelerated aging and the mortality of Japanese A-bomb victims. In *Late biological effects of ionizing radiation*, Vol 1. International Atomic Energy Agency, Vienna.

Beebe, G.W., Kato, H., and Land, C.E. (1978b). Studies of the mortality of A-bomb survivors. 6. Mortality and radiation dose, 1950–74. *Radiat. Res.* **75**, 138–201.

BEIR (1980). *The effects on populations of exposure to low levels of ionizing radiation: 1980.* Committee on the Biological Effects of Ionizing Radiations. National Research Council. National Academy Press, Washington, D.C.

Bithell, J. and Stewart, A. (1975). Prenatal irradiation and childhood malignancy: A review of British data from the Oxford survey. *Brit. J. Cancer* **31**, 271–307.

Boice, J.D. and Hutchison, G.B. (1980). Leukemia following radiotherapy for cervical cancer. 10 year follow up of an international study. *J. nat. Cancer Inst.* **65**, 115–29.

Boice, J.D. Jr and Land, C.E. (1982) Ionizing radiation. In *Cancer epidemiology and prevention* (ed. D. Schottenfeld and J.F. Fraumeni Jr), pp. 231–53. W.B. Saunders Co., Philadelphia.

Boice, J.D., Day, N.E., and 34 others (1984). Cancer risk following radiotherapy of cervical cancer: a preliminary report. In *Radiation carcinogenesis: epidemiology and biological significance* (ed. J.D. Boice and J.F. Fraumeni), pp. 161–79. Raven Press, New York.

Bross, I.D.J. and Natarajan, N. (1972). Leukemia from low-level radiation. Identification of susceptible children. *New Engl. J. Med.* **287**, 107–10.

Court Brown, W.M. and Abatt, J.D. (1955). The incidence of leukaemia in ankylosing spondylitics treated with x-rays. *Lancet* **i**, 1283.

Court Brown, W.M. and Doll, R. (1957). *Leukaemia and aplastic anaemia in patients irradiated for ankylosing spondylitis*. Medical Research Council Special Report Series No. 295. HMSO, London.

Court Brown, W.M. and Doll, R. (1958). Expectation of life and mortality from cancer among British radiologists. *Brit. med. J.* **ii**, 181–7.

Court Brown, W.M. and Doll, R. (1965). Mortality from cancer and other causes after radiotherapy for ankylosing spondylitis. *Brit. med. J.* **ii**, 1327–32.

Court Brown, W.M., Spiers, F.W., Doll, R., Duffy, B.J., and McHugh, M.J. (1960a). Geographical variation in leukaemia mortality in relation to background radiation and other factors. *Brit. med. J.* **i**, 1753–9.

Court Brown, W.M., Doll, R., and Hill, A.B. (1960b). Incidence of leukaemia after exposure to diagnostic radiation in utero. *Brit. med. J.* **iv**, 1539–45.

Doll, R. (1970). Cancer and ageing: the epidemiologic evidence. In *Tenth International Cancer Congress. Oncology 1970.* Year Book Medical Pub. Inc., Chicago.

Doll, R. and Smith, P.G. (1968). The long term effects of x-irradiation in patients treated for metropathia haemorrhagia. *Brit. J. Radiol.* **41**, 362–8.

Folley, J.H., Borges, W., and Yamawaki, T. (1952). Incidence of leukemia in survivors of the atomic bomb in Hiroshima and Nagasaki, Japan. *Amer. J. Med.* **13**, 311–81.

Gray, L.H. (1965). Radiation biology and cancer. In *Cellular radiation biology*, pp. 7–25. Williams and Wilkins, Baltimore.

Hempelmann, L.H., Hall, W.J., Phillips, M., Cooper, R.A., and Ames, W.R. (1975). Neoplasms in persons treated with x-rays in infancy: fourth survey in 20 years. *J. Nat. Cancer Inst.* **55**, 519–30.

Hewitt, D. (1955). Some features of leukaemia mortality. *Brit. J. prev. soc. Med.* **9**, 81–8.

Hutchison, G. B. (1968). Leukemia in patients with cancer of the cervix treated with radiation. A report covering the first 5 years of an international study. *J. nat Cancer Inst.* **40**, 951–82.

ICRP (1977). *Recommendations of the International Commission on Radiological Protection*. Pergamon Press, Oxford. (ICRP Publications 26)

Ichimaru, T.M., Ishimaru, T., and Belsky, J.L. (1978). Incidence of leukaemia in atomic bomb survivors belonging to a fixed cohort in Hiroshima and Nagasaki, 1950–71. *J. Radiat. Res.* **19**, 262–82.

Jablon, S. and Kato, H. (1970). Childhood cancer in relation to prenatal exposure to atomic bomb radiation. *Lancet* **ii**, 1000–3.

Jablon, S. and Kato, H. (1972). Studies of the mortality of A-bomb survivors. 5.

Radiation dose and mortality 1950–1970. *Radiat. Res.* **50**, 649–98.

Jablon, S. and Bailar, J.C. (1980). The contribution of ionizing radiation to cancer mortality in the United States. *Prevent. Med.* **9**, 219–26.

Kato, H. and Schull, W.J. (1982). Studies of the mortality of A-bomb survivors. 7. Mortality, 1950–1978. Part 1: Cancer mortality. *Radiat. Res.* **90**, 395–432.

Kato, H., Brown, C.C., Hoel, D.G., and Schull, W.J., (1982). Studies of the mortality of A-bomb survivors. Report 7: Mortality 1950–1978; Part II: Mortality from causes other than cancer and mortality in early entrants. *Radiat. Res.* **91**, 243–64.

Land, C. (1980). Estimating cancer risks from low doses of ionizing radiation *Science NY* **209**, 1197–203.

Loewe, W.E. and Mendelsohn, E. (1981). Revised dose estimates at Hiroshima and Nagasaki. *Health Phys.* **41**, 663–6.

MacMahon, B. (1962). Prenatal x-ray exposure and childhood cancer. *J. nat. Cancer Inst.* **5**, 1173–91.

Major, I.R. and Mole, R.H. (1978). Myeloid leukaemia in x-ray irradiated CBA mice. *Nature Lond.* **272**, 455–6.

Matanoski, G.M. Risk of cancer associated with occupational exposure in radiologists and other radiation workes. In *Cancer: achievements, challenge and prospectives for the 1980s* (ed. J.H. Burchenal and H.F. Oettgen), Vol. 1, pp. 241–54. Grune and Stratton, New York.

Matanoski, G.M., Seltser, R., Sartwell, P.E., Diamond, E.L., and Elliott, E.E. (1975a). The current mortality rates of radiologists and other physician specialists: deaths from all causes and from cancer. *Amer. J. Epidemiol.* **101**, 188–98.

Matanoski, G.M., Seltser, R., Sartwell, P.E., Diamond, E.L., and Elliott, E.E. (1975b). The current mortality rates of radiologists and other physician specialists: specific cause of death. *Amer. J. Epidemiol.* **101**, 199–210.

McGregor, D.H., Land, C.E., Choi, K., Tokuokas, S., Liu, P.I., Wakabayashi, T., and Beebe, G.W. (1977). Breast cancer incidence among atomic bomb survivors Hiroshima and Nagasaki, 1950–1969. *J. Nat. Cancer Inst.* **59**, 799–811.

Milton, R.C. and Shohoji, T. (1968). *Tentative 1965 radiation dose estimation for atomic bomb survivors: Hiroshima and Nagasaki.* Atomic Bomb Casualty Commission ABCC TR 1–68.

Mole, R. (1973). Late effects of radiation: carcinogenesis. *Brit. med. Bull.* **29**, 78–83.

Mole, R.H. (1974). Antenatal irradiation and childhood cancer: causation or coincidence? *Brit. J. Cancer* **30**, 199–208.

Mole, R.H. (1975). Ionizing radiation as a carcinogen: practical questions and academic pursuits. *Brit. J. Radiol.* **48**, 157–69.

Mole, R.H. and Major, I.R. (1983). Myeloid leukaemia frequency after protracted exposure to ionizing radiation: experimental confirmation of the flat dose response found in ankylosing spondylitis after a single treatment course with x-rays. *Leuk. Res.* **7**, 295–300.

Mole, R.H., Papworth, D.C., and Corp, M.J. (1983). The dose–response for x-ray induction of myeloid leukaemia in male CBA/H mice. *Brit. J. Cancer* **47**, 285–91.

Monson, R.R. and MacMahon, B. (1984). Prenatal x-ray exposure and cancer in children. In *Radiation carcinogenesis: epidemiology and biological significance* (ed. J.D. Boice and J.F. Fraumeni), pp. 97–105. Raven Press, New York.

Ohkita, T. (1975). Review of thirty years study of Hiroshima and Nagasaki atomic bomb survivors. II. Biological effects. A. Acute effects. *J. Radiat. Res.* (Suppl.) 49–66.

Prentice, R.L., Yoshimoto, Y., and Mason, M.W. (1983). Relationship of cigarette smoking and radiation exposure to cancer mortality in Hiroshima and Nagasaki. *J. Nat. Cancer Inst.* **70**, 611–22.

Radford, E.P., Doll, R., and Smith, P.G. (1977). Mortality among patients with ankylosing spondylitis not given x-ray therapy. *New Engl. J. Med.* **297**, 572–6.

Ron, E. and Modan, B. (1980). Benign and malignant thyroid neoplasms after childhood irradiation for tinea capitis. *J. Nat. Cancer Inst.* **65**, 7–11.

Seltser, R. and Sartwell, P.E. (1959). The application of cohort analysis to the study of ionizing radiation and longevity in physicians. *Amer. J. publ. Hlth* **49**, 1610–20.

Seltser, R. and Sartwell, P.E. (1965). The influence of occupational exposure to radiation on the mortality of American radiologists and other medical specialists. *Amer. J. Epidemiol.* **81**, 2–22.

Simon, N., Brucer, M., and Hayes, R. (1960). Radiation and leukaemia in cancer of the cervix. *Radiology* **74**, 905–11.

Smith, P.G. (1977). Leukaemia and other cancers following radiation treatment of pelvic disease. *Cancer* **39**, 1901–5.

Smith, P.G. and Doll, R. (1976). Late effects of x irradiation in patients treated for metropathia haemorrhagica. *Brit. J. Radiol.* **49**, 224–32.

Smith, P.G. and Doll, R. (1981). Mortality from cancer and all causes among British radiologists. *Brit. J. Radiol.* **54**, 187–94.

Smith, P.G. and Doll, R. (1982). Mortality among patients with ankylosing spondylitis after a single treatment course with x rays. *Brit. med. J.* **284**, 449–60.

Smith, P.G., Doll, R., and Radford, E.P. (1977). Cancer mortality among patients with ankylosing spondylitis not given x-ray therapy. *Brit. J. Radiol.* **50**, 728–34.

Stewart, A. and Kneale, G.W. (1968). Changes in the cancer risk associated with obstetric radiography. *Lancet* **i**, 104–7.

Stewart, A.M. and Kneale, G.W. (1970). Radiation dose effects in relation to obstetric x-rays and childhood cancers. *Lancet* **i**, 1185–8.

Stewart, A., Webb, A., Giles, D., and Hewitt, D. (1956). Malignant disease in childhood and diagnostic irradiation in utero. *Lancet* **ii**, 447.

Stewart, A., Webb, J., and Hewitt, D. (1958). A survey of childhood malignancies. *Brit. med. J.* **i**, 1495–1508.

Taylor, F.E. and Webb, G.A.M. (1978). *Radiation exposure of the UK population.* National Radiological Protection Board Report NRPB–R77.

Tokunaga, M., Land, C.E., Yamamoto, T., Asano, M., Tokuoka, S., Ezaki, H., Nishimore, I., and Fujikura, T. (1984). Breast cancer among atomic bomb survivors. In *Radiation carcinogenesis: epidemiology and biological significance* (ed. J.D. Boice and J.F. Fraumeni), pp. 45–56. Raven Press, New York.

UNSCEAR (1977). *Sources and effects of ionizing radiation.* United Nations Scientific Committee on the Effects of Atomic Radiation. United Nations, New York.

Whittlemore, A. and McMillan, A. (1983). Lung cancer mortality among US uranium miners: a reappraisal. *J. Nat. Cancer Inst.* **70**, 489–99.

7 Infections and immune impairment

L.J. Kinlen

Infections

Infections have from the earliest times presented us with the most vivid and widespread model of disease causation. Inevitably, therefore, the notion that cancers might have a similar basis has been a recurring speculation. Nor is this excluded by the lack of evidence of contagion, since we have in leprosy a reminder that an infection may show little sign of contagion. Indeed so many oncogenic viruses have been demonstated in animals that it would be surprising if such a cause of cancer was not represented in man. This view dominated the direction of the tremendous research effort that followed the passing of the U.S. National Cancer Act of 1971. Only a few years ago it was difficult to point to more than a single cancer that was commonly regarded as viral in origin, a series of recent advances has extended the list beyond five.

In this brief review, I have included not only those cancers for which the evidence, both epidemiological and laboratory, of a specific viral cause is strong (such as primary liver cancer) but also those tumours that show similarities with certain infections, such as cervical cancer (with venereal infections) or Hodgkin's disease (with paralytic poliomyelitis) even though the evidence for their causation by any specific virus is far from convincing.

Cervical cancer

The high frequency of cervical cancer in prostitutes and the consistent relationship of the disease with multiple sexual partners have for long pointed to an origin in a venereal infection, though at first these observations were interpreted as indicating pathological sperm or smegma as the probable cause. Latterly, advances in virology have led to an overshadowing of the pathological sperm hypothesis, though without disproving it. Recently, however, additional evidence has emerged that the disease originates in a sexually transmitted infection and in particular, the observation that the partners of affected women, who have had only one sexual partner themselves, tend to have had several (Buckley *et al*. 1981).

But identification of the responsible infective agent continues to be elusive, bedevilled by the fact that the sexual behaviour that encourages one venereal infection inevitably does the same for others, so that strong but indirect relationships are produced. Suspect viruses include herpes simplex type 2 virus (HSV2) and the papilloma virus group, the former being the most favoured until recently. Women with cervical cancer have higher antibody levels to HSV2 antigen than controls (Rawls and Adam 1977; Aurelian *et al.* 1980) and HSV2-specific RNA has been detected in the nuclei of tumour cells (Eglin *et al.* 1981). On the other hand, raised antibody levels are not invariably found in the affected women and HSV2-specific DNA has not been identified in host nuclei (see p. 277).

A common cervical disorder that is receiving renewed attention is human papilloma virus (HPV) infection, which is also the cause of genital warts (condylomata acuminata). A greatly increased incidence of cervical dysplasia and neoplasia has been noted in women with cervical condylomata (Purola and Savia 1977; Meisel and Morin 1981) as well as malignant transformation in the genital warts themselves. Recently, papilloma virus DNA has been identified in cells from cervical cancers, both invasive and *in situ*.

The first epidemiological study aimed at distinguishing different viruses in the aetiology of the disease has only recently been carried out (Francheschi *et al.* 1983). Cervical smears were examined from 415 women with genital warts newly attending a clinic for sexually transmitted diseases, 135 with genital herpes, and 458 with trichomoniasis or gonorrhoea. A significantly greater proportion of the patients with genital warts showed probable early premalignant changes (dyskaryosis) in cervical smears than did the other patients, and indeed among those with genital herpes no relationship with dyskaryosis was apparent. Further elucidation of the relationship is impeded by our present inability to distinguish antibodies in genital HPV infection from those associated with common cutaneous warts, and uncertainty as to whether subclinical cervical lesions such as flat warts and koilocytotic atypia are specific for HPV infection.

In view of the recent evidence that HPV infection may be a cause of cervical cancer, it is interesting to note that it is almost 50 years since Rous and Beard (1935), as a result of their work on the related rabbit papilloma virus, suggested that condylomata might be precursors of cervical cancer.

Burkitt's lymphoma and nasopharyngeal cancer

The delineation by Burkitt (1958, 1962b) of an unusual lymphoma in children with a predilection for the jaw and the abdominal organs and which occurred in a broad belt across tropical Africa led to an enormous surge in research in viral oncology both in the laboratory and the field. This was due to the intriguing relationship shown by this tumour with rainfall and its absence at altitudes over 5000 feet, at first suggesting an origin in an arthropod-borne virus. One outcome was the identification in a culture of Burkitt's lymphoma cells of a new herpes-type virus, named after its discoverers the Epstein–Barr virus. This virus was later found to be the cause of infectious mononucleosis, but its relationship to Burkitt's lymphoma is more complex. All Burkitt's lymphoma patients in endemic areas have Epstein–Barr virus antibodies and at higher levels than controls, and a prospective study has shown that these higher levels predate the development of the lymphoma (de Thé *et al.* 1978). The geographic distribution of Burkitt's lymphoma, however, and also its relative rarity even in the endemic areas, contrast strikingly with the ubiquity of the virus. It is clear that other factors must be involved, and a strong possibility is the holoendemic malaria present in the same areas as Burkitt's lymphoma. The immunological effects of intense malarial infection may not only facilitate oncogenesis but perhaps also through varying attack rates, cause the space–time clustering sometimes observed in Burkitt's lymphoma (Pike *et al.* 1967; Williams *et al.* 1969) (see p. 276).

The existence of a high prevalence of Epstein–Barr virus antibodies in nasopharyngeal cancer was first reported in 1966 by Old and his colleagues and has since been repeatedly confirmed in many parts of the world, including China where the incidence of the disease is particularly high. In addition, the viral genome has been identified in epithelial tumour cells, but not in Epstein–Barr virus-infected lymphocytes present in the tumour tissue. The fact, however, that certain Epstein–Barr virus antibodies (to the capsid antigen) are reported to be raised in patients with carcinomas in other parts of the pharynx prompts caution in accepting as causal the abundant evidence of association with the Epstein–Barr virus (Henderson *et al.* 1977).

But even if Epstein–Barr virus is a cause of the tumour, this alone will not explain the high incidence of the disease in the Chinese. Genetic factors may be involved, as suggested by the HLA differences that have been reported between cases in Chinese patients and controls (Simons *et al.* 1974). HLA differences from controls were also noted among Tunisian and Malay patients, but these were not the same as in the Chinese (Betuel *et al.* 1975; Simons and Day 1977). In addition environmental factors may be important (p. 275).

Hepatocellular carcinoma

Only a few years ago many people hardly suspected hepatocellular carcinoma of having an infective origin, whereas now there is more convincing evidence of its causation by an identified virus than for any other human malignancy. The virus is the hepatitis B virus, and these insights have come from both laboratory and epidemiological work. Hepatocellular cancer has its highest incidence in Africa and Eastern Asia, where it is one of the commonest cancers and where also the prevalence of chronic hepatitis B virus carriers is higher than elsewhere. But, more importantly, there is a significant excess of chronic carriers (as indicated by the presence of hepatitis B virus surface antigen (HBs Ag) in serum) among hepatocellular carcinoma patients than among controls, both in high- and low-incidence areas for the disease (Szmuness 1978). The most arresting epidemiological findings, however, are those of Beasley and his colleagues (1981) who followed up 22 000 male civil servants in Taiwan whose HBs Ag status had been determined at entry to the study. All but one of 41 cases of hepatocellular carcinoma occurred in the 15 per cent of men who were HBs Ag-positive at entry, indicating a more than 200-fold increased risk of this cancer in hepatitis B virus carriers.

Detailed laboratory work also supports the relationship. DNA from the hepatitis B virus can be identified in tissue from primary liver cancer, integrated with cellular host DNA. The story does not stop there. Supporting evidence for this relationship has come from studies of closely related animal viruses. A colony of woodchucks in the Philadelphia zoo with a high mortality rate from primary liver cancer were found also to be infected with what is now named the woodchuck hepatitis virus (Summers *et al.* 1978). In addition, another related virus has been found in Chinese domestic ducks in which there is also a high incidence of liver cancer.

Some indication of the way by which hepatitis B virus infection occurs in high incidence areas for liver cancer was provided by the work of Larouze and his colleagues (1976). They found that whereas among the fathers of hepatocellular carcinoma patients there was no excess of carriers as compared with the control group, there was a significant excess of carriers among the mothers of cases, suggesting that transmission from mothers to newborn or infant children may be an important mode of infection in individuals who later develop hepatocellular carcinoma.

Given the encouraging reports from the first trials of a new hepatitis B vaccine, it is difficult to suppress enormous optimism about the future prevention of this cancer (see p. 273).

Hodgkin's disease

The earliest suspicions that Hodgkin's disease had an infective origin, predating those for cervical cancer, were raised by pathologists who were impressed by the histological resemblance to certain infective lesions of the more granulomatous forms of this malignancy. However, as no organism could be incriminated, the suspicions largely died. It remained for MacMahon (1957, 1966) to marshall the available epidemiological data relevant to the question. He pointed out the bimodal age-distribution of the disease and also data suggesting that the form commoner in young adults might have an infective basis. This possibility was encouraged by periodic reports of clusters of cases of Hodgkin's disease culminating in an extraordinary group of cases in Albany, New York State, in which Vianna and his colleagues (1972) reported that no less than 31 cases, centering on a high school, could be linked directly or through a contact without the disease. The study was largely uncontrolled, but by any reckoning it concerned a remarkable concentration of linked cases. Another study by the same workers (Vianna and Polan 1973; Vianna *et al.* 1974) of pupils and teachers in Long Island high schools found that cases tended to be concentrated in particular schools. It is possible than these differences were at least partly due to under-ascertainment of cases in certain schools, and a series of later studies has with few exceptions failed to confirm these findings or detect more contact among affected individuals than among controls (Smith *et al.* 1977; Grufferman *et al.* 1979; Paffenbarger *et al.* 1977; Zack *et al.* 1977).

Several prospective studies have found an approximately three fold increased risk of Hodgkin's disease among individuals with infectious mononucleosis (Rosdahl *et al.* 1974; Coleman *et al.* 1977; Munoz *et al.* 1978; Kvale *et al.* 1979), raising the possibility that the Epstein–Barr virus may cause this disease. However, although Epstein–Barr virus antibody levels are higher among affected patients than among controls, the proportion of those with detectable levels is similar in both groups. Moreover, the Epstein–Barr virus genome has not been recovered from the cells of Hodgkin's tissue, and some patients with this lymphoma do not have raised antibody levels.

In 1977 Gutensohn and Cole pointed out that paralytic poliomyelitis and Hodgkin's disease share several epidemiological features. Both are similar in their social-class gradient (commoner among the well-off) and in their relationship to small family size, and both show a preponderance of males at ages under five years. It was argued that these features would fit the model that Hodgkin's disease was a rare response to a common infective agent made more likely when exposure was deferred beyond early childhood. This model, which is similar to that proposed for infectious mononucleosis, has received support from more recent work. A study of 225 cases aged 15–39 years, and 450 controls, found that significantly more of the cases were first- or second-born children or came from single-child homes, and had few neighbourhood playmates, all factors that would tend to reduce exposure to an infective pool (Gutensohn and Cole 1981). The specific agent, however, remains to be identified.

Kaposi's sarcoma

The isolation of cytomegalovirus from a culture of cells from a Kaposi's sarcoma in 1972 led Giraldo and his colleagues (1975) to carry out a series of studies of antibody levels to cytomegalovirus, Epstein–Barr virus, and the herpes simplex viruses (HSVI and HSV2) in patients with this malignancy. In cases from Europe and the U.S.A. the antibody levels to cytomegalovirus were higher than in controls but not so in African cases, in which the prevalence of raised titres in both cases and controls was very high. More recently, it has been reported that examination of Kaposi sarcoma tissue using both DNA and RNA probes demonstrated integration of cytomegalovirus-related gene sequences into cellular tumour DNA (Boldogh *et al*. 1981) and this has since been confirmed using more specific molecular probes (Drew *et al*. 1982).

In 1981 an extraordinary outbreak of opportunistic infections and Kaposi's sarcoma began among American homosexuals (Centers for Disease Control 1981). These cases were associated with an immunodeficiency state, now termed the acquired immunodeficiency syndrome (AIDS). The syndrome is not confined to homosexuals, and cases have been reported among drug abusers, haemophiliacs, and people from Haiti as well as the female sexual partners of some of these groups. But the proportion of homosexuals with AIDS who develop Kaposi's sarcoma appears to be much higher than among other groups of AIDS patients. Initially cases were confined to the U.S., but cases have now been reported from other parts of the world, some of these in men who have had contact with homosexuals in the U.S. All this evidence, pointing to causation by a transmissible agent, has stimulated an immense amount of work aimed at identifying the causative agent. This may already have been successful for a retrovirus has been isolated from affected patients by both the Pasteur Institute (Vilmer *et al*. 1984) and the National Cancer Insitute, U.S. (Popovic *et al*. 1984; Galio *et al*. 1984). But even if AIDS is caused by human T-lymphotrophic retrovirus-III (HTLV-III), as the NCI group have named this virus, it does not necessarily follow that the same virus is responsible for Kaposi's sarcoma, since the association could be indirect or contributory by causing additional immunosupression thereby facilitating infection by another agent. In this connection the recent evidence that classical Kaposi's sarcoma in Africa is not associated with the HTLV-III virus appears to be of great relevance (Biggar *et al*. 1984).

This rapid progress promises well for further elucidation of the viral cause of Kaposi's sarcoma, but at present cytomegalovirus seems to be the strongest candidate.

Penis cancer

An excess of cervical cancer among the wives of men with penis cancer was reported by Martinez (1969) and later confirmed by other workers (Graham *et al.* 1979; Smith *et al.* 1980). This evidence of a common aetiological factor is strengthened by a striking correlation between mortality from these diseases in different parts of China (Li *et al.* 1982). But apart from the evidence of a sexually transmitted infection as a cause of cervical cancer, there exists rather more specific evidence for an infective origin of penis cancer. A review of penis cancers concluded that more than 10 per cent of cases showed cytological features suggestive of papilloma virus infection (Hanash *et al.* 1970). More recently, Boxer and Skinner (1977) were able to collect no less than 32 cases of penis cancer occuring in assocation with human papilloma virus infection of the penis.

Work currently in progress in high-incidence areas for this neoplasm may cast additional light on the possible role of the papilloma viruses in its aetiology.

Skin cancer

The earliest experimental evidence of a human tumour virus concerned a neoplasm of the skin, for it was in 1907 that Ciuffo and later Wile and Kingery (1919) transmitted warts from man to man by intradermal innoculation of cell-free filtrates. These neoplasms are of course benign in nature but nonetheless they serve to remind us that viruses may possibly be concerned in the aetiology of malignant skin tumours in man. But more suggestive is the fact that squamous cell cancer of the skin frequently occurs in individuals affected by epidermodysplasia verruciformis (EV), a rare disorder in which the papilloma viruses cause widespread skin lesions. Moreover, in EV patients the viral genome of HPV type 5 has been identified in the cells of complicating squamous carcinomas of the skin (Ostrow *et al.* 1982). It is not impossible therefore that squamous cell skin cancer in the general population may also have a viral aetiology, and in this connection the observation that ultraviolet light converts herpes viruses from an infectious to an oncogenic form is of interest (Matas *et al.* 1975).

Non-Hodgkin's lymphoma in immunodeficiency states

A marked increase in the incidence of non-Hodgkin's lymphomas in organ transplant recipients is now well estabished, and is described in a later section of this chapter. The extraordinarily short latent interval after transplantation shown by many of these lymphomas raised the possibility of a viral origin, so different was the pattern from that shown by cancers caused by chemical agents (Kinlen *et al.* 1979). This has now been confirmed and in all of the eight cases that were recently reported, the genome of the Epstein–Barr virus was identified in the nuclei of the tumour cells (Crawford *et al.* 1981; Hanto *et al.* 1981).

Another immunodeficiency state characterized by an increased incidence of non-Hodgkin's lymphoma is the very rare X-linked lymphoproliferative syndrome first described by Purtilo *et al.* in 1975. Subsequent work has shown that this familial disorder, which affects only males, involves an immunoregulatory defect in which B-cell proliferation in response to Epstein–Barr virus infection is uncontrolled, leading in some cases to lymphomas. Detailed laboratory studies have also produced evidence that lymphomas in two other immunodeficiency states are also caused by the Epstein–Barr virus, namely ataxia telangectasia and severe combined immunodeficiency (Reece *et al.* 1981; Saemundsen *et al.* 1982).

Adult T-cell lymphoma–leukaemia

In 1980 Gallo and his colleagues reported the isolation of a new retrovirus from cultured cells taken from a patient with a particularly aggressive cutaneous T-cell lymphoma (Polesz *et al.* 1980). This virus, which had two core proteins that were serologically distinct from all previously described viruses, bore certain resemblances to the bovine leukosis virus. Later the same group isolated the virus from other patients with lymphomas or leukaemias involving T-cells and also demonstrated that antibodies to the two unique core proteins were detectable in their sera. More recently, Catovsky and his colleagues (1982) were able to find seven patients in Britain, all born in the Caribbean region, who had a distinctive T-cell lymphoma or leukaemia. In these patients also there was a high titre of antibodies to a core protein of the recently described retrovirus, the human T-cell leukaemia–lymphoma virus (HTLV I).

These discoveries have acted as a valuable key in elucidating further the remarkable clustering of cases of T-cell leukaemia in Japan. Uchiyama, Takatsuki, and their colleagues (1977) reported that a high proportion of patients with adult T-cell leukaemia were born or grew up on the west coast of Kyushu. Sera from affected patients were found to show raised antibody levels to the Gallo virus HTLV I.

It is clear that not all T-cell leukaemias can be linked to the new virus, but mainly a subtype that is characterized clinically by an unusual prevalence of hypercalcaemia and cutaneous involvement, a type that appears to be more common in Caribbean people and the Japanese, where also the prevalence of raised serum levels in the general population is much higher than elsewhere. Intensive research now in progress in several countries is likely to result in rapid progress in our understanding of this fascinating disorder.

Immune impairment

Some consideration of immune factors in this review would be justified by the crucial importance of the immune system in relation to infections. But the immune system has other claims for attention in carcinogenesis. Thomas (1959) and Burnet (1965) postulated a role which was explicitly concerned with the elimination of aberrant cells that otherwise would form the starting point of cancer. Their hypothesis of immunosurveillance implied that any significant degree of immunosuppression would tend to increase the incidence of cancer. Fifteen years ago, there was much laboratory support for this view, but among human data there was only the strong hint that cancer was unusually common in individuals with certain rare genetically determined immunodeficiency disorders. But in addition there was speculation that weakening of the immune system with advancing age might also explain the huge increase in the incidence of cancer that ageing brings. Indeed, the possibility was even discussed of stimulating immunosurveillance in order to treat and prevent cancer. Since those days much has been learnt about immune factors and human cancer, mainly from studies of organ-transplant patients, but also of other patients with immunological impairment. Moreover, other evidence strongly suggests that the great increase in malignancy with advancing age reflects the effect not of ageing *per se* (and perhaps any effects this may have on the immune system), but rather the effects of increasing durations of exposure to carcinogens.

Major epithelial cancers

It was the introduction of organ transplantation that provided the first major opportunity for studying the effects of immunosuppression on cancer in man. Initially, the variety of case reports of cancers in transplant patients suggested to some people a confirmation of the immunosurveillance concept. Since then, however, formal studies of the subject have shown that cancers of all types are *not* increased in incidence in states of immune impairment, and neither of the two large prospective studies of renal transplant patients has so far found an excess of any of the commonest types of cancer in Western populations, such as cancers of the lung, breast, and gastrointestinal tract (Hoover and Fraumeni 1973; Kinlen *et al.* 1979).

As with the early reports about transplant recipients, it was also sometimes claimed that patients with chronic renal failure have an increased incidence of cancer of all types. This again was based mainly on uncontrolled observations, and it is notable that the exception concerned a study that found an apparent excess of cases of cancer but no increased mortality from cancer. Furthermore, the observed numbers of cancers were inflated by inclusion of cases diagnosed before entry to the study and perhaps also by cases that were benign or asymptomatic tumours and therefore more likely to be detected in a specialist medical centre (Matas *et al.* 1975). A study that covered both cancer mortality and incidence found no suggestion that cancer of all types was increased (Kinlen *et al.* 1980).

Lymphomas

The malignancy that figures most prominently in studies of individuals with immune impairment is non-Hodgkin's lymphoma. Renal transplant patients have been most studied in this respect, and an almost 50-fold increase in incidence was found in a collaborative U.K.–Australasian study (Kinlen *et al.* 1979, 1982). A smaller excess (28-fold) was found in a study of the data in the International Transplant Registry of the American College of Surgeons (Hoover and Fraumeni 1981), but here it may be relevant that many participating centres stopped contributing data at a relatively early stage and this may have resulted in a lower estimate of risk than would otherwise have been obtained.

An extraordinary feature of the lymphomas in transplant patients is their predilection for the central nervous system. In more than a third of these cases the brain is involved, often exclusively, whereas among lymphomas in the general population the corresponding proportion is less than 2 per cent. Some impression of the contrast in incidence is given by the fact that in the third National Cancer Survey in the U.S., only 15 cases were recorded of cerebral non-Hodgkin's lymphoma over three years in a population of 21 million (Cutler and Young 1975), whereas a larger number were recorded in 4000 transplant patients followed up for an average of less than four years (Kinlen *et al.* 1982). The most persuasive hypothesis to explain the cerebral localization of these tumours has been put forward by Kay (1983), who pointed out that whereas the main effects of immunosuppressive drugs such as azathioprine are felt outside the nervous system (since they do not cross the blood–brain barrier), the consequent stimulus to B-cell regeneration might well cross this barrier. If so, the stimulus would have its effect on B-cells in the brain unchecked by the drugs that continued to limit regeneration outside the nervous system.

All the lymphomas in renal transplant recipients that have been investigated have been of B-cell type and of host origin (Penn 1979), although a single case of lymphoma of donor origin has been recorded in a bone-marrow transplant (Gossett *et al.* 1979). It is of interest that most of the lymphomas that occur in an experimental mice model of graft-versus-host disease have also been of host origin (Gleichmann *et al.* 1975).

No relationship has been found between the risk of lymphoma in renal transplant recipients and the underlying renal disease. However, among cardiac transplant recipients, the risk was much higher when the underlying disorder was idiopathic cardiomyopathy than when it was coronary artery disease, and perhaps the defect in immune regulation that has been reported in the former is relevant here (Anderson *et al.* 1978).

The possible role of the antigenic stimulation by the graft in the development of these lymphomas is a controversial question. No significant difference was detected in the risk of lymphomas in multiple as compared with single transplant recipients in one study (Kinlen *et al.* 1979), but another study has recently found a significant relationship (Hoover and Fraumeni 1984). But several pieces of evidence do suggest that the risk of these lymphomas is influenced by the intensity of immunosuppressive therapy. The highest incidences have been recorded in cardiac transplant recipients (Anderson *et al.* 1978) and in renal transplant recipients treated with both cyclosporin A and other immunosuppressive drugs (Calne *et al.* 1979). Furthermore, a higher incidence was found in association with antilymphocytic globulin, and in patients who received relatively high doses of azathioprine, than in other transplant recipients, though neither of these differences was statistically significant (Kinlen *et al.* 1979). It also seems likely that the decline in the incidence of lymphomas in transplant patients first noted by Hoover, but evident in both major prospective studies, is related in some way to management and most probably to a reduction in the intensity of immunosuppression.

A striking feature of the excess of lymphomas in transplant patients is that it is evident even within six months of transplantation. This abrupt increase in incidence suggested the possibility of viral oncogenesis since, it was tentatively proposed, malignant transformation might occur quickly if a virus was already present in the cell (Kinlen *et al.* 1979). This idea has recently found support in laboratory studies which have shown among other relevant findings that the cells of these lymphomas are positive for Epstein–Barr virus nuclear antigen (Hanto *et al.* 1981; Crawford *et al.* 1981).

Other groups of individuals with immunological impairment also show evidence of an excess of non-Hodgkin's lymphoma. Non-transplant patients treated with azathioprine showed an approximately 10-fold excess of this neoplasm (Kinlen *et al.* 1982). But of the six cases of lymphoma observed, three occurred in patients with rheumatoid arthritis, a disorder that has sometimes been linked with lymphomas in the absence of immunosuppressive therapy. These suggestions have mainly come from case reports, but a threefold excess of non-Hodgkin's lymphoma was reported from a large study of over 30 000 such patients in Finland, though details of treatment were not provided (Isomaki *et al.* 1978). It is possible, therefore, that part of the excess of lymphomas after immunosuppressive therapy in non-transplant patients is due to an increased incidence of these tumours associated with the underlying disorders for which this therapy was prescribed. Some support for this possibility comes from the observation of an excess of lymphomas among patients with Sjogren's disease, irrespective of treatment, but which was more marked after immunosuppressive treatment (100-fold) than in other affected patients (36-fold) (Kassan *et al.* 1978).

There is evidence also that patients with chronic renal failure (who show impaired cell-mediated immunity) also have an increased incidence of non-Hodgkin's lymphoma (Kinlen *et al.* 1980; Slifkin *et al.* 1977). A group of mainly hereditary disorders in which the immunological impairment is more severe than in rheumatoid arthritis, Sjogren's disease or chronic renal failure, includes such rare disorders as agammaglobulinaemia and the Wiscott–Aldrich syndrome. A registry for cases of cancer in such patients is maintained at the University of Minnesota, and it is striking that no less than 49 per cent of all the neoplasms recorded have been of non-Hodgkin's lymphoma (Filipovich *et al.* 1980). This is a higher proportion than in any age group in any cancer registry and strongly suggests a real increase in incidence.

Skin cancer

Skin cancer figures prominently among the early series of cancers recorded in transplant recipients, and an excess was later demonstrated in the U.K.–Australasian prospective study – due to an over 20-fold increase in the incidence of squamous cell skin cancer (Kinlen *et al.* 1979). There also appears to be an increased incidence of melanoma, of about 8-fold in the U.K.–Australasian study, and 2.5-fold in the N.C.I. study (Hoover 1977). Most of the melanomas developed in precursor naevi (Greene *et al.* 1981). Basal cell tumours (rodent ulcers) showed no increase in the first reported analysis of the former study, but more recently an excess has appeared (11 observed; 1.85 expected). Further observations on transplant recipients should clarify whether this excess of rodent ulcers is real or simply due to the combined effects of chance, better and earlier diagnosis of skin lesions in transplant patients, and under-registration of this tumour in cancer registers (from which the expected numbers in these studies are derived).

There have been few observations on the incidence of skin cancer among individuals with other types of immune impairment. An increased incidence, however, was found in patients without transplants treated with immunosuppressive drugs, due as in the transplant patients to an excess of squamous cell cancer (3 observed; 0.1 expected) Kinlen *et al.* 1980).

In view of the above observations in man about squamous cell cancer of the skin in states of immunodeficiency, it is of great interest to see the work which shows the extraordinarily antigenic nature of the ultraviolet light-induced skin tumours in mice, rejected even when transplanted within syngeneic hosts (Kripke 1974). It is possible that squamous cell skin cancers in man are similar and that protection depends to an important extent on an efficient immune system.

Kaposi's sarcoma and other soft tissue sarcomas

An excess of soft tissue sarcomas was noted in both the major prospective studies, but for Kaposi's sarcoma the evidence is particularly strong. Although this neoplasm is represented by only a single case in each of the above-mentioned studies (compared with an expected figure of much less than 0.1), Penn (1982) has collected details of no less than 47 cases of this malignancy in transplant patients, a frequency which for such a rare tumour must indicate a greatly increased incidence.

Observations on these tumours in other states of immune impairment are restricted to non-transplant patients treated with immunosuppressive drugs who showed an excess of mesenchymal tumours (4 observed; $<$ 0.2 expected) (Kinlen *et al.* 1979). None of these cases was a Kaposi's sarcoma, but at least 18 cases of this tumour have been reported in the literature in patients without transplants treated with steroids and other immuno-suppressive drugs (Gange and Jones 1978; Klepp *et al.* 1978; Ilie *et al.* 1981). In view of the extreme rarity of Kaposi's sarcoma in most Western countries, these case reports strongly suggest a greatly increased incidence in association with immunosuppression. This conclusion is supported by the fact that more than 10 per cent of the 53 cases of Kaposi's sarcoma recorded in Norway over a 5-year period had previously received such treatment (Klepp *et al.* 1978).

Other cancers

Both major prospective studies of transplant recipients have found an increased risk of primary liver cancer amounting to 38-fold in one (Kinlen *et al.* 1982) and 20-fold in the other (Hoover and Fraumeni 1984). There have been few observations in other states of immune impairment, although one case was recorded in the study of non-transplant patients treated with immunosuppressive drugs, compared to an expected of less than 0.1. An excess of thyroid cancer was recorded in the U.S.-based study

(Hoover 1977) but not in the other prospective study, and it is possible that at least part of this excess was due to the more complete ascertainment of these often asymptomatic tumours in closely supervised transplant recipients than in the general population.

Both prospective studies of transplant patients have recorded many cases of cervical cancer, but it has not proved possible to evaluate the incidence. This is due to the fact that most of the cases were in the in-situ stage and therefore asymptomatic, so that inevitably their prevalence must at least partly reflect the frequency of performance of cervical smears.

Conclusion

It may be noted that most of the malignancies discussed in the first part of the chapter devoted to infections appear again in the section on cancer after immune impairment. This may not be a coincidence. Indeed, experimental work has indicated that immunosurveillance operates primarily in relation to virus-caused tumours. If we put to one side those virus-linked cancers such as nasopharyngeal cancer, Burkitt's lymphoma, and T-cell lymphoma–leukaemia which have a very restricted distribution, strongly suggesting the operation of additional factors, the degree of correspondence between the remainder of such tumours and those attributable to immunosuppression is striking. And, if we look in the opposite direction for virus-linked neoplasms among those that figure in the section on immunosuppression, only for Hodgkin's disease is there strong evidence against an increase in incidence.

Virus-linked cancers in man include one of the commonest neoplasms in the world, primary liver cancer. For this neoplasm a specific virus has been identified but for several other such tumours, despite circumstantial evidence for an infective and probably viral origin, no specific viruses have been incriminated. But there are grounds for hoping that the next decade will see the identification of the viral causes of Kaposi's sarcoma, cervical cancer – and perhaps also Hodgkin's disease. Much of this evidence is likely to come from laboratory work, and here it is worth bearing in mind that, despite the impressive support for causation that comes from sophisticated techniques such as molecular hybridization, all this still falls short of final proof. For it is conceivable that certain cancers may create such ideal cellular conditions that the most intimate links between certain viruses and tumours are promoted, thereby encouraging the erroneous conclusion that the virus is causal. The ultimate test is not whether there is integration of viral and host DNA but whether intervention directed at the infection will reduce the incidence of the tumour. Already plans are afoot to see if vaccination against hepatitis B virus will reduce the high incidence of primary liver cancer in parts of Africa.

References

Anderson, J.L., Bieber, C.P., Fowles, R.E., and Stinson, E.B. (1978). *Lancet* **ii**, 1174–7.

Aurelian, L., Jariwalla, R.J., Donnenberg, A.D., and Sheridan, J.F. (1980). UBL. *The role of viruses in human cancer* (ed. Giraldo and Beth), p. 75. Elsevier North-Holland Inc.

Beasley, R.P., Whang, L-Y., Lin, C-C., and Chien, C-S. (1981). *Lancet* **ii**, 1129–33.

Betuel, H., Cammoun, M., Columbani, J., *et al.* (1975). *Int. J. Cancer* **16**. 249–54.

Biggar, R.J., Melbye, M., Kestens, L., *et al.* (1984). *New Engl. J. Med.* **311**, 1051–2.

Boldogh, I., Beth, E., Huang, E-S., *et al.* (1981). *Int. J. Cancer* **28**, 469–74.

Boxer, R.J. and Skinner, D.G. (1977). *Urology* **9**, 72–7.

Buckley, J.D., Doll, R., Harris, R.W.C., and Vessey, M.P. (1981). *Lancet* **ii**, 1010–5.

Burkitt, D.P. (1958). *Brit. J. Surg.* **46**, 218–23.

Burkitt, D.P. (1962a). *Brit. J. Cancer* **16**, 279–386.

Burkitt, D.P. (1962b). *Brit. med. J.* **ii**, 1019–23.

Burnet, F.M. (1965). *Brit. med. J.* (i) 338–42.

Calne, R.F., Rolles, K., White, D.J.G., Thiru, S., Evans, D.B., *et al.* (1979). *Lancet* **ii**, 1033–6.

Catovsky, D., Greaves, M.F., Rose, M., *et al.* (1982). *Lancet* **i**, 639–43.

Centers for Disease Control (1981). *Morbidity and mortality weekly report*, Vol. 30, No. 25, pp. 305–8; Vol. 30, No. 33, pp. 409–10.

Ciuffo, G. (1907). *Giorn. Ital. Malat. veneree* **42**, 12–7.

Coleman, C.K., Brown, T.M. Jr, Herbert, J.T., *et al.* (1977). *Amer. J. Epidemiol.* **105**, 30–6.

Crawford, D.H., Edwards, J.M.B., Sweny, P., *et al.* (1981). *Int. J. Cancer* **28**, 705–9.

Cutler, S.J. and Young, J.L. (1975). *Nat. Cancer Inst. Mon.* **41**, 1–454.

de The, G., Geser, A., Day, N.E., *et al.* (1978). *Nature (Lond.)* **274**, 756–61.

Doll, R. and Kinlen, L. (1970). *Brit. med. J.* **4**, 134–6.

Drew, W.L., Conant, M.A., Miner, R.C., *et al.* (1982), *Lancet* **ii**, 125–7.

Eglin, R.P., Gharp, F., Maclean, A.B., *et al.* (1981). *Cancer Res.* **41**, 3597–603.

Filipovich, A.H., Spector, B.D., and Kersey, J. (1980). *J. prevent. Med.* **9**, 252–9.

Francheschi, S., Doll, R., Gallwey, J., *et al.* (1983). *Brit. J. Cancer* **48**, 621–8.

Gallo, R.C., Salahuddin, S.Z., Popovic, M., Shearer, G.M., *et al.* (1984). *Science (N.Y.)* **224**, 500–3.

Gange, R.W. and Jones, E.W. (1978). *Clin. exp. Dermatol.* **3**, 135–46.

Giraldo, G., Beth, E., Kourilsky, F.M., *et al.* (1975). Int. *J. Cancer* **15**, 839–48.

Gleichmann, E., Gleichmann, H., Schwartz, R.S. *et al.* (1975). *J. nat. Cancer Inst.* **54**, 107–16.

Gossett, T.C., Gale, R.P., Fleischman, H., *et al.* (1979). *New Engl J. Med.* **300**, 904–7.

Graham, S., Priore, R., Graham, M., *et al.* (1979). *Cancer* **44**, 1870–4.

Greene, M.H., Young, T.I., and Clark, W.H. Jr (1981). *Lancet* **i**, 1196–9.

Grufferman, S., Cole, P., and Leviton, T.R. (1979). *New Engl. J. Med.* **300**, 1006–11.

Gutensohn, N. and Cole, P. (1977). *Int. J. Cancer* **19**, 595–694.

Gutensohn, N. and Cole, P. (1981). *New Engl. J. Med.* **304**, 135–40.

Hanash, K.A., Furlow, W.L., Utz, D.C., *et al.* (1970). *J. Urol.* **104**, 291–7.
Hanto, D.W., Glauco, F., Purtilo, D.T., *et al.* (1981). *Cancer Res* **41**, 4253–61.
Henderson, B.E., Louie, E.W., Jing, J.S., *et al.* (1977). *J. nat. Cancer Inst.* **59**, 1393–5.
Hoover, R. (1977). In *Origins of human cancer* (ed. H.H. Hiatt, J.D. Watson, and J.A. Winsten), pp. 369–79. Cold Spring Harbor Laboratory, New York.
Hoover, R. and Fraumeni, J.F. Jr. (1973). *Lancet* **ii**, 55–7.
Hoover, R.N. and Fraumeni, J.F. (1985) (in press).
Ilie, B., Brenner, S., Lipitz, R., and Krakowski, A. (1981). *Dermatologica* **163**, 455–9.
Isomaki, H.A., Holulinen, T., and Joutsenlahti, U. (1978). *J. chron. Dis.* **31**, 691–6.
Kassan, S.S., Thomas, T.I., Moutsopoulos, H.M., *et al.* (1978). *Ann. Int. Med.* **89**, 888–92.
Kay, H.E. (1983). *New Engl. J. Med.* **308**, 1099–1100.
Kinlen, L.J., Sheil, A.G.R., Peto, J., and Doll, R. (1979). *Brit. Med. J.* **ii**, 1461–6.
Kinlen, L.J., Eastwood, J. B., Kerr, D.N.S., *et al.* (1980). *Brit. med. J.* **280**, 1401–3.
Klepp, O., Dahl, O., and Stenwig, J.T. (1978). *Cancer* **42**, 2626–30.
Kripke, M.L. (1974). *J. nat. Cancer Inst.* **53**, 1333–6.
Kvale, G., Hoiby, E.A., and Pedersen, E. (1979). *Int. J. Cancer* **23**, 593–7.
Larouze, B., London, W.T., Saimot, G., Werner, B.G., Lustbader, E.D., *et al.* (1976). *Lancet* **ii**, 534–8.
Li, J-Y., Li, F.P., Blot, W.J., *et al.* (1982). *J. nat. Cancer Inst.* **69**, 1063–5.
MacMahon, B. (1957). *Cancer* **10**, 1045–54.
MacMahon, B. (1966). *Cancer Res.* **26**, 1189–200.
Martinez, I. (1969). *Cancer* **24**, 777–80.
Matas, A.J., Simmons, R.L., and Najarian, J.S. (1975). Chronic antigenic stimulations, herpes virus infection, and cancer in transplant recipients. *Lancet* **i**, 1277–9.
Meisels, A. and Morin, C. (1981). *Gynecol. Oncol.* **12**, S111–23.
Munoz, N., Davidson, R.J.L., Witthoff, B., *et al.* (1978). *Int. J. Cancer* **22**, 10–13.
Old, L.J., Boyse, E.A., Oettgen, H.F., *et al.* (1966). *Proc. nat. Acad. Sci. (U.S.A.)* **56**, 1699–704.
Ostrow, R.S., Bender, M., Nimura, M., *et al.* (1982). *Proc. nat. Acad. Sci. (U.S.A.)* **79**, 1634–8.
Paffenbarger, R.S., Jr, Wing, A.L., and Hyde, R.T. (1977). *J. nat. Cancer. Inst.* **58**, 1489–91.
Penn, I. (1979). *Transplantation* **27**, 214.
Penn, I. (1982). *Curr. Prob Cancer* **6**, No. 10.
Pike, M.C., Williams, E.H., and Wright, B. (1967). *Brit. med. J.* **ii**, 395–9.
Poiesz, B.J., Ruscetti, F.W., Gazdar, A.F., *et al.* (1980). *Proc. nat. Acad. Sci. (U.S.A.)* **77**, 7415–9.
Purola, E. and Savia, E. (1977). *Acta Cytol.* **21**, 26–31.
Purtilo, D.T., Cassel, C., Yang, J.P.S., *et al.* (1975). *Lancet* **i**, 935–41.
Rawls, W.E. and Adam, E. (1977). In *Origins of human cancer* (ed. H.H. Hiatt, J.D. Watson, and J.A. Winsten) p. 1133. Cold Spring Harbor Laboratory, New York.
Reece, E.R., Gartner, J.G., Seemayer, T.A., *et al.* (1981). *Cancer Res.* **41**, 4243–7.
Rosdahl, N., Larsen, S.O., and Clemmesen, J. (1974). *Brit. med. J.* **ii**, 253–6.
Rous, P. and Beard, J.W. (1935). *J. exp. Med.* **62**, 523–48.

Saemundsen, A.K., Purtilo, D.T., Sakamoto, K., *et al.* (1981). *Cancer Res.* **41**, 4237–42.
Simons, J.J. and Day, N.E. (1977). *Nat. Cancer Inst. Mon.* **47**, 143–6.
Simons, M.J., Wee, G.B., and Day, W.E. (1974). *Int. J. Cancer* **13**, 122–34.
Slifkin, R.F., Goldberg, J., Neff, M.S., Baez, A., Mattoo, N., and Gapta, S. (1977). *Trans. Amer. Soc. artif. Int. Org.* **23**, 34–9.
Smith, P.G., Pike, M.C., Kinlen, L.J., *et al.* (1977). *Lancet* **ii**, 59–62.
Smith, P.G., Kinlen, L.J. White, G.C., Adelstein, A.M., and Fox, A.J. (1980). *Brit. J. Cancer* **41**, 422–8.
Summers, J., Smolec, J.M., and Snyder, R.A. (1978). *Proc. nat. Acad. Sci. (U.S.A.)* **75**, 4533–7.
Szmuness, W. (1978). *Prog. med. Virol.* **24**, 40–69.
Thomas, L. (1959). In *Cellular and humoral aspects of the hypersensitive states* (ed. H.S. Larence), pp. 529–32.
Vianna, N.J. and Polan, A.K. (1973). *New Engl. J. Med.* **289**, 499–502.
Vianna, N.J., Greenwald, P., Brady, J., *et al.* (1972). *Ann. intern. Med.* **77**, 169–80.
Vianna, N.J., Polan, A.K., Keogh, M.D., and Greenwald, P. (1974). *Lancet* **ii**, 131–3.
Vilmer, E., Barre-Sinoussi, F., Rouzioux C., *et al.* (1984). *Lancet* **i**, 753–7.
Wile, U.J. and Kingery, L.B. (1919). *J. Amer. med. Ass.* **73**, 970–3.
Williams, E.H., Spit, P., and Pike, M.C. (1969). *Brit. J. Cancer* **23**, 235–46.
Zack, M.M. Jr, Heath, C.W. Jr, Andrews, M.D., *et al.* (1977). *J. nat. Cancer Inst.* **59**, 1343–9.

8 Exogenous hormones

Martin Vessey

Introduction

During the last two decades, there has been great interest in the effects of administered hormones on the risk of cancer. Most attention has been focused on synthetic female sex hormones given (1) during pregnancy to try to prevent miscarriage and late pregnancy toxaemia, (2) around the time of the menopause and thereafter to try to relieve the 'menopausal syndrome' and to prevent the development of osteoporosis, and (3) during the childbearing years to prevent pregnancy. In this chapter, I intend to concentrate on these three problems, dealing briefly with the first two (which are of lesser importance) and in more detail with the third (which is of great importance). At the outset, it should be stressed that both animal experimental work (see International Agency for Research on Cancer 1979) and epidemiological, clinical, and laboratory research on the effects of endogenous hormones in the human (see Chapter 9 by Pike in this volume) have made it clear that some influence of administered female sex hormones on the risk of certain cancers would be expected; as we shall see, this has turned out to be the case.

Administration of hormones during pregnancy

Stilboestrol, a non-steroidal oestrogen, was first synthesized about 45 years ago. In the 1940s, Smith and Smith promoted use of this drug during pregnancy for the treatment of habitual abortion and threatened abortion (Smith 1948). It was later claimed that stilboestrol treatment also had a beneficial effect on other pregnancy complications (Smith and Smith 1949) and, as a result, the drug was widely used during pregnancy in the U.S. The dosages recommended were large, up to 15 g of the drug being given between the 7th and 35th weeks of pregnancy.

In the early 1950s, a large randomized controlled trial of stilboestrol therapy was conducted at the University of Chicago, including 840 women who received stilboestrol and 806 who received placebo (Dieckmann *et al.* 1953). The results showed no beneficial effect of stilboestrol on pregnancy outcome – indeed, a recent reanalysis of the data has indicated that treatment with stilboestrol actually increased the risk of spontaneous abortion, neonatal death, and premature birth (Brackbill and Berendes 1978). As a consequence of this trial and one or two others with similar results (e.g. Ferguson 1953; Swyer and Law 1954), there was a general reduction in the use of stilboestrol during pregnancy, but even as late as 1970 some obstetricians were still prescribing the drug (or closely related substances such as dienoestrol). No accurate data are available concerning how many women in the U.S. were given stilboestrol during pregnancy, but the total has been estimated as between two and three million. There is evidence that large numbers also received the drug in a number of other countries (e.g. Holland, see Stolk *et al.* 1982), but in the U.K. it seems that fewer than 10 000 women were involved (Kinlen *et al.* 1974).

In 1971, it became apparent that girls born to mothers who had taken stilboestrol during pregnancy were at an increased risk of clear-cell adenocarcinoma of the vagina and cervix. The first report to this effect was of a case-control study including 8 young women with clear-cell adenocarcinoma of the vagina and 32 matched controls (Herbst *et al.* 1971). Seven of the 8 mothers of the girls with cancer had taken stilboestrol in pregnancy in comparison with none of the mothers of the controls. Supporting evidence appeared subsequently from many additional sources. Of particular importance has been the special registry established by Herbst and his colleagues which has shown the absolute risk of clear-cell cancer to be much smaller than had been feared – the best current estimate indicates a cumulative risk of between 1.4 and 14 per 10 000 exposed up to the age of 24 years (Herbst 1981). The tumours probably arise in areas of vaginal or cervical adenosis which are more common and much more extensive in young women exposed to stilboestrol *in utero* than in other women (Scully and Welch 1981). These areas of adenosis gradually become replaced with metaplastic squamous epithelium during the teens and twenties, so there is reason to hope that the risk of clear-cell cancer will diminish or even disappear with increasing age (Noller *et al.* 1983). Anxieties about an increased risk of *squamous* cancer of the vagina or cervix have not yet proved justified, nor is there evidence that exposed girls suffer a greater chance than usual of developing any other kind of cancer. Fortunately, as might be expected from drug usage data, stilboestrol-associated clear-cell cancers of the vagina or cervix in young British women are very few, but at least three have been reported (Monaghan and Sirisena 1978; Dewhurst *et al.* 1980; Davis *et al.* 1981).

While girls exposed *in utero* to stilboestrol have been the subject of many studies, far less attention has been paid to boys. There is, however, no doubt that certain minor structural abnormalities of the genital tract (especially epididymal cysts and cryptorchidism) are appreciably more common in stilboestrol-exposed males than in unexposed males. Case-control studies done in Los Angeles have also strongly suggested that exposed males may be at an increased risk of testicular tumours (Henderson *et al.* 1979; Depue *et al.* 1983), but this cannot yet be regarded as established (Gill 1981).

It is, of course, also possible that exposure to stilboestrol in pregnancy, especially in the vast doses used in the Smith regimen, might involve a cancer hazard for the mother herself. Published work on this topic is very limited, but if there is an increased risk of breast or reproductive cancer in the exposed mothers, the available data suggest that it is unlikely to be large (Hubby *et al.* 1981; Brian *et al.* 1980; Beral and Colwell 1980; Vessey *et al.* 1983a)

Comment

Although the stilboestrol story is now largely over in that use of the drug during pregnancy ceased more than 10 years ago, the consequences of this medical mistake are still becoming apparent and, in the U.S. at least, vast sums of money are being spent on surveillance of exposed subjects, especially female offspring. Litigation too is still in full swing, a key issue being whether or not it was reasonable to use stilboestrol in the way in which it was used given the state of knowledge at the time.

The question arises as to whether adenosis and adenocarcinoma of the vagina and cervix might follow exposure *in utero* to progestogens or, more importantly, to oral contraceptives. Certainly there are substantial numbers of young people around who were conceived while their mothers were taking 'the pill' (often as a result of inconsistent tablet taking) and who were exposed to contraceptive steroids for weeks, or even months, before the pregnancy was recognized. The available data on this topic are extremely sparse, but so far as they go, they seem to be reassuring (Scully and Welch 1981). Further work on this problem is, in my view, a research priority since this type of exposure to administered hormones *in utero* remains common.

Administration of hormones around the time of the menopause

Oestrogens have long been given around the time of the menopause and beyond (1) to try to relieve the cluster of symptoms (notably hot flushing, sweating, and dyspareunia) often loosely termed 'the menopausal syndrome', (2) to try to prevent the occurrence of bony fractures by slowing down the development of postmenopausal osteoporosis, and (3) to try to enable women to remain 'feminine' into old age by the maintenance of skin elasticity, breast firmness, strong hair growth, libido, and so on (Vessey and Bungay 1982). The practice has been far more popular in the U.S.

(especially along the West Coast) and in certain European continental countries than in the U.K. In the U.S., until recently the 'replacement therapy' market was entirely dominated by one drug – Premarin (conjugated equine oestrogens) – and most of the available data about the cancer risks associated with administration of oestrogens to menopausal women relate to this product.

Endometrial cancer

Evidence that 'oestrogen replacement therapy' is an important cause of endometrial cancer has been derived from two main sources – studies of trends in endometrial cancer incidence in the U.S. and case-control studies. These will be considered briefly in turn.

During the 30 years up to 1970, the incidence of endometrial cancer in the U.S. remained fairly stable. Thereafter, however, a marked rise was noted by Weiss *et al.* (1976) for the period 1969–73 in data from a number of cancer registries. The increase in incidence exceeded 10 per cent per year in some areas and was most marked among women aged 45–74 years. Weiss and his colleagues suggested that the increase might be related to the use of oestrogens (notably Premarin) as 'replacement therapy' as sales of such drugs had risen fourfold during the interval 1963–73.

Subsequently, Walker and Jick (1979) confirmed the rising incidence of endometrial cancer in the U.S. over the period 1970–75 by study of a national 1 per cent sample of hospital discharges. These authors have also shown that a fall in the number of prescriptions for Premarin from 1976 onwards was followed closely by a fall in the incidence of endometrial cancer (Jick *et al.* 1980a). A detailed analysis of data from the Connecticut Tumor Registry has recently produced closely similar results (Marrett *et al.* 1982).

Since January 1975, the results of a large number of case-control studies of the relationship between oestrogen use and endometrial cancer have been published. Some details about 18 of these investigations (the list is probably not exhaustive) are given in Table 1. Only one study, that of Salmi (1979) has given a negative result. Salmi's work, however, was largely concerned with women who had used oestrogens only in the past and for short periods of time and her findings do not weigh heavily against the rest.

In most studies in which the relevant data were available, the risk was found to rise with increasing duration of oestrogen use and with increasing oestrogen dose (see Vessey and Bungay 1982). These effects explain much of the variation in the relative risks shown in Table 1 which (for the sake of simplicity) deals only with 'ever use' of oestrogens. Some of the low relative risks in Table 1 are, however, attributable to an unsatisfactory

Table 1. Case-control studies of oestrogen therapy and endometrial cancer

Authors	Years cases diag-nosed	No. of cases	Relative risk associated with 'ever-use' of oestrogens
Smith *et al.* (1975); Seattle	1960–72	317	7.5
Ziel & Finkle (1975); Los Angeles	1970–74	94	7.6
Mack *et al.* (1976); Los Angeles	1971–75	63	8.0
McDonald *et al.* (1977); Rochester	1945–74	145	2.3 (use for 6 months or more)
Gray *et al.* (1977); Louisville	1947–76	205	2.6
Wigle *et al.* (1978); Alberta (Canada)	1971–73	202	2.2
Horwitz & Feinstein (1978); Hew Haven	974–76	268	(i) 12.0 (ii) 1.7
Antunes *et al.* (1979); Baltimore	1973–77	451	(i) 6.0 (ii) 2.1
Jick *et al.* (1979); Seattle	1975–77	67	11.2
Weiss *et al.* (1979); King County	1975–76	322	8.7 (current use)
Salmi (1979); Turku (Finland)	1970–76	318	0.8
Jelovsek *et al.* (1980); Durham	1940–75	431	2.4
Hulka *et al.* (1980); Chapel Hill	1970–76	256	3.6 (use for 3½ years or more)
Shapiro *et al.* (1980); Many U.S. centres	1976–79	149	3.9 (conjugated oestrogens)
Stavraky *et al.* (1981); Ontario (Canada)	1976–78	206	(i) 4.8 (ii) 1.5
Spengler *et al.* (1981); Toronto (Canada)	1977–78	88	2.9
Öbrink *et al.* (1981); Stockholm (Sweden)	1974–77	622	3.7 (use for 3 years or more)
La Vecchia *et al.* (1982); Milan (Italy)	1979–80	179	2.3

method of selecting the control group. This applies particularly to the studies by Gray *et al.* (1977), Horwitz and Feinstein (1978) estimate (ii), Antunes *et al.* (1979) estimate (ii), and Stavraky *et al.* (1981) estimate (ii).

Few of the studies have provided information about the risk of endometrial cancer after discontinuation of therapy and there is considerable variation in the results which are available. Hulka *et al.* (1980), for example, found that, on average, a two-year oestrogen-free interval was sufficient to eliminate the excess risk of endometrial cancer while in the study by Shapiro *et al.* (1980), long-term users of oestrogens still had a nearly threefold elevation of risk five or more years after stopping.

A large number of criticisms have been levelled at the case-control studies, but in my view, only two have any real substance. First, Horwitz and Feinstein (1978) and Horwitz *et al.* (1981) have postulated that endometrial cancer is a much more common condition than is generally supposed and that many women have the disease without being aware of it. They have further postulated that the administration of oestrogens may cause occult cancers to bleed, thus leading to the detection of neoplasms which would otherwise have gone undetected. Secondly, it is known that oestrogens can induce atypical endometrial hyperplasia and it is postulated that this condition accounts for a substantial proportion of the 'cancer' cases in case-control studies. Space precludes a detailed consideration of the former criticism and the interested reader who wishes to review the evidence which, in my opinion, has refuted it is referred to publications by

Crombie and Tomenson (1981), Merletti and Cole (1981), and Vessey and Bungay (1982). The latter criticism has been shown to be invalid by careful independent histological review of the pathological material in a number of the studies. Having said this, it is important to stress that endometrial cancers occurring in women using oestrogens tend to be less advanced at detection, of a more favourable grade, and to carry a better prognosis than tumours occurring in other women (Collins *et al.* 1980).

As well as demonstrating the fact that oestrogen therapy is a cause of endometrial cancer, epidemiological studies have also given clues as to how to reduce, or even eliminate, the risk – for example, by ensuring that therapy is of as short a duration and at as low a dose as possible. Of particular importance is the suggestion that the addition of progestogen to the oestrogen will eliminate the risk – this idea is strongly supported by careful clinical research (Sturdee *et al.* 1978; Whitehead *et al.* 1981), by cohort studies reported by Gambrell *et al.* (1979) and by Persson (1983) and by studies indicating that combined oral contraceptives protect against endometrial cancer (see p. 182).

Cancer of the breast

As we have seen, cancer registry data in the U.S. strongly support the view that oestrogen replacement therapy is an important cause of endometrial cancer. The same does not appear to be true of registry data for cancer of the breast. Early case-control and cohort studies of the possible association between oestrogen use and breast cancer (like those relating to endometrial cancer) had too many shortcomings to be of much value, but since the mid-1970s a number of more satisfactory reports have started to appear. The first of these (Hoover *et al.* 1976) concerned 1891 women in Louisville, Kentucky, who had been given long-term treatment with conjugated oestrogens and followed up for an average of 12 years. In total, 49 cases of breast cancer were observed while 39.1 would have been expected on the basis of rates in the general population. The relative risk increased with follow-up duration, progressing to 2.0 after 15 years. In addition, after 10 years of follow-up, two factors normally related to a low risk of breast cancer, multiparity and oophorectomy, no longer imparted a protective effect.

Most of the remaining recent studies (all of which were carried out in the U.S.) are of the case-control type. Some of their main features are summarized in Table 2 – note once again that the list of studies is probably not exhaustive. On balance, there is reasonably strong evidence of a moderate increase in breast cancer risk when oestrogens are administered at high doses for long periods of time but there are discrepancies between the studies.

In addition to the investigations listed in Table 2, special mention should be made of (1) a cohort study reported from the Wilford Hall Medical Center by Gambrell *et al.* (1983) including 5563 postmenopausal women followed for a total of 37 000 person-years in which some evidence was obtained that the addition of progestogen to oestrogen replacement therapy significantly decreases the risk of breast cancer and (2) a cohort study reported by Thomas *et al.* (1982) of women with biopsy-proven benign breast disease in which there was evidence of an unfavourable interaction between certain types of histopathological abnormality and oestrogen administration. Thomas (1982) has also prepared an excellent review of oestrogen therapy and breast cancer to which the reader is referred for greater detail than is provided here.

Table 2. Recent case-control studies of oestrogen replacement therapy and cancer of the breast

Authors	Cases studied	Results
Ross *et al.* (1980); Los Angeles	138 women with breast cancer aged 50–74	Relative risk for a total cumulative dose in excess of 1500 mg Premarin estimated to be 2.5 in women with intact ovaries. Increase in risk inconsistent at low doses and not present in oophorectomized women.
Brinton *et al.* (1981); 28 centres throughout U.S.	881 postmenopausal women with breast cancer	Overall relative risk for users of 1.2. Relationship with dose. Effects mostly seen in those with bilateral oophorectomy (relative risk 1.5). In this group, risk increased with years of use and in those with other risk factors.
Jick *et al.* (1980b); Seattle	97 postmenopausal women with breast cancer aged 45–64	Principally concerned with current use. Little association in those with a previous hysterectomy (ovarian status not given). Positive association in those with natural menopause (relative risk 3.4).
Hoover *et al.* (1981); Portland	345 women with breast cancer, mean age 57	Overall relative risk for users 1.4. Effects seen in those with intact ovaries and those with ovaries removed. Increased risk with long duration of use and high dose.
Kelsey *et al.* (1981); Connecticut	332 women with breast cancer aged 45–74	Overall relative risk for users 0.9. Data analysed in same way as by Ross *et al.* (1980) but no effects apparent.
Hulka *et al.* (1982a); North Carolina	199 postmenopausal women with breast cancer	No increase in risk for those with ovaries removed, relative risk of 1.7 for those with ovaries intact. Little evidence of dose–response relationship. Risk especially associated with injected oestrogens.
Sherman *et al.* (1983); Iowa	113 postmenopausal women with breast cancer	No general association, but evidence of interaction between obesity and oestrogen use.

Ovarian cancer

Weiss *et al.* (1982) have suggested that oestrogen replacement therapy may increase the risk of endometrioid tumours of the ovary, but this observation requires confirmation.

Comment

Oestrogen replacement therapy has received a great deal of adverse publicity during the last few years and, as a result, its use has declined, at least in the U.K. (Hunt and Vessey 1983). There is, however, little evidence of any harmful effect of therapy on cardiovascular disease (indeed, the risk of ischaemic heart disease may even be reduced by such medication) while the prevention of postmenopausal osteoporosis and its complications is of great importance (see Vessey and Bungay 1982). In my view, work should continue to try to identify a form of replacement therapy which retains the beneficial effects and minimizes adverse effects. This may be difficult to achieve, but at least it is worth remembering that women who have undergone hysterectomy and bilateral oophorectomy, who are at special risk of severe osteoporosis, are not susceptible to any carcinogenic effect of oestrogens on the organs which have been removed.

Administration of hormones to prevent pregnancy

Oral contraceptives first became available in the U.S. in 1959 and since that time they have been widely adopted by women in many different countries. Well over 50 million women worldwide are currently 'on the pill' while many millions more have used oral contraceptives in the past. Accordingly, a proper assessment of the possible relationship between oral contraceptive use and cancer is of great public-health importance.

In this section, attention is concentrated on combined oral contraceptives, although there are also a few references to sequential preparations. Reliable human data on progestogen-only pills and on injectable progestogen contraceptives (medroxyprogesterone acetate and norethisterone oenanthate) are sparse, and these preparations are not discussed here.

A number of important general considerations need to be borne in mind when studying the literature on the relationship between oral contraceptives and cancer (some of what follows is also relevant to studies of the effects of oestrogen replacement therapy):

Latent period. There is usually an appreciable 'latent period' between first exposure to a carcinogen and the development of overt malignant disease. In addition, the cumulative effects of prolonged exposure or repeated exposure are likely to be of importance. Steroid contraceptives have only been in widespread use for about 20 years; relatively few women have had both the prolonged exposure and the extended period of follow-up required to evaluate carcinogenic effects with confidence. It should be noted, however, that if oral contraceptives were to alter the rate of growth of occult tumours, or were to affect the rate of change from a premalignant state to malignancy, an effect should now be apparent.

Changes in preparation. The types and doses of steroid in common use have changed markedly since the introduction of the pill. For example, (1) the dosages of both oestrogens and progestogens have been progressively reduced; (2) some new progestogens (e.g. levonorgestrel, desogestrel) have been introduced; (3) other progestogens (e.g. chlormadinone acetate, megestrol acetate) have been withdrawn; and (4) sequential preparations have largely disappeared while triphasic and biphasic preparations have been developed. From this, it follows that even recent studies of the possible carcinogenic effects of oral contraceptives largely relate to discontinued products.

Time of exposure. Exposure to contraceptive steroids at particular times of life, such as during adolescence, during pregnancy, or during the perimenopausal years might be of special importance. In this context, it must be remembered that over the years women have tended to adopt the pill at younger and younger ages and to use hormonal contraception to delay the first birth as well as to space or limit later births. Again, during the last five years there has been a sharp fall in the numbers of women over 35 years of age who use the pill. It is important not to extrapolate the results of epidemiological studies to groups of women to whom they do not relate. For example, data derived from women who first started to use the pill in their mid-twenties may not be relevant to women who first started to use the pill in their mid-teens.

High-risk groups. It is possible that oral contraceptives might have no relationship with a particular cancer in the generality of women but, nonetheless, might have an effect on risk in those with predisposing factors: for example, in the case of breast cancer, in those with a history of benign disease or a positive family history. To draw a well-known analogy from another field, it seems that the pill has an important effect on the risk of acute myocardial infarction only in the presence of other risk factors such as cigarette smoking.

Breast cancer

The use of oral contraceptives seems to be associated with a protective effect against clinically detectable *benign breast disease*. This topic has been reviewed in detail by Vessey (1983). The protective effect increases with duration of use; is probably confined to current or very recent users; is probably attributable to the progestogen component of the pill; and may be restricted to the less serious forms of disease in which epithelial atypia are minimal or absent. The last-mentioned observation provides a possible explanation for the apparent paradox that oral contraceptives protect against benign breast disease, but not (as we shall see) against breast cancer.

As oral contraceptives are used by more and more women, any major effect on the risk of *breast cancer* might be reflected in temporal trends in age-specific incidence rates or mortality rates. To the best of my knowledge, no changes in trend have yet been reported which might be attributed to the influence of the pill. Mortality data for England and Wales are given in Table 3. As can be seen, the biggest increase in mortality has been in women aged 45–64 years among whom the trend in rates has been steadily upward during the last 25 years.

Table 3. Breast cancer mortality, England and Wales 1955–80

Year	Rate per 100 000 population				
	15–24 years	25–44 years	45–64 years	65–74 years	75+ years
1955	0.04	12	64	106	164
1960	0.20	12	66	105	161
1965	0.12	13	70	104	161
1970	0.23	14	78	109	158
1975	0.21	14	80	120	174
1980	0.05	13	83	122	183

Vital statistical data, however, have obvious limitations and to make further progress we need to examine the results of analytical epidemiological studies. Many such studies have been carried out, and those published before mid-1983 have been reviewed in detail by Kalache *et al.* (1983) and Vessey (1985). Unfortunately, at the time of writing (January 1984), controversy is raging about the possible adverse effects of early oral contraceptive use on breast cancer risk and new data are rapidly appearing in the literature. Accordingly, the account I have presented here is bound to be out of date by the time these words are published.

Case-control studies The main design features of the five largest case-control studies conducted to date are given in Table 4, and Table 5 summarizes the overall findings in these studies about breast cancer risk in relation to total duration of oral contraceptive use. The data are clearly reassuring and the same is true for analyses relating risk to interval since first oral contraceptive use (Vessey 1984).

Table 4. Main features of major case-control studies

Authors	Age range (y)	Time cases diagnosed	No. of cases	Nature of cases	No. of controls	Nature of controls	Matching criteria	Method of data collection
Paffenbarger *et al*. (1979); San Francisco, U.S.	All ages	1973–7	1432	Newly diagnosed at participating hospitals	2560	Hospital patients	Age, race, hospital, admission date	Home interview
Brinton *et al*. (1982); multicentre, U.S.	All ages 35 up	1973–7	963	Newly diagnosed in BCDDP† Those with artificial menopause excluded White only.	858	Screening participants	Age, centre, time of entry to project, continuation in project	Home interview by trained nurses
Centers for Disease Control (1983a); multicentre, U.S.	20–54	1980–1	689	Newly diagnosed – identified by cancer registries	1077	Population based	Not individually matched. Selected in same age group within same geographical areas	Home interview
Vessey *et al*. (1983b); London and Oxford, U.K.	16–50	1968–80	1176	Newly diagnosed at 9 hospitals. Married only	1176	Hospital patients	Age, parity, hospital, admission date	Interviewed in hospital by trained nurse or social worker
Rosenberg *et al*. (1984); multicentre, U.S. and Canada	20–59	1976–81	1191	Newly diagnosed at participating hospitals	5026	Hospital patients	Not individually matched. Selected in same age group within same hospitals	Interviewed in hospital by trained nurse

† BCDDP = Breast Cancer Detection Demonstration Project.

Table 5. Breast cancer risk in case-control studies in relation to total duration of oral contraceptive use (the listing of 19 years as the upper limit of use is arbitrary)

Total duration oral contraceptive use (y)	Paffenbarger *et al.* (1979)		Brinton *et al.* (1982)		Centers for Disease Control (1983a)		Vessey *et al.* (1983b)		Rosenberg *et al.* (1984)	
	Rel. risk	No. cases	Rel. risk	No. cases	Rel. risk	No. cases	Rel. risk	No. cases	Rel. risk	No. cases
0	1.0	1106	1.0	738	1.0	294	1.0	639	1.0	794
1	1.1	112			0.9	147	0.9	203	0.9	97
2	1.2	39	0.9	113						
3	1.4	49					1.0	145	1.0	127
4					1.2	125				
5			1.2	36						
6	1.3	33								
7					1.0	36	1.2	123		
8			1.5	35					1.3	88
9					0.7	29				
10										
11										
12										
13	1.4	72								
14			1.0	29			1.0	66	0.8	25
15					0.9	35				
16										
17										
18										
19										

The published reports of three of the five studies shown in Table 4 include no data on types of oral contraceptive used. Brinton *et al.* (1982) provide a fairly detailed analysis by oestrogen content, with some suggestion of an elevated risk for users of high oestrogen dose (100 μg or more) preparations. However, these authors did not find any 'distinct trend' when risk was related to cumulative lifetime oestrogen dose. Vessey *et al.* (1983b) were unable to detect any association between breast cancer risk and oral contraceptive type although their analysis was limited to looking at the proportions of breast cancer cases and controls who had ever used particular individual preparations or groups of preparations. It is clear that work on the relationship between pill type and breast cancer is handicapped not only by the inadequate recall of brand names by study participants but also by the lack of any satisfactory way of grouping different oral contraceptives together, taking into account both the oestrogen and the progestogen components.

Oral contraceptive use in high-risk groups. Most attention has been concentrated on women with a family history of breast cancer or with a history of benign breast disease. Brinton *et al.* (1982) reported rather worrying findings for oral contraceptive users in both of these high-risk groups, although their results were not statistically significant. A similar elevation in risk (also not statistically significant) was described by Paffenbarger *et al.* (1979) in women with a maternal history of breast cancer, but not in those with a history of benign breast disease. Negative results for both high-risk groups were reported in the studies by the Centers for Disease Control (1983a), Vessey *et al.* (1983b), and Rosenberg *et al.* (1984).

Oral contraceptive use at different times of life. Analyses of the relationship between oral contraceptive use and breast cancer risk in subgroups defined by age and parity were carried out in four of the studies shown in Table 5 and by menopausal status in all five. In general, the results were unrevealing although Brinton *et al.* (1982) found that premenopausal women who used the pill after the age of 40 had an approximately 50 per cent increase in risk and suggested that this might be due to 'artificial prolongation of a premenopausal rate of disease incidence'. It is of interest that Jick *et al.* (1980c), in a much smaller study, had previously reported a positive association between current oral contraceptive use and breast cancer risk in premenopausal women over 45 years of age. Vessey *et al.* (1983b) also found some elevation of risk in women aged 46–50 years (but not in those aged 41–45 years), but this was not confined to current users, nor was it influenced by menopausal status.

Anxiety about a possible harmful effect of prolonged oral contraceptive use before first time pregnancy followed publication of the data shown in Table 6 by Pike *et al.* (1981). The study involved 163 women in Los Angeles County in whom breast cancer had been diagnosed at age 32 years or less. Unfortunately, the five case-control studies listed in Table 4 provide few data about this extremely important issue, although Vessey *et al.* (1982) and the Centers for Disease Control (1983a) subsequently published limited results which did not support the Californian findings. In October 1983, however, Pike *et al.* published a further report from Los Angeles. Their series of cases now included 314 women with breast cancer aged 36 years or less and their primary analyses concerned oral contraceptive use before age 25 years rather than before first term pregnancy. Their main findings, which are clearly extremely worrying, are summarized in Table 7. Pike *et al.* (1983) also related breast cancer risk in their study to the 'progestogen potency' of the oral contraceptives used as measured by the delay of menses test, claiming that the adverse effect was largely attributable to pills with a 'potency score' of 5 or more. Subsequent correspondence about the paper by Pike *et al.* (see, for example, Swyer 1983) has made it clear that the classification of progestogen potency used by the Los Angeles group is invalid, but this, of course, does not alter the basic findings shown in Table 7!

At the time of writing, preliminary results from a new case-control study conducted by my department in Oxford and in London since 1980, have just been published (McPherson *et al.* 1983). In contrast to our earlier findings (Vessey *et al.* 1982) the present results (which are still based on small numbers) suggest an increased risk of breast cancer in young women who have prolonged oral contraceptive use before first pregnancy – indeed, the data closely resemble those published by Pike *et al.* in 1981. It is, however, widely rumoured that the Centers for Diseae Control Study, which now includes some 4000 women with breast cancer, replicates

Table 6. Risk of breast cancer in relation to use of oral contraceptives before first full-term pregnancy (modified from Pike *et al.* 1981)

Duration of oral contraceptive use (months)	Cases		Controls		Relative risk
	No.	%	No.	%	
0	79	48.5	141	52.2	1.0
1–48	53	32.5	103	38.2	1.0
49–96	24	14.7	22	8.1	2.2
97–	7	4.3	4	1.5	3.5
Total	163	100.0	270	100.0	

Test for linear trend: $p = 0.009$.

Table 7. Risk of breast cancer in relation to use of oral contraceptives before age 25 (modified from Pike *et al.* 1983)

Duration of oral contraceptive use (months)	Cases		Controls		Relative risk
	No.	%	No.	%	
0	65	20.7	93	29.6	1.0
1–24	106	33.8	118	37.7	1.3
25–48	79	25.2	67	21.3	1.7
49–72	40	12.7	29	9.2	2.0
73–	24	7.6	7	2.2	4.9
Total	314	100.0	314	100.0	

neither these findings nor those of Pike *et al.* The situation is, therefore, extremely confused and it may be some years yet before a conclusive answer about the possible effects of early pill use on breast cancer risk becomes available.

Cohort studies Data on oral contraceptive use and breast cancer have been reported from four large cohort studies: (1) the Royal College of General Practitioners Study which includes 46 000 British women recruited by 1400 family doctors (Royal College of General Practitioners 1981), (2) the Oxford–Family Planning Association Contraceptive Study which includes 17 000 British women recruited at 17 family planning centres (Vessey *et al.* 1981), (3) the Walnut Creek Contraceptive Drug Study which includes 16 500 North American women who joined the study by having a general health check in an automated multitest laboratory (Ramcharan *et al.* 1981), and (4) a study conducted in Eastern Massachussets which includes 96 000 women who were identified from residence lists and mailed a questionnaire in 1970 (Trapido 1981). The findings have, in general, been reassuring but the numbers of cases involved are rather small. In the Royal College of General Practitioners Study (1981), however, there was some evidence that breast cancer risk might be increased in oral contraceptive users under 35 years of age (relative risk; ever-users to never-users 2.8 to 1, $p = 0.05$). There was no indication of any such effect in the other three studies. Trapido (1981) found the relative risk associated with oral contraceptive use in nulliparous women to be 2.1, but the figure was not statistically significantly different from unity.

The Royal College of General Practitioners Study and the Oxford–Family Planning Association Contraceptive Study, both of which are still continuing, will eventually yield a very large amount of information about the risk of breast cancer in oral contraceptive users. Neither study, however, will be able to provide much data about women starting to use the pill at a very young age and much of the exposure information will inevitably relate to pills which are no longer used.

Oral contraceptive use and prognosis of breast cancer Spencer *et al.* (1978) compared 44 newly diagnosed breast cancer patients with recent oral contraceptive use with 44 other newly diagnosed breast cancer patients who were non-users of the pill, and found prognosis to be better in the former group. Similar findings were later reported by the same workers in an investigation involving an additional 93 breast cancer patients who had been taking the pill and 93 'controls', studied in an identical way (Mathews *et al.* 1981).

Vessey *et al.* (1983) have reported on clinical stage of breast cancer at diagnosis in 572 breast cancer patients included in their case-control study. As shown in Table 8, women who had never used oral contraceptives presented with more advanced tumours than those who had used them during the year before detection of cancer, while past users were in an intermediate position. These differences in staging were reflected in the pattern of survival.

Possible explanations for these observations include 'surveillance bias' among oral contraceptive users leading to earlier diagnosis (although Vessey *et al.* (1983b) found little evidence to support this suggestion) or a beneficial effect of oral contraceptives on tumour growth and spread.

Table 8. Stage classification of 572 patients with breast cancer (modified from Vessey *et al.* 1983)

Clinical stage	Use of oral contraceptives†					
	Never used		Used only in past		Used recently	
	No.	%	No.	%	No.	%
I	196	55.9	83	64.3	66	74.2
II	74	20.8	23	17.8	11	12.4
III–IV	84	23.8	23	18.0	12	13.4
Total	354	100.0	124	100.0	89	100.0

† 'Used recently' indicates use during year before detection of lump. 'Used only in past' indicates use only before that time.

Ovarian cancer

The first data to suggest that oral contraceptives might protect against epithelial ovarian cancer appeared in a paper from the U.K. by Newhouse *et al.* (1977). Among 300 women with the disease (the great majority with epithelial tumours), only 19 (6.3 per cent) had ever used the pill while in each of two control groups of 300 women, 31 (10.3 per cent) had done so. Since then, at least eight additional case-control studies have been published and, as can be seen from Table 9, all have yielded results pointing in the same direction. As epithelial ovarian tumours tend to be more common in less fertile women, it was at first thought that the apparent protective effect of the pill might be attributable to confounding, but the more recent studies make it clear that this explanation is extremely unlikely.

Table 9. Case-control studies of oral contraceptive use and ovarian cancer

Authors	Ovarian cancer cases		Relative risk: ever-use to never-use of pill
	Age range	Number	
Newhouse *et al.* (1977);U.K.	All ages	300	0.6
Casagrande *et al.* (1979);U.S.	25–49	150	0.7†
Weiss *et al.* (1981);U.S.	35–54	112	0.6
Willett *et al.* (1981);U.S.	30–55	47	0.8 (0.4–1.5)‡
Hildreth *et al.* (1981);U.S.	45–74	62	0.5 (0.2–1.5)
Franceschi *et al.* (1982);Italy	–69	161	0.7 (0.4–1.1)
Rosenberg *et al.* (1982);U.S.	–59	136	0.6 (0.4–0.9)
Cramer *et al.* (1982);U.S.	–59	144	0.4 (0.2–1.0)
Centers for Disease Control (1983b);U.S.	20–54	179	0.6 (0.4–0.9)

† Use for more than 6 months.
‡ Figures in brackets indicate 95 per cent confidence limits (not always given by author).

Ovarian cancer is rare below the age of 40 years. Present teaching about oral contraceptive use recommends discontinuation of medication in the majority of women at about age 35 years because of the risk of cardiovascular adverse effects. For the protective effect of the pill against ovarian cancer to be of any practical value, it follows that it must persist in ex-users, and persist for many years. Table 10 summarizes the available findings on this point and also provides information about the effect of duration of contraceptive use. The results so far look encouraging, but clearly more extensive data are required.

The major cohort studies concerned with the long-term effects of oral contraceptive use still include too few cases of ovarian cancer for firm conclusions to be drawn. Such data as are available, however, are in support of the findings in the case-control studies (Vessey, unpublished; C.R. Kay, personal communication; Ramcharan *et al.* 1981).

Endometrial cancer

In view of the fact that oestrogen replacement therapy is a well-established cause of endometrial cancer (see page 169), it is not surprising that the

Table 10. Case-control studies of oral contraceptive use and ovarian cancer. Data on duration of use and recency of use

Authors	Increasing protection with duration of use?	Persistent protection after stopping use?
Newhouse *et al.* (1977)	Not stated	Not stated
Casagrande *et al.* (1979)	Yes	Not stated
Weiss *et al.* (1981)	Not after 3 y use	Not stated
Willett *et al.* (1981)	No	Not stated
Hildreth *et al.* (1981)	No data	No data
Franceschi *et al.* (1982)	Not stated	Not stated
Rosenberg *et al.* (1982)	Yes	For at least 10 y
Cramer *et al.* (1982)	Not after 3 y use	For at least 10 y
Centers for Disease Control (1983b)	Yes	For at least 10 y

highly oestrogenic sequential oral contraceptives also have this effect (Silverberg and Makowski 1975; Weiss and Sayvetz 1980; Centers for Disease Control 1983c). The earliest data to indicate that combined preparations might protect against this disease were reported by Weiss and Sayvetz in 1980. These workers, in a case-control study including 117 women aged 35–54 years with endometrial cancer and 395 healthy controls, found combined oral contraceptives to reduce the risk of cancer by 50 per cent. As Table 11 shows, six other case-control studies published since then have produced equally encouraging results. As with ovarian cancer, it seems clear that the apparent protective effect is not merely a reflection of the fact that women at risk of endometrial cancer are less fertile than other women.

Table 11. Case-control studies of combined oral contraceptive use and endometrial cancer

Authors	Endometrial cancer cases		Relative risk: ever-use to never-use combined pills
	Age	Number	
Weiss and Sayvetz (1980); U.S.	35–54	117	0.5 (0.1–1.0)†
Kaufman *et al.* (1980); U.S.	–59	154	0.5 (0.3–0.8)
Kelsey *et al.* (1982); U.S.	45–74	167	0.6
Hulka *et al.* (1982b); U.S.A.	–59	79	0.4
La Vecchia *et al.* (1982); Italy	–84	173	0/173 cases and 12/347 controls exposed
Centers for Disease Control (1983c); U.S.	20–54	187	0.5 (0.3–0.8)
Henderson *et al.* (1983a); U.S.	–45	127	0.5

† Figures in brackets indicate 95 per cent confidence limits (not always given by author).

Endometrial cancer is rare below the age of 45 years, so the comments made previously about the public health importance of a persistent protective effect against ovarian cancer in ex-users of the pill apply even more strongly for this tumour. The data summarized in Table 12 offer a certain amount of encouragement in this respect.

Table 12. Case-control studies of combined oral contraceptive use and endometrial cancer. Data on duration of use and recency of use of pills

Authors	Increasing protection with duration of use?	Persistent protection after stopping use?
Weiss and Sayvetz (1980)	Not after 1 y use	For a year or two
Kaufman *et al.* (1980)	Yes	For at least 5 y
Kelsey *et al.* (1982)	Yes	Not stated
Hulka *et al.* (1982b)	Yes	Effect wanes
La Vecchia *et al.* (1982)	No data	No data
Centers for Disease Control (1983c)	Not after 1 y use	For at least 10 y
Henderson *et al.* (1983)	Yes	Not stated

Some authors have found that the protective effect against endometrial cancer is more prominent with the strongly progestogenic pills and that use of oestrogen replacement therapy can eliminate the benefit. Henderson *et al.* (1983a) found clear evidence of reduced risk only in women who had had less than three livebirths and who weighed less than 170 lb.

As with ovarian cancer, the preliminary results from the large cohort studies are generally encouraging (Kay 1980; Ramcharan *et al.*1981).

Cancer of the cervix uteri

Studies attempting to relate the risk of neoplasia of the cervix uteri to the use of oral contraceptives are beset by many difficulties (Swan and Pettiti 1982). First, it is extremely difficult to make adequate allowance for the effect of confounding variables, especially age at first sexual intercourse and number of sexual partners, which are powerful predictors of cervical neoplasia risk. Secondly, it is reasonably well established that occlusive methods of contraception offer some protection against cervical neoplasia. Thirdly, since almost all pre-invasive lesions and many invasive ones are detected by cervical cytology, any substantial difference in the pattern of smear examinations between groups being compared may easily lead to incorrect conclusions. Fourthly, histopathologists vary greatly in their interpretation and classification of pre-invasive lesions of the cervix, and this can lead to serious bias if any one pathologist receives a disproportionate amount of material from women using a particular contraceptive method.

Perhaps not surprisingly, almost all published studies of the possible relationship between oral contraceptive use and cancer of the cervix deal with the pre-invasive lesions, dysplasia or carcinoma *in situ*. Many investigations have been based on data derived from routine cervical cytology screening programmes. Such studies are difficult to interpret and have yielded conflicting results. Most of the remaining studies (which have dealt with histologically diagnosed lesions) have been well reviewed by a World Health Organization Scientific Group (1978). Of the case-control studies, those by Worth and Boyes (1972), Thomas (1972) and Boyce *et al.*(1977) indicated no relation, while those by Ory *et al.* (1977) and Harris *et al.* (1980) showed a positive association between risk and duration of use. Cohort studies of cervical neoplasia and the pill have tended to produce positive results. Thus in the Walnut Creek Study a statistically significant association between the incidence of carcinoma *in situ* and duration of pill use was reported (Peritz *et al.* 1977), although it was subsequently suggested that this result was, to some extent, attributable to confounding by differences in sexual activity, both between users and non-users of oral contraceptives and among women with different durations of oral contraceptive use (Swan and Brown 1981). Again, in a large cohort study conducted in Los Angeles, rates of progression from cervical dysplasia to carcinoma *in situ* were much higher in women using Ovulen than in women using intrauterine devices (Stern *et al.* 1977).

The most recent cohort data come from the Oxford–Family Planning Association Contraceptive Study (Vessey *et al.* 1983c, 1983d). In this analysis, the incidence of biopsy-proven cervical neoplasia during a 10-year follow-up period was determined in 6838 parous women who entered the study while using oral contraceptives and 3154 parous women who entered the study while using an intrauterine device. Risk factors for cervical neoplasia and frequency of examination by cervical cytology were similar in the two groups. All 13 cases of invasive cancer occurred in women in the oral contraceptive group; 9 had more than six years' use of the pill. Both carcinoma-in-situ and dysplasia also occurred more frequently in the oral contraceptive group than in the intrauterine device group, and when the two conditions were considered together there was a trend in incidence with duration of oral contraceptive use. The incidence of all these forms of neoplasia combined rose from 0.9 per 1000 woman-years in those with up to two years' pill use to 2.2 per 1000 woman-years in those with more than eight years' pill use. Amongst the IUD users there was no such trend in incidence with duration of use; the rate fluctuated around 1.0 per 1000 woman-years.

Other tumours

There is little doubt that hepatocellular adenomas occur much more frequently in oral contraceptive users than in other women, although their incidence among the former is still extremely low (perhaps 1–2 per 100 000 users per annum). Evidence in support of this association has been derived from numerous case-reports and (more importantly) from two case-control studies (Edmondson *et al.* 1976; Rooks *et al.* 1979). The risk seems to be greatest in older women using oral contraceptives of high hormonal potency over a long period of time (Rooks *et al.* 1979). The suspicion that oral contraceptive use may also, on very rare occasions, lead to the occurrence of hepatocellular carcinoma is supported by the findings in a recent case-control study from Los Angeles (Henderson *et al.* 1983b).

The possibility that oral contraceptive use might increase the risk of malignant melanoma of the skin was first raised by Beral *et al.* in 1977 on the basis of data collected in the Walnut Creek area in California. Subsequent studies have given conflicting results (Adam *et al.* 1981; Bain *et al.* 1982; Holly *et al.* 1983). However, no investigation has yet been reported which includes a sufficiently large number of cases with long-term oral contraceptive use for any firm conclusions to be drawn.

For many years, it has been widely held that oral contraceptive use increases the risk of certain benign tumours of the pituitary gland, particularly prolactinoma. Two recently reported case-control studies have provided strong evidence against this association (Shy *et al.* 1983; Pituitary Adenoma Study Group 1983). Shy *et al.* (1983) have suggested that previous reports of an association between pill use and prolactinoma may have resulted from oral contraceptive treatment of menstrual irregularity in women with an undiagnosed tumour.

Comment

As anticipated, oral contraceptives are proving to have effects on a wide variety of tumours. The risks of benign breast lumps, endometrial cancer, and epithelial cancer of the ovary are almost certainly reduced by the use of combined preparations. Protection against cancer of the ovary, in particular, is of great potential importance since this terrible disease commonly presents at an advanced stage and the results of treatment are extremely depressing. On the other hand, the evidence that early use of oral contraceptives may increase breast cancer risk and that prolonged use generally may increase cervical cancer risk, while certainly not conclusive, is none the less disturbing. In comparison, the known risk of occasionally inducing hepatocellular adenoma and, perhaps, extremely rarely, hepatocellular carcinoma is of minor consequence.

Further research into the effects of oral contraceptive use on cancer is obviously of great importance. It should focus on defining the risks and benefits according to patterns of use and types of preparations. Clearly, the long-term aim must be to develop a pill or pills which will retain the known benefits of existing preparations, but not be associated with serious hazards. A major handicap at present for epidemiologists working in this field is the absence of useful information from the laboratory and from clinical research about the ways in which different oral contraceptives might be grouped together when attempting to assess their effects on certain end-organs, particularly the breast. Perhaps the attempt by Pike *et al.* (1983) to stimulate interest in this kind of approach, while having caused confusion for the pharmaceutical industry, the medical profession, and the public alike, will encourage appropriate basic research in the future.

References

Adam, S.A., Sheaves, J.K., Wright, N.H., Mosser, G., Harris, R.W., and Vessey, M. (1981). A case-control study of the possible association between oral contraceptives and malignant melanoma. *Brit. J. Cancer* **44**, 45–50.

Antunes, C.M.F., Stolley, P.D., Rosenshein, N.B., Davies, J.L., Tonascia, J.A., Brown, C., Burnett, L., Rutledge, A., Pokempner, M., and Garcia, R. (1979). Endometrial cancer and estrogen use. *New Engl. J. Med.* **300**, 9–13.

Bain, C., Hennekens, C.H., Speizer, F.E., Rosner, B., Willett, W., and Belanger, C. (1982). Oral contraceptive use and malignant melanoma. *J. nat. Cancer Inst.* **68**, 537–9.

Beral, V. and Colwell, L. (1980). Randomised trial of high doses of stilboestrol and ethisterone in pregnancy: long-term follow-up of mothers. *Brit. med. J* **ii**, 1098–101.

Beral, V., Ramcharan, S., and Faris, R. (1977). Malignant melanoma and oral contraceptive use among women in California. *Brit. J. Cancer* **36**, 804–9.

Boyce, J.G., Lu, T., Nelson, J.H., and Fruchter, R.G. (1977). Oral contraceptives and cervical carcinoma. *Amer. J. Obstet Gynecol.* **128**, 761–6.

Brackbill, Y. and Berendes, H.W. (1978). Dangers of diethylstilboestrol: review of a 1953 paper. *Lancet* **ii**, 520.

Brian, D.D., Tilley, B.C., Labarthe, D.R. O'Fallon, W.M., Noller, K.L., and Kurland, L.T. (1980). Breast cancer in DES-exposed mothers. Absence of association. *Mayo Clin. Proc.* **55**, 89–93.

Brinton, L.A., Hoover, R.N. Szklo, M., and Fraumeni, J.F. (1981). Menopausal estrogen use and risk of breast cancer. *Cancer* **47**, 2517–22.

Brinton, L.A., Hoover, R., Szklo, M., and Fraumeni, J.F. (1982). Oral contraceptives and breast cancer. *Int. J. Epidemiol.* **11**, 316–22.

Casagrande, J.T., Louie, E.W., Pike, M.C., Roy, S., Ross, R.K., and Henderson, B.E. (1979). "Incessant ovulation" and ovarian cancer. *Lancet* **ii**, 170–4.

Centers for Disease Control. (1983a). Long term oral contraceptive use and the risk of breast cancer. *J. Amer. med. Assoc.* **249**, 1591–5.

Centers for Disease Control (1983b). Oral contraceptive use and the risk of ovarian cancer. *J. Amer. med. Assoc.* **249**, 1596–9.

Centers for Disease Control (1983c). Oral contraceptive use and the risk of endometrial cancer. *J. Amer. med. Assoc.* **249**, 1600–4.

Collins, J., Donner, A., Allen, L.H., Adams, O. (1980). Oestrogen use and survival in endometrial cancer. *Lancet* **ii**, 961–4.

Cramer, D.W., Hutchinson, G.B., Welch, W.R., Scully, R.E., and Knapp, R.C. (1982). Factors affecting the association of oral contraceptives and ovarian cancer. *New Engl. J. Med.* **307**, 1047–51.

Crombie, I.K. and Tomenson, J. (1981). Detection bias in endometrial cancer. *Lancet* **ii**, 308–9.

Davis, J.A., Wadehra, V., McIntosh, A.S., and Monaghan, J.M. (1981). A case of clear cell adenocarcinoma of the vagina in pregnancy. *Brit J. Obstet. Gynaecol.* **88**, 322–6.

Depue, R.H., Pike, M.C., and Henderson, B.E. (1983). Estrogen exposure during gestation and risk of testicular cancer. *J. nat. Cancer Inst.* **71**, 1151–5.

Dewhurst, J., Ferreira, H.P., Dalley, V.M., and Staffurth, J.F. (1980). Stilboestrol-associated vaginal carcinoma treated by radiotherapy. *J. Obstet. Gynaecol.* **1**, 63–4.

Dieckmann, W.J., Davis, M.E., Rynkiewicz, S.M., and Pottinger, R.E. (1953). Does the administration of diethylstilbestrol during pregnancy have therapeutic value? *Amer. J. Obstet. Gynecol.* **66**, 1062–75.

Edmonson, H.A., Henderson, B., and Benton, B. (1976). Liver cell adenomas associated with use of oral contraceptives. *New Engl. J. Med.* **294**, 470–2.

Ferguson, J.H. (1953). Effect of stilbestrol on pregnancy compared to the effect of a placebo. *Amer J. Obstet. Gynecol.* **65**, 592–601.

Franceschi, S., La Vecchia, C., Helmrich, S.P., Mangioni, C., and Tognoni, G. (1982). Risk factors for epithelial ovarian cancer in Italy. *Amer. J. Epidemiol.* **115**, 714–9.

Gambrell, R.D., Maier, R.C., and Sanders, B.I. (1983). Decreased incidence of breast cancer in postmenopausal estrogen-progestogen users. *Obstet. Gynecol.* **62**, 435–43.

Gambrell, R.D., Massey, F.M., Castaneda, T.A., Ugenas, A.J., and Ricci, C.A. (1979). Reduced incidence of endometrial cancer among postmenopausal women treated with progestogens. *J. Amer. Geriat. Soc.* **27**, 389–94.

Gill, W.B., Schumacher, G.F.B., Hubby, M.M., and Blough, R.R. (1981). Male genital tract changes in humans following intrauterine exposure to diethylstilbestrol. In *Developmental effects of diethylstilbestrol (DES) in pregnancy* (ed. A.L. Herbst and H.A. Bern), pp. 103–19. Thieme Stratton, New York.

Gray, L.A., Christopherson, W.M., and Hoover, R.N. (1977). Estrogens and endometrial carcinoma. *Obstet. Gynecol.* **49**, 385–9.

Harris, R.W.C., Brinton, L.A., Cowdell, R.H., Skegg, D.C.G., Smith, P.G., Vessey, M.P., and Doll, R. (1980). Characteristics of women with dysplasia or carcinoma-in-situ of the cervix uteri. *Brit. J. Cancer* **42**, 359–69.

Henderson, B.E., Benton, B., Jing, J., Yu, M.C., and Pike, M.C. (1979). Risk factors for cancer of the testis in young men. *Int. J. Cancer* **23**, 598–602.

Henderson, B.E., Casagrande, J.T., Pike, M.C., Mack, T., Rosario, I., and Duke, A. (1983a). The epidemiology of endometrial cancer in young women. *Brit. J. Cancer* **47**, 749–56.

Henderson, B.E., Preston-Martin, S., Edmondson, H.A., Peters, R.L., and Pike,

M.C. (1983b). Hepatocellular carcinoma and oral contraceptives. *Brit. J. Cancer* **48**, 437–40.

Herbst, A.L. (1981). The epidemiology of vaginal and cervical clear cell adenocarcinoma. In *Developmental effects of diethylstilbestrol (DES) in pregnancy* (ed. A.L. Herbst and H.A. Bern), pp. 63–70. Thieme Stratton, New York.

Herbst, A.L., Ulfelder, H., and Poskanzer, D.C. (1971). Adenocarcinoma of the vagina. Association of maternal stilbestrol therapy with tumor appearance in young women. *New Engl. J. Med.* **284**, 878–81.

Hildreth, N.G., Kelsey, J.L., Li Volsi, V.A., Fischer, D.B., Holford, T.R., Mostow, E.D., Schwartz, P.E., and White, C. (1981). An epidemiological study of epithelial carcinoma of the ovary. *Amer. J. Epidemiol.* **114**, 398–405.

Holly, E.A., Weiss, N.S., and Liff, J.M. (1983). Cutaneous melanoma in relation to exogenous hormones and reproductive factors. *J. nat. Cancer Inst.* **70**, 827–31.

Hoover, R., Glass, A., Finkle, W.D., Azevedo, D., and Milne, K. (1981). Conjugated estrogens and breast cancer risk in women. *J. nat. Cancer Inst.* **67**, 815–20.

Hoover, R., Gray, L.A., Cole, P., and MacMahon, B. (1976). Menopausal estrogens and breast cancer. *New Engl. J. Med.* **295**, 401–5.

Horwitz, R.I. and Feinstein, A.R. (1978). Alternative analytic methods for case-control studies of estrogens and endometrial cancer. *New Engl. J. Med.* **299**, 1089–94.

Horwitz, R.I., Feinstein, A.R., Horwitz, S.M., and Robboy, S.J. (1981). Necropsy diagnosis of endometrial cancer and detection-bias in case/control studies. *Lancet* **ii**, 66–8.

Hubby, M.M., Haenszel, W.M., and Herbst, A.L. (1981). Effects on the mother following exposure to diethylstilbestrol in pregnancy. In *Developmental effects of diethystilbestrol (DES) in pregnancy* (ed. A.L. Herbst and H.A. Bern), pp. 120–8. Thieme Stratton, New York.

Hulka, B.S., Chambless, L.E., Deubner, D.C., and Wilkinson, W.E. (1982a). Breast cancer and estrogen replacement therapy. *Amer. J. Obstet. Gynecol.* **143**, 638–44.

Hulka, B.S., Chambless, L.E., Kaufman, D.G., Fowler, W.C., and Greenberg, B.G. (1982b). Protection against endometrial carcinoma by combination-product oral contraceptives. *J. Amer. med. Assoc.* **247**, 475–7.

Hulka, B.S., Fowler, W.C., Kaufman, D.G., Grimson, R.C., Greenberg, B.G., Hogue, C.J.R., Berger, G.S., and Pulliam, C.C. (1980). Estrogen and endometrial cancer: cases and two control groups from North Carolina. *Amer. J. Obstet. Gynecol.* **137**, 92–101.

Hunt, K. and Vessey, M.P. (1983). Long-term effects of oestrogen therapy – preliminary report of a Medical Research Council survey. Presented at the Symposium on Advances in the Management of the Menopause, Royal College of Obstetricians and Gynaecologists, Dec 1983.

IARC (1979). IARC Monographs on the Evaluation of the Carcinogenic Risk of Chemicals to Humans. *Sex hormones* (II). International Agency for Research on Cancer, Lyon.

Jelovsek, F.R., Hammond, C.B., Woodard, B.H., Draffin, R., Lee, K.L., Creasman, W.T., and Parker, R.T. (1980). Risk of exogenous estrogen therapy and endometrial cancer. *Amer. J. Obstet. Gynecol.* **137**, 85–91.

Jick, H., Walker, A.M., and Rothman, K.J. (1980a). The epidemic of endometrial cancer: a commentary. *Amer. J. publ. Health* **70**, 264–7.

Jick, H., Walker, A.M., Watkins, R.N., D'Ewart, D.C., Hunter, J.R., Danford,

A., Madsen, S., Dinan, B.J., and Rothman, K.J. (1980b). Replacement estrogens and breast cancer. *Amer. J. Epidemiol.* **112**, 586–94.

Jick, H., Walker, A.M., Watkins, R.N., D'Ewart, D.C., Hunter, J.R., Danford, A., Madsen, S., Dinan, B.J., and Rothman, K.J. (1980c). Oral contraceptives and breast cancer. *Amer. J. Epidemiol.* **112**, 577–85.

Jick, H., Watkins, R.N., Hunter, J.R., Dinan, B.J., Madsen, S., Rothman, K.J., and Walker, A.M. (1979). Replacement estrogens and endometrial cancer. *New Engl. J. Med.* **300**, 218–22.

Kay, C.R. (1980). Progestogens before and after the menopause. *Lancet* **ii**, 811–2.

Kalache, A., McPherson, K., Barltrop, K., and Vessey, M.P. (1983). Oral contraceptives and breast cancer. *Brit. J. Hosp. Med.* **30**, 278–83.

Kaufman, D.W., Shapiro, S., Slone, D., Rosenberg, L., Miettinen, O.S., Stolley, P.D., Knapp, R.C., Leavitt, T., Watring, W.G., Rosenshein, N.B., Lewis, J.L. Schottenfeld, M.D., and Engle, R.L. (1980). Decreased risk of endometrial cancer among oral contraceptive users. *New Engl. J. Med.* **303**, 1045–7.

Kelsey, J.L., Fischer, D.B., Holford, T.R., Li Volsi, V.A., Mostow, E.D., Goldenberg, I.S., and White, C. (1981). Exogenous estrogens and other factors in the epidemiology of breast cancer. *J. nat. Cancer Inst.* **67**, 327–33.

Kelsey, J.L., Li Volsi, V.A., Holford, T.R., Fischer, D.B., Mostow, E.D., Schwartz, P.E., O'Connor, T., and White, C. (1982). A case-control study of cancer of the endometrium. *Amer. J. Epidemiol.* **116**, 333–42.

Kinlen, L.J. Badaracco, M.A., Moffett, J., and Vessey, M.P. (1974). A survey of the use of oestrogens during pregnancy in the United Kingdom and of the genito-urinary cancer mortality and incidence rates in young people in England and Wales. *J. Obstet. Gynaecol. Brit. Commonwlth* **81**, 849–55.

La Vecchia, C., Franceschi, S., Gallus, G., Decarli, A., Colombo, E., Mangioni, C., and Tognoni, G. (1982). Oestrogens and obesity as risk factors for endometrial cancer in Italy. *Int. J. Epidemiol.* **11**, 120–6.

McDonald, T.W., Annegers, J.F., O'Fallon, W.M., Dockerty, M.B., Malkasian, G.D., and Kurland, L.T. (1977). Exogenous estrogen and endometrial carcinoma: case-control and incidence study. *Amer. J. Obstet. Gynecol.* **127**, 572–80.

McPherson, K., Neil, A., Vessey, M.P., and Doll, R. (1983). Oral contraceptives and breast cancer. *Lancet* **ii**, 1414–5.

Mack, T.M., Pike, M.C., Henderson, B.E., Pfeffer, R.I., Gerkins, V.R., Arthur, M., and Brown, S.E., (1976). Estrogens and endometrial cancer in a retirement community. *New Engl. J. Med.* **294**, 1262–7.

Marrett, L.D., Meigs, J.W., and Flannery, J.T. (1982). Trends in the incidence of cancer of the corpus uteri in Connecticut, 1964–79, in relation to consumption of exogenous estrogens. *Amer. J. Epidemiol.* **116**, 57–67.

Mathews, P.N., Millis, R.R., and Hayward, J.L. (1981). Breast cancer in women who have taken contraceptive steroids. *Brit. med. J.* **282**, 774–6.

Merletti, F. and Cole, P. (1981). Detection bias and endometrial cancer. *Lancet* **ii**, 579–80.

Monaghan, J.M. and Sirisena, L.A.W. (1978). Stilboestrol and vaginal clear-cell adenocarcinoma syndrome. *Brit. med. J.* **i**, 1588–90.

Newhouse, M.L., Pearson, R.M., Fullerton, J.M., Boesen, E.A.M., and Shannon, H.S. (1977). A case control study of carcinoma of the ovary. *Brit. J. prev. soc. Med.* **31**, 148–53.

Noller, K.L., Townsend, D.E., Kaufman, R.H., Barnes, A.B., Robboy, S.J.,

Fish, C.R., Jefferies, J.A., Bergstralh, E.J., O'Brien, P.C., McGorray, S.P., and Scully, R. (1983). Maturation of vaginal and cervical epithelium in women exposed *in utero* to diethylstilbestrol (DESAD Project). *Amer. J. Obstet. Gynecol.* **146**, 279–85.

Öbrink, A., Bunne, G., Collen, J., and Tjernberg, B. (1981). Estrogen regimen of women with endometrial carcinoma. *Acta Obstet. Gynecol. scand.* **60**, 191–7.

Ory, H.W., Conger, S.B., Naib, Z., Tyler, C.W., and Hatcher, R.A. (1977). Preliminary analysis of oral contraceptive use and risk of developing premalignant lesions of the uterine cervix. In *Pharmacology of steroid contraceptive drugs* (ed. S. Garratini and H.W. Berendes), pp. 211–24. Raven Press, New York.

Paffenbarger, R.S., Kampert, J.B., and Chang, H-G. (1979). Oral contraceptives and breast cancer risk. Eds *l'INSERM* **83**, 93–114.

Peritz, E., Ramcharan, S., Frank, J., Brown, W.L., Huang, S., and Ray, R. (1977). The incidence of cervical cancer and duration of oral contraceptive use. *Amer. J. Epidemiol.* **106**, 462–9.

Persson, I. (1983). Climacteric treatment with estrogens and estrogen-progestogen combinations: the risk of endometrial neoplasia. Results of a cohort study. Abstracts of Uppsala Dissertations from the Faculty of Medicine, No 471.

Pike, M.C., Henderson, B.E., Casagrande, J.T., Rosario, I., and Gray, G.E. (1981). Oral contraceptive use and early abortion as risk factors for breast cancer in young women. *Brit. J. Cancer* **43**, 72–6.

Pike, M.C., Henderson, B.E., Krailo, M.D., Duke, A., and Roy, S. (1983). Breast cancer in young women and use of oral contraceptives: possible modifying effect of formulation and age at use. *Lancet* **ii**, 926–30.

Pituitary Adenoma Study Group (1983). Pituitary adenomas and oral contraceptives: a multicenter case-control study. *Fertil. Steril.* **39**, 753–60.

Ramcharan, S., Pellegrin, F.A., Ray, R., and Hsu, J-P. (1981). The Walnut Creek contraceptive drug study: a prospective study of the side effects of oral contraceptive use. *The Walnut Creek Contraceptive Drug Study*, Vol. III. US Government Printing Office, Washington, DC.

Rooks, J.B., Ory, H.W., Ishak, K.G., Strauss, L.T., Greenspan, J.R., Paganini-Hill, A., and Tyler, C.W. (1979). Epidemiology of hepatocellular adenoma. The role of oral contraceptive use. *J. Amer. med. Assoc.* **242**, 644–8.

Rosenberg, L., Miller, D.R., Kaufman, D.W., Helmrich, S.P., Stolley, P.D., Schottenfeld, D., and Shapiro, S. (1984). Breast cancer and oral contraceptive use. *Amer. J. Epidemiol.* **119**, 167–76.

Rosenberg, L., Shapiro, S., Slone, D., Kaufman, D.W., Helmrich, S.P., Miettinen, O.S., Stolley, P.D., Rosenshein, N.B., Schottenfeld, D., and Engle, R.L. (1982). Epithelial ovarian cancer and combination oral contraceptives. *J. Amer. med. Assoc.* **247**, 3210–12.

Ross, R.K., Paganini-Hill, A., Gerkins, V.R., Mack, T.M., Pfeffer, R., Arthur, M., and Henderson, B.E. (1980). A case-control study of menopausal estrogen therapy and breast cancer. *J. Amer. med. Assoc.* **243**, 1635–9.

Royal College of General Practitioners (1981). Breast cancer and oral contraceptives: findings in Royal College of General Practitioners Study. *Brit. med. J.* **282**, 2089–93.

Salmi, T. (1979). Risk factors in endometrial carcinoma with special reference to the use of estrogens. *Acta Obstet. Gynecol. scand.* Suppl. **86**, 1–119.

Scully, R.E. and Welch, W.R. (1981). Pathology of the female genital tract after prenatal exposure to diethylstilbestrol. In *Developmental effects of diethylstil-*

bestrol (DES) in pregnancy (ed. A.L. Herbst and H.A. Bern), pp. 26–45. Thieme Stratton, New York.

Shapiro, S., Kaufman, D.W., Slone, D., Rosenberg, L., Miettinen, O.S., Stolley, P.D., Rosenshein, N.B., Watring, W.G., Leavitt, T., and Knapp, R.C. (1980). Recent and past use of conjugated estrogens in relation to adenocarcinoma of the endometrium. *New Engl. J. Med.* **303**, 485–9.

Sherman, B., Wallace, R., and Bean, J. (1983). Estrogen use and breast cancer. Interaction with body mass. *Cancer* **51**, 1527–31.

Shy, K.K., McTiernan, A.M., Daling, J.R., and Weiss, N.S. (1983). Oral contraceptive use and the occurrence of pituitary prolactinoma. *J. Amer. med. Assoc.* **249**, 2204–7.

Silverberg, S.G. and Makowski, E.L. (1975). Endometrial carcinoma in young women taking oral contraceptive agents. *Obstet. Gynecol.* **46**, 503–6.

Smith, D.C., Prentice, R., Thompson, D.J., and Herrmann, W.L. (1975). Association of exogenous estrogen and endometrial carcinoma. *New Engl. J. Med.* **293**, 1164–7.

Smith, O.W. (1948). Diethylstilbestrol in the prevention and treatment of complications of pregnancy. *Amer. J. Obstet. Gynecol.* **56**, 821–34.

Smith, O.W. and Smith, G. van S. (1949). The influence of diethylstilbestrol on the progress and outcome of pregnancy as based on a comparison of treated with untreated primigravidas. *Amer. J. Obstet. Gynecol.* **58**, 994–1005.

Spencer, J.D., Millis, R.R., and Hayward, J.L. (1978). Contraceptive steroids and breast cancer. *Brit. med. J.* **i**, 1024–6.

Spengler, R.F., Clarke, E.A., Woolever, C.A., Newman, A.M., and Osborn, R.W. (1981). Exogenous estrogens and endometrial cancer: a case-control study and assessment of potential biases. *Amer. J. Epidemiol.* **114**, 497–506.

Stavraky, K.M., Collins, J.A., Donner, A., and Wells, G.A. (1981). A comparison of estrogen use by women with endometrial cancer, gynecologic disorders, and other illnesses. *Amer. J. Obstet. Gynecol.* **141**, 547–55.

Stern, E., Forsythe, A.B., Youkeles, L., and Coffelt, C.F. (1977). Steroid contraceptive use and cervical dysplasia: increased risk of progression. *Science, N.Y.* **196**, 1460–2.

Stolk, J.G., Vooijs, G.P., Aartsen, E.J., and Heintz, A.P. (1982). Het teratogene effect van diethylstilbestrol in de zwangerschap; de omvang van het DES-probleem in Nederland. *Ned. Tijdschr. Geneesk.* **126**, 1350–8.

Sturdee, D.W., Wade-Evans, T., Paterson, M.E.L., Thom, M., and Studd, J.W.W. (1978). Relations between bleeding pattern, endometrial histology, and oestrogen treatment in menopausal women. *Brit. med. J.* **i**, 1575–7.

Swan, S.H. and Brown, W.L. (1981). Oral contraceptive use, sexual activity and cervical carcinoma. *Amer. J. Obstet. Gynecol.* **139**, 52–7.

Swan, S.H. and Pettiti, D.B. (1982). A review of problems of bias and confounding in epidemiologic studies of cervical neoplasia and oral contraceptive use. *Amer. J. Epidemiol.* **115**, 10–18.

Swyer, G.I.M. (1983). Oral contraceptives and cancer. *Lancet* **ii**, 1019.

Swyer, G.I.M. and Law, R.G. (1954). An evaluation of the prophylactic ante-natal use of stilboestrol. Preliminary report. *J. Endocrinol.* **10**, vi.

Thomas, D.B. (1972). Relationship of oral contraceptives to cervical carcinogenesis. *Obstet. Gynecol.* **40**, 508–18.

Thomas, D.B. (1982). Non-contraceptive exogenous estrogens and risk of breast cancer: a review. *Breast Cancer Res. Treat.* **2**, 203–11.

Thomas, D.B., Persing, J.P., and Hutchinson, W.B. (1982). Exogenous estrogens and other risk factors for breast cancer in women with benign breast diseases. *J. nat. Cancer Inst.* **69**, 1017–25.

Trapido, E.J. (1981). A prospective cohort study of oral contraceptives and breast cancer. *J. nat. Cancer Inst.* **67**, 1011–5.

Vessey, M.P. (1983). Contraception and benign breast disease. Epidemiological studies. *Contraception et sein* (ed. R. Renaud and B. Gairard), pp. 63–9. Masson, Paris.

Vessey, M.P. (1985). Oral contraceptives and breast cancer. In *Proceedings of the Symposium on Interpretation of Epidemiological Evidence* (ed. N. Wald). IARC, Lyon. (In press.)

Vessey, M.P. and Bungay, G.T. (1982). Benefits and risks of hormone therapy in the menopause. In *Recent Advances in Community Medicine*, Vol. 2 (ed. A. Smith), pp. 77–94. Churchill Livingstone, Edinburgh.

Vessey, M., Baron, J., Doll, R., McPherson, K., and Yeates, D. (1983b). Oral contraceptives and breast cancer: final report of an epidemiological study. *Brit. J. Cancer* **47**, 455–62.

Vessey, M.P., Fairweather, D.V.I., Norman-Smith, B., and Buckley, J. (1983a). A randomized double-blind controlled trial of the value of stilboestrol therapy in pregnancy: long-term follow-up of mothers and their offspring. *Brit. J. Obstet. Gynaecol.* **90**, 1007–17.

Vessey, M.P., Lawless, M., McPherson, K., and Yeates, D. (1983c). Neoplasia of the cervix uteri and contraception – a possible adverse effect of the pill. *Lancet* **ii**, 930–4.

Vessey, M.P., Lawless, M., McPherson, K., and Yeates, D. (1983d). Oral contraceptives and cervical cancer. *Lancet* **ii**, 1358–9.

Vessey, M.P., McPherson, K., and Doll, R. (1981). Breast cancer and oral contraceptives: findings in the Oxford–Family Planning Association contraceptive study. *Brit. med. J.* **287**, 2093–4.

Vessey, M.P., McPherson, K., Yeates, D., and Doll, R. (1982). Oral contraceptive use and abortion before first term pregnancy in relation to breast cancer risk. *Brit. J. Cancer* **45**, 327–31.

Walker, A.M. and Jick, H. (1979). Cancer of the corpus uteri: increasing incidence in the United States, 1970–1975. *Amer. J. Epidemiol.* **110**, 47–51.

Weiss, N.S., Lyon, J.L., Krishnamurthy, S., Dietert, S.E., Liff, J.M., and Daling, J.R. (1982). Noncontraceptive estrogen use and the occurrence of ovarian cancer. *J. nat. Cancer Inst.* **68**, 95–8.

Weiss, N.S., Lyon, J.L., Liff, J.M., Vollmer, W.M., and Daling, J.R. (1981). Incidence of ovarian cancer in relation to the use of oral contraceptives. *Int. J. Cancer* **28**, 669–71.

Weiss, N.S. and Sayvetz, T.A. (1980). Incidence of endometrial cancer in relation to the use of oral contraceptives. *New Engl. J. Med.* **302**, 551–4.

Weiss, N.S., Szekely, D.R., and Austin, D.F. (1976). Increasing incidence of endometrial cancer in the United States. *New Engl. J. Med.* **294**, 1259–62.

Weiss, N.S., Szekely, D.R., English, D.R., and Schweid, A.I. (1979). Endometrial cancer in relation to patterns of menopausal estrogen use. *J. Amer. med. Assoc.* **242**, 261–4.

Whitehead, M.I., Townsend, P.T., Pryse-Davies, J., Ryder, T.A., and King, R.J.B. (1981). Effects of estrogens and progestins on the biochemistry and morphology of the postmenopausal endometrium. *New. Engl. J. Med.* **305**, 1599–1605.

WHO Scientific Group (1978). *Steroid contraception and the risk of neoplasia.* Technical Report Series, No 619.

Wigle, D.T., Grace, M., and Smith, E.S.O. (1978). Estrogen use and cancer of the uterine corpus in Alberta. *Can. med. Assoc. J.* **118**, 1276–8.

Willett, W.C., Bain, C., Hennekens, C.H., Rosner, B., and Speizer, F.E. (1981). Oral contraceptives and risk of ovarian cancer. *Cancer* **48**, 1684–7.

Worth, A.J. and Boyes, D.A. (1972). A case-control study into the possible effects of birth control pills on pre-clinical carcinoma of the cervix. *J. Obst. Gynecol. Brit. Commonwlth* **79**, 673–9.

Ziel, H.K. and Finkle, W.D. (1975). Increased risk of endometrial carcinoma among users of conjugated estrogens. *New Engl. J. Med.* **293**, 1167–70.

9 Endogenous hormones

M.C. Pike

Hormone-related cancers, in particular those of the breast, endometrium, ovary, and prostate, figure prominently in the category of cancers affected by 'life-style', and these tumours account for approximately 10 per cent of all cancer cases in men and 40 per cent of all cancer cases in women in the U.K. (see Table 1). Normal growth and function of each of the endocrine target organs shown in the Table are controlled by one or more steroid or polypeptide hormones, and, in line with the concept that hormones can cause, i.e. increase the incidence of, neoplasia which was developed by Bittner (1947), Huggins (1967), and Furth (1975), it has been shown in experimental animals that the incidence of neoplasia at the majority of these sites can be raised by an increase in hormonal stimulation of the target organ. There is a progressive transition from normal growth to hyperplasia to neoplasia; the neoplasms produced are initially hormone-responsive, but they beome autonomous with time. Primary prevention of these neoplasms should be possible by modifying the factors (mostly unknown) which directly affect the secretion and metabolism of the responsible hormones and since such hormones affect cell division rates of normal, hyperplastic, and even early neoplastic cells, understanding these

Table 1. Age-adjusted† annual incidence rates of hormone-related malignant neoplasms (Birmingham and West Midlands Region 1973–1976)

Site	Men	Women
Breast	0.5	56.4
Prostate	18.6	
Ovary		11.0
Endometrium		9.4
Testis	2.9	
Thyroid	0.6	1.2
Bone	0.8	0.7
Total	23.4	78.7
All sites‡	246.9	193.6

† Age-adjusted to 'world population' (Waterhouse *et al.* 1982)
‡ Excluding non-melanoma skin

factors should lead to effective intervention even late along the course of transition from normal-functioning cells to hormone-responsive neoplastic cells.

In this review the evidence relevant to an 'increased hormonal stimulus' hypothesis for cancers of each of the sites shown in Table 1 is discussed. For cancer of the endometrium, breast, prostate, thyroid, and bone the hypothesis is straightforward, and simply states that increased bioavailable levels of the steroid and polypeptide hormones, which increase mitotic activity in the organ, increase the risk of each of these cancers. For ovarian carcinoma the hypothesized mode of action of the responsible hormone is indirect and the ovarian epithelial cell proliferation is in response to the 'injury' to the ovarian surface caused by ovulation. For germ-cell cancer of the testis the excess hormone hypothesis is fundamentally different and refers to the mother's hormone status during the relevant pregnancy: evidence is presented suggesting that excessive bioavailable oestrogen during the first few weeks of gestation affects testicular differentiation, and altered germ cells are then stimulated to form testicular cancers after puberty in response to pituitary gonadotropins.

Endometrial cancer will be discussed first, as the relationships between the responsible hormones and this cancer are the most completely understood.

Cancer of the endometrium

Proliferation of endometrial tissue is induced by oestrogen 'unopposed' by progesterone: this is clearly seen in histological studies of the endometrium over the duration of the normal menstrual cycle. Animal studies have found that the risk of endometrial cancer can be increased by administration of stilboestrol in rabbits and of oestrone sulphate in mice (Meissner *et al.* 1957; Papadaki *et al.* 1979).

The importance of oestrogens in the aetiology of endometrial cancer has long been recognized; early studies of women with endometrial cancer demonstrated evidence of high levels of circulating oestrogens, including ovarian stromal hyperplasia and a high vaginal cornification index (Ayre and Bauld 1946; Sommers and Meissner 1957). The importance of oestrogens is also suggested by the observation that obesity is a major risk factor for endometrial cancer in postmenopausal women (see Judd *et al.* 1980 and references therein). The level of circulating oestrogens in a postmenopausal woman is determined to an important degree by her body weight (Siiteri and MacDonald 1973); plasma oestrone is largely derived by extraglandular conversion of the adrenal androgen androstenedione, and the rate of this conversion increases with body weight. The biologically more active oestradiol is then derived from peripheral conversion of oestrone. This last step may be particularly important, since, although the concentration of oestrone is two to three times that of oestradiol in postmenopausal women, oestradiol is more strongly bound to cytosol receptors in the endometrium, and there is some evidence that oestrone has no effect on this organ (Gurpide 1978).

Circulating oestradiol is either bound to sex-hormone-binding globulin, more loosely bound to albumin, or is in a 'free' state. There is debate as to which fraction is available to tissue, but it is generally accepted that the sex-hormone-binding globulin-bound fraction is not, and high levels of sex-hormone-binding globulin generally imply a low percentage of free oestradiol. The plasma concentration of sex-hormone-binding globulin is lower in obese women (de Moor and Joossens 1970; O'Dea *et al.* 1979). Obese women thus not only have greater concentrations of circulating oestradiol, but the oestradiol is more available to tissue.

The few published studies which directly measured plasma oestrogen levels in cases of endometrial cancer and controls all showed increased levels in the cases (Aleem *et al.* 1976; Benjamin and Deutsch 1976; MacDonald *et al.* 1978; Judd *et al.* 1980). Three of these studies considered whether the higher levels in cases were only a reflection of the greater average weight of the cases; two concluded that the higher oestrogen levels in cases did merely reflect their greater weight (Macdonald *et al.* 1978; Judd *et al.* 1980), but Benjamin and Deutsch (1976) found increased oestrogen levels in cases even after adjusting for differences in weight. The oestrogen-excess hypothesis would clearly be greatly strengthened if the oestrogen levels adjusted for weight had been increased in all three studies: further studies of cases and controls matched for weight (and certain other endometrial cancer risk factors) are needed to clarify this important issue. These studies need to consider the quantity and binding constants of each of the various oestradiol fractions in the blood, i.e. sex-hormone-binding globulin-bound, albumin-bound, and free. Recent results comparing the quality of the binding of albumin to oestradiol in the U.K. and Japan suggests that this binding may be of very variable strength (Moore *et al.* 1983).

The oestrogen-excess hypothesis predicts, of course, that menopausal oestrogen replacement therapy would increase the risk of endometrial cancer. The risk ratios observed in case-control studies have been high, usually in the range of three to eight, and in most, increasing risk with increasing dose and duration of treatment has been apparent (see Vessey, Chapter 8 of this book).

Progesterone and other progestogens have profound effects on the endometrium and are therapeutically useful in treating both endometrial hyperplasia and carcinoma. In the endometrium progestogens have two anti-oestrogenic effects: they increase the activity of the dehydrogenase that converts oestradiol to the biologically less active oestrone (Tseng and

Gurpide 1976), and they decrease the concentration of oestradiol receptors (Hsueh *et al.* 1975). For these reasons, there is considerably more endometrial mitotic activity in the follicular phase, during which circulating oestrogen is 'unopposed' by progesterone, compared with the luteal phase of the menstrual cycle. One would therefore predict that a high frequency of anovulatory cycles, during which time no progesterone 'opposes' the circulating oestrogen, would increase the risk of endometrial cancer. Premenopausal endometrial cancer cases do have an increased rate of amenorrhoea (Henderson *et al.* 1983) and hence one may presume a higher frequency of anovulatory cycles; the situation is, however, confounded by the fact that this is commonly found in association with obesity, but when adjustment is made for weight there is still a much increased risk in women with amenorrhea. A protective role for progestogens is also supported by the increased risk of endometrial cancer in users of sequential oral contraceptives, with a high dose of 'unopposed' oestrogen being given for two of every four weeks, and the decreased risk in users of combined oral contraceptives, with an oestrogen and a progestogen always being given in combination (see p. 187).

Breast cancer

The breast cancer risk factors of early age at menarche and delayed age at menopause indicate that ovarian activity is an important determinant of risk of this cancer.

The mitotic activity of breast epithelium varies markedly during the normal menstrual cycle, with the peak activity occurring late in the luteal phase (Ferguson and Anderson 1981), suggesting that, in addition to oestrogen and prolactin, progesterone may be important in inducing mitotic activity in breast epithelium. This effect of progesterone would be in sharp distinction to its effect on endometrial tissue, where the peak mitotic activity is in the follicular phase of the cycle. It agrees however with the experimental finding that progesterone induces ductal growth in rodent breast tissue (see Dulbecco *et al.* 1982 and references therein).

Factors contributing to elevated endogenous levels of oestrogen would be expected to elevate risk. Thus, increased body weight, by contributing to elevated endogenous oestrogen levels as we discussed above, should elevate risk in postmenopausal women. This effect has been found in the studies of de Waard *et al.* (1977) and in the long-term follow-up study of the American Cancer Society (Lew and Garfinkel 1979).

A few studies of oestrogen levels in premenopausal breast cancer patients and controls have been reported. England *et al.* (1974) found an average elevation of 15 per cent in total plasma oestrogens in a small study of 40–49-year-old patients. A similar increase was reported by Cole *et al.* (1978) for total urinary oestrogens. England *et al.* (1974) also studied oestradiol levels in postmenopausal breast cancer cases and controls and found that, on average, the levels were 30 per cent higher in cases; no data were given on the weight of these women. Moore *et al.* (1982) studied blood levels of oestradiol in postmenopausal cases and controls as well, and found that not only was the average level of oestradiol some 27 per cent higher in the cases, but also that both their sex-hormone-binding globulin and albumin levels were depressed so that their average non-protein bound oestradiol level was approximately 3½ times higher than that in the controls. There have been several studies on urinary oestrogens in postmenopausal cases and controls; most, however, included very few subjects. Data on total oestrogens from four of the five studies (Brown 1958; Persson and Risholm 1964; Marmorston *et al.* 1965; Gronroos and Aho 1968; Arguelles *et al.* 1973) suggest increased levels of oestrogen in the cases; weights of the women in these studies were not given.

A number of studies of prolactin levels in breast cancer patients and controls have been reported. Many of these studies have had small numbers of patients and controls, and it is not always clear that the investigators have controlled carefully for the marked variation in prolactin levels that occurs during a 24-hour period. Nevertheless, of six patient-control comparisons of premenopausal women (Sheth *et al.* 1975; Hill *et al.* 1976; Cole *et al.* 1977; Malarkey *et al.* 1977), five showed higher levels in the patients, and, on the average, the values for the breast cancer patients were elevated some 1.5 to 2-fold. The results of a similar study in postmenopausal women by Hill *et al.* (1976) also showed a clear elevation of prolactin levels in U.S. white breast cancer patients and in Japanese patients, but not in South African black patients, when compared with controls. A number of other studies of postmenopausal women have not found any differences (see Henderson *et al.* 1982 for references).

If progesterone increases breast cancer risk, then regular and short ovulatory cycles should be more common in breast cancer patients than in controls. There are not many studies which address this issue; but Henderson *et al.* (1981), in their study of young breast cancer cases, found that the rapid onset of regular cycles after menarche was associated with a doubling of breast cancer risk, and the recent paper by Olsson *et al.* (1983) found that breast cancer patients had shorter cycles than controls. MacMahon *et al.* (1982) found that the rapid onset of regular cycles was more common in countries with a high breast cancer rate.

There is some evidence that the increased risk of breast cancer in family members of breast cancer cases may be partly mediated by higher levels of oestrogens, progesterone, and prolactin. Henderson *et al.* (1975) found elevated serum levels of all three hormones in daughters of young breast cancer cases. Urinary oestrogens and progesterone in teenage daughters of breast cancer patients have also been shown to be elevated in a recent study by Trichopoulos *et al.* (1981), and Levin and Malarkey (1981) found elevated mean 24-hour serum prolactin levels in daughters, mostly nulliparous, of breast cancer cases. Fishman *et al.* (1978), however, did not find high values for oestrogens or prolactin when they studied women with a mean age of 32 and a mean parity of 1.8 from breast cancer families.

The results of Henderson *et al.* (1975) and Trichopoulos *et al.* (1981) suggest that the teenage daughters of breast cancer patients were ovulating more frequently than were other girls of their age even after allowing for age at menarche. Such differences in ovulation frequency may well disappear with increasing age and, probably more importantly, after a pregnancy. This may be the explanation for the different results reported by Fishman *et al.* (1978).

A major decrease in breast cancer risk may be achieved by early first full-term pregnancy (MacMahon *et al.* 1973). The protective effect of early full-term pregnancy could be due, at least in part, to a reduction in prolactin levels in the long term (i.e. when the woman is not pregnant or actually lactating). This notion was suggested by the steady decrease with age in mean prolactin levels of women but not of men (Vekemans and Robyn 1975; del Pozo and Brownell 1979), and Pike *et al.* (1979) published some preliminary evidence that prolactin levels are lower in parous than in nulliparous women. Yu *et al.* (1981) confirmed the finding by showing that a group of nuns and their nulliparous sisters had early-morning prolactin levels some 35 per cent higher than their parous sisters of the same age, and Kwa *et al.* (1981) have reported similar results. The protective effect of first full-term pregnancy could also be partly mediated by a permanent increase in sex-hormone-binding globulin levels induced by such a pregnancy – preliminary evidence suggesting this effect has been reported by Bernstein *et al.* (1985). They report, however, that the position is confused by the fact that nulliparous women tend to have longer cycles than parous women.

Cancer of the prostate

Although prostatic cancer is currently the second most common cancer in men in the U.K., little is known about the aetiology of the disease. The principle growth-regulating hormones of the prostate are testosterone and its metabolite dihydrotestosterone (O'Malley 1971; Wilson 1972); a testosterone-excess hypothesis for prostate cancer is therefore suggested, i.e. that elevated levels of testosterone and/or dihydrotestosterone over the course of many decades lead to prostate gland hyperplasia and carcinoma.

The strongest evidence in favour of this hormonal hypothesis has been provided by Noble (1977) and Brown *et al.* (1979). Noble showed that testosterone alone can produce prostatic adenocarcinoma in rats, and Brown and his colleagues induced adenocarcinoma of the prostate in male rats by raising their circulating testosterone levels by parabiosing them to castrated males. These findings are of particular importance since adenocarcinoma of the prostate has apparently not been induced experimentally by any other means.

There have been a few epidemiological studies which have compared circulating testosterone levels in prostate cancer cases and controls. Ghanadian *et al.* (1979) found that prostatic cancer cases had a higher mean serum testosterone level than did healthy controls of the same age. Prostate cancer cases in this study had a clear excess of high values: 7 of the 33 cases but only 1 of the 42 controls had a serum testosterone level greater than 30 nmol/100 ml. Ahluwalia *et al.* (1981) also found significantly higher levels of serum testosterone in U.S. black prostatic cancer cases compared with age-matched black controls, but they did not find any difference between prostatic cancer cases and controls in African blacks. Hammond *et al.* (1978) did not find any difference in androgen levels in their case-control study, but they studied only 11 cases of cancer of the prostate.

Other epidemiological data relevant to the elevated testosterone hypothesis are sparse, but what information is available is generally supportive. Autopsy studies show that patients with cirrhosis of the liver have lower rates of cancer of the prostate than do controls of the same age (Glantz 1964), and alcohol depresses circulating testosterone levels (Gordon *et al.* 1976). Castration produces a palliative effect on advanced prostatic cancer (Huggins and Hodges 1941), and prostatic cancer is seemingly unknown in castrates (Hovenian and Deming 1948).

Epithelial ovarian cancer

The hypothesis that this tumour is caused by an excess of growth-regulating hormone differs in a fundamental way from the above hypotheses for cancer of the endometrium, breast, and prostate. In this instance, the responsible hormones, namely gonadotrophins, are not directly stimulatory to the ovarian epithelial cells, but instead, the epithelial cells replicate after each ovulation to cover the exposed surface of the ovary. This indirect hormone-excess hypothesis predicts that any respite from the normal cyclic gonadotrophin stimulation of the ovary would be protective.

The hypothesis is supported by compelling evidence from a number of case-control studies showing that the risk of ovarian cancer progressively declines with each succeeding pregnancy (Annegers *et al.* 1979; and see

Casagrande *et al.* 1979 and references therein), and that oral contraceptive use protects against the disease (see p. 181).

Cancer of the testis

The age-specific incidence curve of cancer of the testis shows a broad peak between ages 20 and 40, with a decline to low levels with increasing age. This suggests that gestational, and/or early childhood, events are probably critical in the pathogenesis of the disease. This is also strongly suggested by the fact that the major known risk factor for testicular cancer is a history of an undescended testis, i.e. cryptorchidism (see Depue *et al.* 1983 and references therein).

A number of epidemiological studies which investigated gestational factors and events directly, by questioning the mothers of testicular cancer cases and mothers of controls, have recently been reported (Henderson *et al.* 1979; Schottenfeld *et al.* 1980; Depue *et al.* 1983). Increasing maternal weight immediately before the index pregnancy was found to be associated with an increasing risk of cancer of the testis (Depue *et al.* 1983). The clearest gradient of risk was obtained when weight was expressed in terms of Quetelet's index (QI = (weight in kg)/(square of height in metres)) – an increase in QI from 18.5 to 22.5 increased the risk of testicular cancer approximately 2.5-fold: for a 1.68-metre (5ft 6in) woman this is an increase of only 12kg from approximately 52 to 64kg.

Hormone administration during the first trimester of pregnancy was consistently found to be associated with an increased risk of cancer of the testis. The hormones implicated were stilboestrol and other oestrogens, and in particular pregnancy tests (Depue *et al.* 1983). The implication of pregnancy tests is particularly interesting because they generally employed a mixture of an oestrogen and a progestogen and were given as a single injection.

Both these risk factors – increasing maternal weight and hormone administration during early pregnancy – have also been identified as risk factors for cryptorchidism (Rothman and Louik 1978; Depue 1984).

'Excessive' nausea of pregnancy, as indicated by treatment with drugs, was also found to be a risk factor for testicular cancer in first-born pregnancies (Depue *et al.* 1983). It is difficult to separate the effect of severe nausea from the effect of the drugs used to treat it, but the fact that the risk appears to be confined to first births argues strongly that the severe nausea itself is the risk factor. The cause of nausea of pregnancy is not definitely known, but it almost invariably starts in the first two months of gestation when oestrogen levels rise rapidly in the mother. This rise has been suggested as the event inciting nausea because exogenous oestrogens commonly produce nausea when first administered, and nausea in pregnancy may similarly be due to the abrupt rise in the level of oestrogen. Nausea as a risk factor may thus be related to the risk factor of hormone administration. That the mother's nausea should be a risk factor only in first-born sons suggests that the first pregnancy is endocrinologically different from subsequent pregnancies. It is the mother's first experience of very high oestrogen levels, and her sex-hormone-binding globulin levels rise 5 to 10-fold by mid-pregnancy to bind the increased levels of oestradiol. It is possible that the production of sex-hormone-binding globulin lags behind the increasing oestrogen synthesis in some women for about the first 12 weeks of pregnancy, the critical period for urogenital differentiation. Such an effect would be expected to be greatest and most frequent at a first pregnancy, and would lead to an especially increased level of bioavailable oestrogen.

Increasing weight has a strong inhibitory effect on sex-hormone-binding globulin production, so that increased bioavailability of oestrogens during the first trimester of pregnancy may also be the mode of action of the increasing risk of testicular cancer with increasing maternal weight.

The risk factors discussed above are probably all related to events in the first trimester of pregnancy when the testis is being formed. The other main risk factor identified for cancer of the testis was early delivery, as measured by a low birthweight (Depue *et al.* 1983): this suggests that events in the last few weeks of pregnancy are also important in the aetiology of testicular cancer.

There is roughly a 7-fold increased risk of testicular cancer in a person with cryptorchidism (an approximately 12-fold increased risk in the affected testis and an approximately 3-fold increased risk in the unaffected testis (Henderson *et al.* 1979; Schottenfeld *et al.* 1980)). Cryptorchidism must partly predispose to testicular cancer because of the defect itself, but the increased risk in the contralateral testis suggests that the increased levels of follicle-stimulating hormone (the hormone responsible for germ cell proliferation) associated with both unilateral and bilateral cryptorchidism (Werder *et al.* 1976; van Vliet *et al.* 1980) may lead to increased activity in the normal testis and hence to an increased risk of cancer. Microscopic examination of the contralateral descended testis in infants and young boys does reveal, however, defects similar to those found in the undescended testis (Mengel *et al.* 1974). The difference in the rates of cancer in the two testes may therefore merely reflect a quantitative difference in frequency of the (unknown) precursor lesion.

Boys born underweight also have a higher risk of being cryptorchid (Swerdlow *et al.* 1983; Depue 1984). It is not clear whether the cryptorchidism related to events in the first trimester carries the same, or higher or lower, risk of subsequent testicular cancer, than cryptorchidism related to short gestation.

Thyroid cancer

The pituitary hormone, thyroid stimulating hormone, is the principal hormone regulating the growth and function of the thyroid gland, and we therefore suggest, following the same line of reasoning we have used above, a thyroid stimulating hormone-excess hypothesis for thyroid cancer. This hypothesis is supported by the observation that growth of some thyroid cancers is dependent on thyroid stimulating hormone secretion so that suppression of thyroid stimulating hormone release by administration of thyroxine is often an effective treatment for thyroid carcinomas (Crile 1966). The hypothesis is also supported by experimental work. Sustained elevation of thyroid stimulating hormone induces thyroid tumours in rodents (Axelrad and Leblond 1955), and the mechanism by which such elevated thyroid stimulating hormone levels are achieved appears to be unimportant.

Thyroid cancer is roughly 2.5 times more common in women than in men. Under age 10, however, the ratio is quite close to one; it then changes abruptly around puberty so that the ratio of girls to boys is roughly 3 in the 10–19-year-old age group. The ratio remains at about 3 until the menopause in women when it begins to decline steadily, reaching 1.5 by age 65. The relative risk for radiation-induced thryoid cancer appears to be independent of sex (Hempelmann *et al.* 1975; Ron and Modan 1980), so that in absolute terms, women are more susceptible to radiation-induced thyroid cancer. The age distribution of occurrence in the infancy-irradiated series of Hempelmann *et al.* (1975) again shows the pattern described above, namely, near equality of cancer rates in females and males until puberty and only thereafter a preponderance of female cases.

These observations suggest that sex hormones may also play an important role in the development of thyroid cancer. The thyroxine-binding globulin level in normal females is 10–20 per cent higher than in males, and in pregnancy, a 50 per cent increase in the level of thyroxine-binding globulin results in a similar magnitude increase in the level of thyroid stimulating hormone. It therefore appears likely that thyroid stimulating hormone levels in non-pregnant normal women will be elevated above the level in men at some point in the menstrual cycle although not necessarily throughout the cycle. It has been claimed that there are changes in size and activity of the thyroid during the course of a normal menstrual cycle (Robbins 1979), and this would also suggest transient changes in thyroid stimulating hormone levels.

Osteosarcoma

The age-specific incidence curve of osteosarcoma peaks in the adolescent period and again in old age, but the disease rarely occurs in middle age. Epidemiological findings strongly suggest that the adolescent peak in incidence is associated with the pattern of childhood skeletal growth. Skeletal growth results from a combination of factors, but hormonal activity is a primary stimulus. Pituitary growth hormone, thyroid hormone, androgens, and oestrogens are all involved. The excess-growth hypothesis first proposed by Johnson (1953), namely, that the incidence of osteosarcomas is simply a function of the amount of cellular activity in the bones, explains most of the known facts about this tumour.

During the pre-adolescent period from about age 5–11, girls grow faster than boys, but their growth stops earlier so that, by the middle to late teenage years, boys are considerably taller. The age-specific incidence curves for osteosarcoma follow the same pattern. The osteosarcoma rates for girls up to about age 13 are roughly 30 per cent higher than are the rates in boys, but after this age, the incidence rates for girls declines sharply while the rate for boys continues to rise. In the age group 15–24, the rate in men exceeds that in women by some 140 per cent. Maximal skeletal growth preceeds the adolescent peak in incidence by 3–4 years in each sex. The higher peak in men appears simply to reflect the greater overall size of men compared with women.

Osteosarcomas in adolescents occur most frequently in the epiphyses of long bones, sites of maximal bone growth (Price 1958). Fraumeni (1967) compared the height of children with osteosarcoma to that of children with other cancers and to national standards. The two comparisons gave similar answers. The average differences in height were quite small, but by expressing the data in relative risk terms, it could be shown that the risk of osteosarcoma in children above the 75th percentile of height for age was 2.6 times the risk in children of average height. Children above the 97th percentile had 7.2 times the risk of children of average height.

The excess-growth hypothesis is also supported by clinical studies of osteosarcomes in older people, in whom the sarcomas often occur in conjunction with benign bone pathology, primarily Paget's disease (Price 1958). The common denominator of these benign conditions appears to be excessive bone turnover, either as part of a reparative process or as part of the pathological condition itself.

Discussion

The evidence linking 'increased hormonal stimulus' to various human cancers has steadily accumulated over the last two decades; and the general validity of the concept of increased hormonal stimulus being associated with increased cancer rates must be considered as established. However, as we have seen, further research is still needed to establish the precise hormonal milieux that are most closely associated with increased cancer rates at the various affected sites. Although epidemiological research has a continuing important role to play in establishing these precise conditions of maximal (and minimal) risk, its most exciting future role may well be in helping to establish the relationship between truly modifiable environmental factors, such as diet and exercise, and the circulating levels (and metabolism) of the various responsible hormones.

References

Ahluwalia, B., Jackson, M.A., Jones, G.W., Williams, A.O., Rao, M.S., and Rajguru, S. (1981). Blood hormone profiles in prostate cancer patients in high-risk and low-risk populations. *Cancer* **48**, 2267–73.

Aleem, F.A., Moukhtar, M.A., Hung, H.C., and Romney, S. (1976). Plasma estrogen in patients with endometrial hyperplasia and carcinoma. *Cancer* **38**, 2101–4.

Annegers, J.F., Strom, H., Decker, D.G., Dockerty, M.B., and O'Fallon, W.M. (1979). Ovarian cancer: incidence and case-control study. *Cancer* **43**, 723–9.

Arguelles, A.E., Hoffman, C., Poggi, U.L., Chekherdemian, M., Sasborida, C., and Blanchard, O. (1973). Endocrine profiles and breast cancer. *Lancet* **i**, 165–8.

Axelrad, A.A. and Leblond, C.P. (1955). Induction of thyroid tumors in rats by a low iodine diet. *Cancer* **8**, 339–67.

Ayre, J.E. and Bauld, W.A.G. (1946). Thiamine deficiency and high estrogen findings in uterine cancer and in menorrhagia. *Science N.Y.* **102**, 441–5.

Benjamin, F. and Deutsch, S. (1976). Plasma levels of fractionated estrogens and pituitary hormones in endometrial carcinoma. *Amer. J. Obstet. Gynecol.* **126**, 638–47.

Bernstein, L., Pike, M.C., Ross, R.K., Judd, H.L., Brown, J.B., and Henderson, B.E. (1985). Estrogen and sex-hormone-binding globulin levels in nulliparous and parous women. *J. nat. Cancer Inst.* (In press).

Bittner, J.J. (1947). The causes and control of mammary cancer in mice. *Harvey Lect.* **42**, 221–46.

Brown, C.E., Warren, S., Chute, R.N., Ryan, K.J., and Todd, R.B. (1979). Hormonally induced tumours of the reproductive system of parabiosed male rats. *Cancer Res.* **39**, 3971–5.

Brown, J.B. (1958). Urinary oestrogen excretion in the study of mammary cancer. In *Endocrine aspects of breast cancer* (ed. A.R. Curie), pp. 197–207. E. & S. Livingstone Ltd, Edinburgh.

Casagrande, J.T., Pike, M.C., Ross, R.K., Louie, E.W., Roy, S., and Henderson, B.E. (1979). "Incessant ovulation" and ovary cancer. *Lancet* **ii**, 170–3.

Cole, E.N., England, P.C., Sellwood, R.A., and Griffiths, K. (1977). Serum prolactin concentration throughout the menstrual cycle of normal women and patients with recent breast cancer. *Eur. J. Cancer* **13**, 677–84.

Cole, P., Cramer, D., Yen, S., Paffenbarger, R., MacMahon, B., and Brown, J. (1978). Estrogen profiles of premenopausal women with breast cancer. *Cancer Res.* **38**, 745–8.

Crile, G. (1966). Endocrine dependency of papillary carcinomas of the thyroid. *J. Amer. med. Assoc.* **195**, 721–4.

del Pozo, E. and Brownell, J. (1979). Prolactin, I. Mechanism of control, peripheral actions, and modifications by drugs. *Hormone Res.* **10**, 143–74.

de Moor, P. and Joossens, J.V. (1970). An inverse relationship between body weight and the activity of the steroid binding beta-globulin in human plasma. *Steroidologia* **1**, 129–36.

Depue, R.H. (1984). Maternal and gestational factors affecting the risk of cryptorchidism and inguinal hernia. *Int. J. Epidemiol.* **13**, 311–8.

Depue, R.H., Pike, M.C., and Henderson, B.E. (1983). Estrogen exposure during gestation and risk of testicular cancer. *J. nat. Cancer Inst.* **71**, 1151–5.

de Waard, F., Cornelis, J.P., Aoki, K., and Yoshida, M. (1977). Breast cancer incidence according to weight and height in two cities of the Netherlands and in Aichi Prefecture, Japan. *Cancer* **40**, 1269–75.

Dulbecco, R., Henahan, M., and Armstrong, B. (1982). Cell types and morphogenesis in the mammary gland. *Proc. nat. Acad. Sci. U.S.A.,* **79**, 7346–50.

England, P.C., Skinner, L.G., Cottrell, K.M., and Sellwood, R.A. (1974). Serum oestradiol-17 (beta) in women with benign and malignant breast disease. *Brit. J. Cancer* **30**, 571–6.

Ferguson, D.J.P. and Anderson, T.J. (1981). Morphological evaluation of cell turnover in relation to the menstrual cycle in the "resting" human breast. *Brit. J. Cancer* **44**, 177–81.

Fishman, J., Fukushima, D., O'Connor, J., Rosenfeld, R.S., Lynch, H.T., Lynch, J.F., Guirgis, H., and Maloney, K. (1978). Plasma hormone profiles of young women at risk for familial breast cancer. *Cancer Res.* **38**, 4006–11.

Fraumeni, J.F. (1967). Stature and malignant tumors of bone in childhood and adolescence. *Cancer* **20**, 967–73.

Furth, J. (1975). Hormones as etiological agents in neoplasia. In *Cancer, a comprehensive treatise* (ed. F.F. Becker), Vol. 1, pp. 75–120. Plenum, New York.

Ghanadian, R., Puah, K.M. and O'Donoghue, E.P.M. (1979). Serum testosterone and dihydrotestosterone in carcinoma of the prostate. *Brit. J. Cancer* **39**, 696–9.

Glantz, G.M. (1964). Cirrhosis and carcinoma of the prostate gland. *J. Urol.* **91**, 291–3.

Gordon, G.G., Altman, K., Southern, A.L., Rubin, E., and Lieber, C.S. (1976). Effect of alcohol (ethanol) administration on sex-hormone metabolism in normal men. *New Engl. J. Med.* **295**, 793–7.

Gronroos, M. and Aho, A.J. (1968). Estrogen metabolism in postmenopausal women with primary and recurrent breast cancer. *Eur. J. Cancer* **4**, 523–7.

Gurpide, E. (1978). Enzymatic modulation of hormonal action at the target tissue. *J. Toxicol. environ. Hlth* **4**, 249–68.

Hammond, G.L., Kontturi, M., Vihko, P., and Vihko, R. (1978). Serum steroids in normal males and patients with prostatic diseases. *Clin. Endocrinol.* **9**, 113–21.

Hempelmann, L.H. and Furth, J. (1978). Etiology of thyroid cancer. In *Thyroid cancer* (ed. L.D. Greenfeld), pp. 37–49. CRC Press, Florida.

Hempelmann, L.H., Hall, W.J., Phillips, M., Cooper, R.A., and Ames, W.R. (1975). Neoplasms in persons treated with X-rays; fourth survey in 20 years. *J. nat. Cancer Inst.* **55**, 519–30.

Henderson, B.E., Gerkins, V., Rosario, I., Casagrande, J.T., and Pike, M.C. (1975). Elevated serum levels of estrogen and prolactin in daughters of patients with breast cancer. *New Engl. J. Med.* **293**, 790–5.

Henderson, B.E., Benton, B., Jing, J., Yu, M., and Pike, M.C. (1979). Risk factors for cancer of the testis in young men. *Int. J. Cancer* **23**, 598–601.

Henderson, B.E., Pike, M.C., and Casagrande, J.T. (1981). Breast cancer and the oestrogen window hypothesis. *Lancet* **ii**, 363.

Henderson, B.E., Ross, R.K., Pike, M.C., and Casagrande, J.T. (1982). Endogenous hormones as a major factor in human cancer. *Cancer Res.* **42**, 3232–9.

Henderson, B.E., Casagrande, J.T., Pike, M.C., Mack, T., Rosario, I. and Duke, A. (1983). The epidemiology of endometrial cancer in young women. *Brit. J. Cancer* **47**, 749–756.

Hill, P., Wynder, E.L., Kumar, H., Helman, P., Rona, G., and Kuno, K. (1976). Prolactin levels in populations at risk of breast cancer. *Cancer Res.* **36**, 4102–6.

Hovenian, M.S. and Deming, C.L. (1948). The heterologous growth of cancer of the human prostate. *Surg. Gynecol. Obstet.* **86**, 29–35.

Hsueh, A.J.W., Peck, E.J., and Clark, J.H. (1975). Progesterone antagonism of the oestrogen receptor and oestrogen-induced uterine growth. *Nature (Lond.)* **254**, 337–9.

Huggins, C. (1967). Enocrine-induced regression of cancers. *Science (N.Y.)* **156**, 1050–4.

Huggins, C. and Hodges, C.V. (1941). Studies on prostatic cancer: effect of castration, of estrogen, and of androgen injection on serum phosphatases in metastatic carcinoma of the prostate. *Cancer Res.* **1**, 293–7.

Johnson, L.C. (1953). A general theory of bone tumors. *Bull. N.Y. Acad. Med.* **29**, 164–71.

Judd, H.L., Davidson, B.J., Frumar, A.M., Shamonki, I.M., Lagasse, L.D., and Ballon, S.C. (1980). Serum androgens and estrogens in postmenopausal women with and without endometrial cancer. *Amer. J. Obstet. Gynecol.* **136**, 859–71.

Kwa, H.G., Engelsman, E., De Jong-Bakker, M., and Cleton, F.J. (1974). Plasma prolactin in human breast cancer. *Lancet* **i**, 433–5.

Kwa, H.G., Cleton, F., Bulbrook, R.D., Wang, D.Y., and Hayward, J.L. (1981). Plasma prolactin levels and breast cancer: relation to parity, weight and height, and age at first birth. *Int. J. Cancer* **28**, 31–4.

Levin, P.A., and Malarkey, W.B. (1981). Daughters of women with breast cancer have elevated mean 24-hour prolactin (PRL) levels and a partial resistance of PRL to dopamine suppression. *J. Clin. Endocrinol. Metab.* **53**, 179–83.

Lew, E.A. and Garfinkel, L. (1979). Variations in mortality by weight among 750,000 men and women. *J. chron. Dis.* **32**, 563–76.

MacDonald, P.C., Edman, C.D., Hemsell, D.L., Porter, J.C., and Siiteri, P.K. (1978). Effect of obesity on conversion of plasma androstenedione to estrone in postmenopausal women with and without endometrial cancer. *Amer. J. Obstet. Gynecol.* **130**, 448–55.

MacMahon, B., Cole, P., and Brown, J. (1973). Etiology of human breast cancer: a review. *J. nat. Cancer Inst.* **50**, 21–42.

MacMahon, B., Trichopoulos, D., Brown, J., *et al.* (1982). Age at menarche, probability of ovulation and breast cancer risk. *Int. J. Cancer* **29**, 13–6.

Malarkey, W.B., Schroeder, L.L., Stevens, V.C., James, A.G., and Lanese, R.R. (1977). Disordered nocturnal prolactin regulation in women with breast cancer. *Cancer Res.* **37**, 4650–4.

Marmorston, J., Crowley, L.G., Myers, S.M., Stern, E., and Hopkins, C.E. (1965). Urinary excretion of estradiol and estriol by patients with breast cancer and benign breast disease. *Amer. J. Obstet. Gynecol.* **92**, 460–7.

Meissner, W.A., Sommers, S.C., and Sherman, B.M. (1957). Endometrial hyperplasia, endometrial carcinoma, and endometriosis produced experimentally by estrogen. *Cancer* **10**, 500–9.

Mengel, W., Heinz, H.A., Sippe, W.G., and Hecker, W.C. (1974). Studies on cryptorchidism: a comparison of histologic findings in the germinative epithelium before and after the second year of life. *J. pediat. Surg.* **9**, 445–50.

Moore, J.W., Clark, G.M.G., Bulbrook, R.D., Hayward, J.L., Murai, J.T., Hammond, G.L., and Siiteri, P.K. (1982). Serum concentrations of total and non-protein bound oestradiol in patients with breast cancer and in normal controls. *Int. J. Cancer* **29**, 17–21.

Moore, J.W., Clark, G.M.G., Takatani, O., Wakabayashi, Y., Hayward, J.L., and Bulbrook, R.D. (1983). Distribution of 17(beta)-estradiol in the sera of normal British and Japanese women. *J. nat. Cancer Inst.* **71**, 749–54.

Noble, R.L. (1977). The development of prostatic adenocarcinoma in Nb rats following prolonged sex hormone administration. *Cancer Res.* **37**, 1929–33.

O'Dea, J.P., Wieland, R.G., Hallberg, M.C., Llerena, L.A., Zorn, E.M., and Genuth, S.M. (1979). Effect of dietary weight loss of sex steroid binding, sex steroids, and gonadotropins in obese menopausal women. *J. Lab. clin. Med.* **39**, 1004–8.

Olsson, H., Landin-Olsson, M., and Gullberg, B. (1983). Retrospective assessment of menstrual cycle length in patients with breast cancer, in patients with benign breast disease, and in women without breast disease. *J. nat. Cancer Inst.* **70**, 17–20.

O'Malley, B.W. (1971). Mechanism of action of steroid hormones. *New Engl. J. Med.* **284**, 370–7.

Papadaki, L., Beilby, J.O.W., Chowaniec, J., Coulson, W.F., Darby, A.J., Newman, J., O'Shea, A., and Wykes, J.R. (1979). Hormone replacement therapy in the menopause: a suitable animal model. *J. Endocrinol.* **83**, 67–77.

Persson, B.H. and Risholm, L. (1964). Oophorectomy and cortisone treatment as a method of eliminating estrogen production in patients with breast cancer. *Acta Endocrinol.* **47**, 15–26.

Pike, M.C., Gerkins, V.R., Casagrande, J.T., Gray, G.E., Brown, J., and Henderson, B.E. (1979). The hormonal basis of breast cancer. *Nat. Cancer Inst. Mon.* **53**, 187–93.

Price, C.H.G. (1958). Primary bone-forming tumors and their relationship to skeletal growth. *J. Bone Jt Surg. Br.* **40**, 574–93.

Robbins, S.L. (1979). The thyroid gland. In *Pathological basis of disease* (ed. S.L. Robbins and R.S. Cotran), pp. 1350–79. W.B. Saunders, Philadelphia.

Ron, E. and Modan, B. (1980). Benign and malignant thyroid neoplasms after childhood irradiation for tinea capitis. *J. nat. Cancer Inst.* **65**, 7–11.

Rothman, K.J. and Louik, C. (1978). Oral contraceptives and birth defects. *New Engl. J. Med.* **299**, 522–4.

Schottenfeld, D., Warshaner, M.E., Sherlock, S., Zauber, A.G., Leder, M., and Payne, R. (1980). The epidemiology of testicular cancer in young adults. *Amer. J. Epidemiol.* **112**, 232–46.

Sheth, N.A., Ranadive, K.J., Suraiya, J.N., and Sheth, A.R. (1975). Circulating levels of prolactin in human breast cancer. *Brit. J. Cancer* **32**, 160–7.

Siiteri, P.K. and MacDonald, P.C. (1973). Role of extraglandular estrogen in human endocrinology. In *Handbook of physiology*, Sect. 7, Vol. 2, part 1, pp. 615–29. American Physiological Society, Washington D.C.

Sommers, S.C. and Meissner, W.A. (1957). Endocrine abnormalities accompanying human endometrial cancer. *Cancer* **10**, 516–21.

Swerdlow, A.J., Wood, K.H., and Smith, P.G. (1983). A case-control study of the aetiology of cryptorchidism. *J. Epidemiol. comm. Hlth* **37**, 238–44.

Trichopoulos, D., Brown, J.B., Garas, J., Papaioannou, A., and MacMahon, B. (1981). Urine estrogen and pregnanediol levels of daughters of breast cancer patients. *J. nat. Cancer Inst.* **67**, 603–6.

Tseng, L. and Gurpide, E. (1976). Induction of human endometrial estradiol dehydrogenase by progestins. *Endocrinology* **97**, 825–33.

van Vliet, G., Canfriez, A., Robyn, C., and Wolter, R. (1980). Plasma gonadotropin values in prepubertal cryptorchid boys: similar increase of FSH secretion in uni- and bilateral cases. *J. Pediat.* **39**, 253–5.

Vekemans, M. and Robyn, C. (1975). Influence of age on serum prolactin levels in women and men. *Brit. med. J.* **ii**, 738–9.

Waterhouse, J., Muir, C., Shanmugaratnam, K., and Powell, J. (1982). *Cancer incidence in five continents*. International Agency for Research on Cancer, Lyon.

Werder, E.A., Illig, R., Torresani, T., Zachmann, M., Baumann, P., Ott, F., and Prader, A. (1976). Gonadal function in young adults after surgical treatment of cryptorchidism. *Brit. med. J.* **ii**, 1357–9.

Wilson, J.D., (1972). Recent studies on the mechanism of action of testosterone. *New Engl. J. Med.* **287**, 1284–91.

Yu, M.C., Gerkins, V.R., Henderson, B.E., Brown, J.B., and Pike, M.C. (1981). Elevated levels of prolactin in nulliparous women. *Brit. J. Cancer* **43**, 826–31.

10 Other drugs

David Skegg

When we turn attention from hormones to other drugs, the opportunities for cancer induction seem limitless. The taking of medicines is almost universal and many people consume the same drugs for months or years. There were 36 000 medicines on the market in Britain 10 years ago (*The Lancet* 1975), though some of these have been withdrawn since the Committee on Review of Medicines began its work. Some drugs may themselves be capable of initiating or promoting tumours; some may alter the metabolism of other carcinogens; some may facilitate the production of carcinogens within the body; and some may suppress the body's immune response to abnormal cells. Apart from their active principles, medicines usually also contain excipients, dyes, and other ingredients that could produce their own effects (Coustou 1979).

It is surprising, therefore, that medicines do not appear to be a common cause of cancer. Although at least a couple of dozen drugs are thought to be carcinogenic, Doll and Peto (1981) estimated that less than 1 per cent of all cancers were due to known effects of drugs. Smith and Jick (1977), analysing data from the Boston Collaborative Drug Surveillance Program, reached a similar conclusion.

Despite these estimates, there are several reasons why the carcinogenicity of drugs is an important field of study. First, although the overall picture is reassuring, certain groups of patients have a substantial risk. Secondly, our methods of drug surveillance are so inadequate that important hazards could have escaped detection. Thirdly, the continual development of new drugs means that new problems are likely to emerge. Fourthly, physicians have a particular responsibility to ensure the safety of treatments they prescribe and iatrogenic cancers should, in principle, be easier to prevent than cancers due to personal habits such as smoking. Finally, research on drug-induced cancers may provide clues about the nature of carcinogenesis.

Drugs that have been shown to be carcinogenic in humans

Students of this subject owe a great debt to the International Agency for Research on Cancer (IARC) which, since 1971, has brought together groups of scientists to evaluate the carcinogenic risk of chemicals and to prepare monographs on them. In 1982 a special Working Group reviewed the evidence concerning 155 chemicals and industrial processes included in the first 29 IARC Monographs and for which some data on carcinogenicity in humans were available (IARC 1982). Apart from the epidemiological evidence, the group scrutinized evidence for carcinogenicity in animals and for activity in short-term laboratory tests. Each chemical was assigned to one of three groups: (1) carcinogenic in humans, (2) *probably* carcinogenic in humans, or (3) not classifiable as to carcinogenicity in humans. The first category, which was used only when there was sufficient evidence from human epidemiological studies, included the 11 drugs or treatments in Table 1.

Table 1. Drugs that have been shown to be carcinogenic in humans†

Drug or treatment	Site of cancer
Analgesic mixtures containing phenacetin	Renal pelvis
Arsenic	Skin
Azathioprine	Reticulo-endothelial system, skin, etc.
Cytotoxic drugs:	
busulphan ('Myleran')	Marrow
chlorambucil	Marrow
chlornaphazine	Bladder
combined chemotherapy for lymphomas	Marrow (and other sites)
cyclophosphamide	Bladder
melphalan	Marrow
treosulphan	Marrow
Methoxsalen with ultraviolet A (PUVA)	Skin

† Hormones and radiopharmaceuticals are not included.

Exogenous hormones have been omitted from this and subsequent tables (see Chapter 8). The IARC Working Group also did not consider *radioactive compounds* which, not surprisingly, can induce cancers. For example, thorium dioxide ('thorotrast'), which was formerly used as an X-ray contrast medium, has caused haemangioendotheliomas of the liver, leukaemia, and other malignancies (da Silva Horta *et al*. 1965; Baxter *et al*. 1980). With the exception of hormones and radiopharmaceuticals, Table 1 includes the drugs for which there is the strongest evidence of carcinogenicity in man.

Analgesic mixtures containing phenacetin

During the last 30 years, there has been increasing recognition of the syndrome of analgesic nephropathy in people who have habitually consumed large quantities of analgesic mixtures containing phenacetin

(Kincaid-Smith 1978). Patients with this syndrome characteristically develop renal papillary necrosis and chronic interstitial nephritis. In 1965, Hultengren and his colleagues reported that four women from a series of 103 patients with renal papillary necrosis had developed carcinoma of the renal pelvis. There were no cases of hypernephroma, despite the fact that this is usually much commoner than cancer of the renal pelvis. Since this observation, evidence has accumulated that people who abuse analgesic mixtures have an increased risk of transitional cell carcinomas of the renal pelvis and (possibly) the lower urinary tract.

Much of the evidence has come from Scandinavia and Australia, where analgesic nephropathy seems to be particularly common. Grimlund (1963), the medical officer to a factory in the small Swedish town of Huskvarna, gave a fascinating account of the occurrence of renal failure in workers who habitually took 'Hjorton's powder'. This consisted of caffeine, phenacetin, and phenazone. Taking the powder was thought to increase the workers' productivity, so that their earnings could be increased. Six years later, Angervall *et al.* (1969) described a cluster of patients with renal pelvic carcinoma in Huskvarna. Of ten patients affected, nine had been employees at the factory.

While the possibility of an occupational carcinogen had to be considered, the combination of analgesic nephropathy and renal pelvic carcinoma was being observed in quite different groups, including housewives (Bengtsson *et al.* 1978). The association was confirmed in analytical studies. For example, Bengtsson *et al.* (1968) followed up 192 patients with chronic non-obstructive pyelonephritis for an average of five years. Among 104 abusers of analgesics, eight developed renal pelvic tumours, whereas no such tumours were found in the other 88 patients.

Phenacetin is carcinogenic in rats (IARC 1982), but it is not certain that this component of the analgesic mixtures has been responsible for the carcinogenic effect in humans.

Arsenic

The link between treatment with inorganic arsenic compounds and skin cancer should now be mainly of historical interest, but it illustrates how much time can elapse between recognition of an iatrogenic problem and its control. Arsenical drugs have been used for at least 2500 years for treating diverse conditions, including skin diseases. They were also often prescribed as 'tonics'. Hutchinson (1887) was the first to implicate prolonged arsenic treatment as a cause of skin cancer. He described five patients in whom cancers had developed at unusual sites, such as on the palms and soles, following the appearance of chronic lesions of the skin. Although his suggestion was at first disputed, many similar cases were soon described.

By 1947, Neubauer was able to review more than 100 patients with chronic skin arsenicism (including hyperpigmentation and keratoses) and squamous cell or basal cell carcinomas of the skin.

The skin cancers associated with arsenic treatment were characteristically multifocal, involving atypical sites unexposed to sunlight. Patients tended to be relatively young when the cancers were diagnosed (one-third under 40 years of age), and the period from the commencement of treatment to the appearance of tumours ranged from 5 to 60 years (average 18 years). A dose–response relationship with total arsenic dose was found (IARC 1980a). Although a number of malignancies apart from skin cancer have been reported in patients treated with arsenic, causal associations have not been proven.

Medicines containing inorganic arsenic compounds have been abandoned in many countries. Nevertheless, despite long awareness of their hazards and the availability of alternative treatments, Schmähl *et al.* (1977) cited evidence that, as recently as 1968, 73 per cent of German dermatologists were prescribing arsenicals. In 1979, the German register of proprietary drugs still listed seven preparations containing inorganic arsenic compounds (Reinicke 1982).

Arsenic is also an occupational carcinogen, causing cancers of the lung as well as the skin (IARC 1980a). Interestingly, carcinogenicity studies of arsenic compounds in experimental animals have generally been negative (IARC 1980a, 1982).

Azathioprine

Azathioprine is an immunosuppressive agent which, together with corticosteroids, is used after transplantation. It is also prescribed for a variety of diseases in which autoimmunity is thought to play a role, such as rheumatoid arthritis and systemic lupus erythematosus.

The risk of malignancies associated with immunosuppression has been discussed by Kinlen in Chapter 7 of this book. Renal transplant recipients have an increased incidence of non-Hodgkin's lymphoma (often involving the brain), skin cancer, mesenchymal tumours, and primary liver cancer. In striking contrast to other iatrogenic cancers, the increased risk of lymphomas appears within the first year after transplantation. Patients without transplants treated with azathioprine and other immunosuppressive drugs also experience an excess of the malignancies mentioned, although to a lesser extent (Kinlen 1982).

Cytotoxic drugs

The treatment of neoplastic diseases has been revolutionized during the past two decades by increasing use of various cytotoxic drugs. As the number of patients treated has increased and as many have survived longer, it has become clear that second neoplasms can develop as a complication of chemotherapy. Malignancies have also been observed in patients who have received cytotoxic drugs for non-neoplastic diseases such as rheumatoid arthritis and glomerulonephritis (IARC 1981).

The carcinogenic potential of different classes of cytotoxic drugs varies greatly (Schmähl and Habs 1980). The six single cytotoxic drugs listed in Table 1 are all *alkylating agents*. These drugs form electrophilic reactants and damage cells by binding to nucleophilic cellular macromolecules, including DNA (Harris 1976). In short-term tests, they cause chromosomal aberrations, mutations, and transformation of cultured cells; and they are carcinogenic in laboratory animals (IARC 1982). Although, as will be discussed later, several other types of cytotoxic drugs are also probably carcinogenic in humans, the alkylating agents appear to be the most important in this respect.

Chlornaphazine was found to be so hazardous that its use was abandoned. This alkylating agent was employed, particularly in Scandinavian countries, in the treatment of leukaemia, Hodgkin's disease, and polycythaemia vera. In 1964, Thiede *et al.* reported that 7 of 61 polycythaemia patients treated with chlornaphazine had developed bladder tumours; by 1969, 10 of the 61 had tumours and a further 5 had abnormal urinary cytology (Thiede and Christensen 1969). The latent period from administration of chlornaphazine to diagnosis of bladder cancer ranged from three to ten years. Nine of the ten patients had also been treated with radioactive phosphorus (P-32 as sodium phosphate injections), but no bladder tumours were found among 46 patients treated with [^{32}P]sodium phosphate alone (Thiede *et al.* 1964).

Another drug that can cause bladder cancer is cyclophosphamide (IARC 1981). Presumably the production of bladder tumours reflects the concentration of the drug in the urinary tract (Griffin 1979). But the commonest malignancy caused by the other alkylating agents is leukaemia, which is usually of an acute non-lymphocytic type.

Rosner *et al.* (1982) recently reviewed the problem of acute myeloid leukaemia and its variants in patients treated with alkylating agents. The risk is higher in patients given multiple drug chemotherapy. Radiotherapy also increases the risk, especially if it precedes the chemotherapy. The period from treatment to occurrence of leukaemia tends to be shorter with more intensive chemotherapy or radiotherapy; the average period is about four to six years. Although the risk for an individual is often not very large, some surprisingly high rates have been observed. For example, the results of a study of 5455 patients who received alkylating agents for treatment of advanced ovarian cancer suggested that leukaemia would develop in 5–10 per cent of a group of patients surviving for ten years after treatment (Reimer *et al.* 1977).

Patients given chemotherapy for Hodgkin's disease and non-Hodgkin's lymphoma have been some of the most intensively studied groups. These patients often receive combined chemotherapy, such as in the MOPP regime – comprising 'Mustargen' (nitrogen mustard), 'Oncovin' (vincristine), procarbazine, and prednisone. Patients given such chemotherapy have a much greater risk of leukaemia than those treated with radiation alone (Coleman *et al.* 1982).

The occurrence of iatrogenic malignancies in patients given cytotoxic drugs is likely to be an increasing problem as patients receiving cancer chemotherapy survive longer (especially in the case of children) and as these drugs are prescribed more widely for non-fatal diseases. Since the induction period for most solid tumours would be expected to be much longer than the latent periods observed for leukaemia, other types of malignancy may appear in patients treated with alkylating agents. Possible control measures will be mentioned later in this chapter.

Methoxsalen with ultraviolet A (PUVA)

Methoxsalen (8-methoxypsoralen) is a photosensitizing drug that is taken orally before exposure to long-wavelength ultraviolet radiation (UV-A) in the treatment of psoriasis known as photochemotherapy (Parrish *et al.* 1974). This form of treatment is also called PUVA (an acronym from 'psoralen' and 'UV-A'). Since its description in 1974, PUVA has become widely used for treating psoriasis and for maintenance therapy after lesions have cleared.

PUVA causes DNA damage and mutations in bacteria and in mammalian and human cells exposed *in vitro*; it also produces chromosomal aberrations in mammalian cells *in vitro* and *in vivo* (IARC 1980b). In mice, methoxsalen and long-wave ultraviolet light increase the incidence of epidermal and dermal tumours (IARC 1980b). These experimental findings, together with studies in Man, were recently reviewed by Bridges *et al.* (1981). There are a number of case reports and one cohort study suggesting that PUVA increases the risk of skin cancer in humans (Stern *et al.* 1979). Although the epidemiological data are still rather inadequate, the recent IARC Working Group (1982) concluded that there was sufficient evidence that PUVA therapy is carcinogenic in humans. The effects of methoxsalen could not be distinguished from those of long-wave ultraviolet light or of the combination of the two.

Only a few years have elapsed since PUVA therapy became widely used and further data are needed to evaluate its risks in comparison with those of other treatments for psoriasis. Surveillance should be for other effects as well as skin cancer, since Bridges *et al.* (1981) postulated that the irradiation of circulating stem cells could possibly lead to malignant disease of the reticulo-endothelial system.

Drugs that are probably carcinogenic in humans

The IARC Working Group (1982) also classified a number of chemicals as 'probably carcinogenic' in humans. These included the drugs listed in Tables 2 and 3. The tables show, for each drug, the IARC assessments of the degrees of evidence for carcinogenicity in humans and in experimental animals, and for activity in short-term tests that are believed to predict potential carcinogenicity. Full definition of the terms 'sufficient', 'limited', and 'inadequate', are given in the IARC report. It should be mentioned that the evidence of carcinogenicity in humans may be described as 'inadequate' because (1) there were few pertinent data; (2) the available studies, while showing evidence of association, did not exclude chance, bias or confounding; or (3) studies were available that did not show evidence of carcinogenicity.

Table 2. Other cytotoxic drugs classified by the IARC as 'probably carcinogenic' in humans†

Drug	Evidence for carcinogenicity in humans	Evidence for carcinogenicity in animals	Evidence for activity in short-term tests
Actinomycin D	Inadequate	Limited	Sufficient
Adriamycin	Inadequate	Sufficient	Sufficient
BCNU	Inadequate	Sufficient	Sufficient
CCNU	Inadequate	Sufficient	Sufficient
Cisplatin	Inadequate	Limited	Sufficient
Dacarbazine	Inadequate	Sufficient	Limited
Nitrogen mustard	Inadequate	Sufficient	Sufficient
Procarbazine	Inadequate	Sufficient	Sufficient
Triaziquone	Inadequate	Limited	Sufficient
Thiotepa	Inadequate	Sufficient	Sufficient
Uracil mustard	Inadequate	Sufficient	Sufficient

† Adapted from IARC (1982)

Two-thirds of the drugs in this category were *cytotoxic drugs* (Table 2). While the evidence for their carcinogenicity in humans is still inadequate, most of these drugs produce malignant tumours in experimental animals and are active in short-term tests. Nitrogen mustard, triaziquone, thiotepa, and uracil mustard are all alkylating agents. Actinomycin D and adriamycin are antibiotics. BCNU (bischloroethyl nitrosourea) and CCNU chloroethylcyclohexyl nitrosourea) are nitrosoureas. The other three agents are miscellaneous compounds.

Table 3. Other drugs (apart from cytotoxic drugs and hormones) classified by the IARC as 'probably carcinogenic' in humans†

Drug	Evidence for carcinogenicity in humans	Evidence for carcinogenicity in animals	Evidence for activity in short-term tests
Chloramphenicol	Limited	Inadequate	Inadequate
Metronidazole	Inadequate	Sufficient	Limited
Phenazopyridine	Inadequate	Sufficient	No data
Phenytoin	Limited	Limited	Inadequate
Propylthiouracil	Inadequate	Sufficient	No data

† Adapted from IARC (1982)

Table 3 shows the other drugs that were regarded as probably carcinogenic in humans. *Metronidazole* (an antiprotozoal), *phenazopyridine* (a urinary tract analgesic), and *propylthiouracil* (an antithyroid agent) produce tumours in mice and rats, but epidemiological evidence for any effects in humans is lacking. In the case of metronidazole ('Flagyl'), Roe (1983) has questioned the relevance of the experimental findings. Two epidemiological studies involving follow-up of patients treated with metronidazole provided reassuring results (Beard *et al.* 1979; Friedman and Ury 1980). Unfortunately, however, the first study was rather small and the second involved follow-up for only three to seven years. Metronidazole is often prescribed in short courses of about one week for treatment of trichomoniasis. From a theoretical point of view, this drug would have to be a very potent carcinogen to produce cancer after such a short exposure. Nevertheless, metronidazole is used for treating a variety of diseases and some patients receive prolonged therapy. There is a particular need for further studies involving long-term follow-up of people exposed to large doses for prolonged periods.

Chloramphenicol is suspected of having caused leukaemia in a small number of people; there are several case reports of leukaemia occurring in patients who developed aplastic anaemia after taking this antibiotic (IARC 1976). In a follow-up study of 126 patients who had been reported to registries because of bone-marrow depression following treatment with chloramphenicol, three developed leukaemia (Fraumeni 1967). Nevertheless, this study had certain limitations and Fraumeni concluded that there was still insufficient evidence that chloramphenicol was leukaemogenic.

Phenytoin has been linked with the occurrence of lymphomas in a number of case reports, but two cohort studies did not confirm this association (White *et al.* 1979; Clemmesen and Hjalgrim-Jensen 1981). More impressive are the occasional reports of cancers, mainly neuroblastoma and tumours of neural crest origin, in children with the fetal hydantoin syndrome – a congenital syndrome thought to be caused by intra-uterine exposure to phenytoin (IARC 1977; 1982). Although the number of reports is small, the coincidence of rare events suggests that phenytoin might act as a transplacental carcinogen.

Drugs that have been suspected of causing cancer in humans

Many other medicines have been suspected of causing cancer. Such suspicions can arise from clinical observations, from the results of animal experiments or short-term tests, or from theoretical considerations. Often there is great difficulty in determining whether a drug does, in fact, affect the risk of cancer. Two recent examples will be mentioned.

In 1979, Horrobin and his colleagues suggested that *diazepam* might have a tumour-promoting effect. Their hypothesis, which was based mainly on the results of certain animal experiments, led them to speculate that 'tranquillizer use may be a major contributor to the development of some types of cancer' (Horrobin and Trosko 1981). Given the ubiquitous prescribing of diazepam and other benzodiazepines, any tumour-promoting properties would certainly be of great public-health significance.

Attention has been focused mainly on breast cancer – partly because some of the original experiments were on mammary tumours in rats, and partly because Horrobin interpreted some observations on a group of women with breast cancer as supportive of his hypothesis. Two case-control studies (Kleinerman *et al.* 1981; Kaufman *et al.* 1982) and a cohort study (Danielson *et al.* 1982) showed no association between use of diazepam and breast cancer. Friedman and Ury (1980) recorded cancers of all types among 12 961 people who had received diazepam. There were 324 cases, which was slightly fewer than the 'expected' number of 335. The period of follow-up was short (about three to seven years), but this should have been less of a problem for studying tumour promotion than tumour initiation. On present evidence, it seems unlikely that diazepam is involved in the causation of human cancer.

Another concern that has been raised in both the scientific and lay press is the possibility that *cimetidine* might cause gastric cancer. This fear has arisen from case reports of gastric cancer in patients taking cimetidine and from the theoretical prediction that treatment with cimetidine would lead to the formation of carcinogenic *N*-nitroso compounds in the stomach. It has been postulated that, by reducing gastric acidity, cimetidine would encourage the bacterial reduction of nitrates to nitrites in the stomach.

Nitrites can react with amines, such as dietary amino acids and even cimetidine itself, to form *N*-nitroso compounds. Some of the latter are carcinogenic in animals, although they have not been proved to be involved in the genesis of human gastric cancer. The evidence for the view that cimetidine might cause gastric cancer was summarized recently (*Drug and Therapeutics Bulletin* 1983).

Considering the very large numbers of patients with symptoms of peptic ulceration who receive cimetidine, it is not surprising that some of them are subsequently diagnosed as having gastric cancer. Apart from chance associations, it seems clear that cimetidine is not infrequently prescribed for symptoms of an undiagnosed gastric cancer (Colin-Jones *et al.* 1982). Colin-Jones *et al.* reported the preliminary results of a study of 9504 patients who had been followed up for at least a year after taking cimetidine. Their findings were fairly reassuring, but studies involving much longer surveillance will be needed before the theoretical concerns about cimetidine can be laid to rest.

These two examples – and many others could have been chosen – illustrate the need for reliable data about the effects of drugs on cancer incidence in humans. When alarms are raised about the safety of a drug, there is often little relevant information to enable any risks to be evaluated. For example, the possibility that diazepam might be carcinogenic had been considered by an IARC Working Group (1977) before Horrobin and his colleagues published their hypothesis about tumour promotion. In the only animal study available to the Working Group, oxazepam (a major metabolite of diazepam) was carcinogenic in mice after oral administration. As far as human data were concerned, 'no case reports or epidemiological studies were available to the Working Group'. This was a highly unsatisfactory situation, considering that diazepam is dispensed to at least 6 per cent of the entire population each year (Skegg *et al.* 1977).

We need to be capable not merely of investigating suspicions about the carcinogenicity of particular drugs, but also of obtaining positive evidence for the safety of others. Possible methods for achieving this will be discussed in the next section.

Detection of carcinogenic risks

Drug hazards should be easier to detect than most other suspected causes of cancer – such as dietary factors – since the agents concerned are relatively pure substances and details of exposure can often be obtained from medical records or from people's own recollections. Despite such advantages, current methods for surveillance of drug hazards are still very imperfect. Ideally, of course, we would like to be able to predict any carcinogenic risk posed by a new medicine before it is given to patients.

Reference has already been made in this chapter to animal experiments and short-term laboratory tests that have been designed for this purpose.

Prediction from laboratory experiments

Many drugs that are on the market have not been tested for possible carcinogenicity. Since the thalidomide experience in 1961, however, increasing attention has been paid to possible teratogenic, carcinogenic, or mutagenic effects (World Health Organization 1975). The emphasis that is given to studies aimed at predicting the carcinogenicity of new drugs is often influenced by theoretical considerations. For example, if a drug (or one of its metabolites) has structural similarities to a known carcinogen, suspicion is aroused. Medicines that are intended for long-term use in humans also receive special attention.

The laboratory methods available for predicting likely carcinogenicity have been well reviewed in an IARC publication (1980c) and critically discussed by Doll and Peto (1981). In the standard *'long-term' tests* in animals, the test drug is administered at high doses (by an appropriate route) for most of the life-span of a group of small animals such as rats or mice. The incidence of tumours is compared with that in a control group. It is customary to test a drug in more than one animal species. Since these animal experiments are extremely time-consuming and expensive, a variety of *short-term tests* have been introduced to supplement them. New short-term tests are being developed continually, but the most useful involve testing either effects of the drug on the genetic material (DNA) of cultured cells, or effects on DNA in the cells of living animals, or effects on the behaviour of cultured cells.

There appears to be a fairly good *qualitative* correlation between the results of long-term tests in animals and effects in humans. For example, a review of chemicals for which both animal and human data were available showed that most of the chemicals known to be carcinogenic in humans were also carcinogenic in one or, in most cases, more than one animal species (Tomatis *et al.* 1982). In several instances, experimental evidence of carcinogenicity preceded the human observations and could have predicted them. Short-term tests also have predictive value, especially if an appropriate range of tests is employed. Nevertheless, some chemicals (e.g. certain hormones) that have been proved to be carcinogenic in animals are inactive in tests that use DNA or chromosomal damage as their end-points. There are still no well-validated short-term tests for tumour promoters, although attempts are being made to fill this gap.

Laboratory testing has undoubtedly prevented the development and marketing of some drugs that would have produced cancers in Man. Unfortunately, however, it is not yet possible to use data from long-term or short-term tests to make a *quantitative* evaluation of human risk (Doll and Peto 1981; Tomatis *et al.* 1982). This is a particular problem in assessing drugs. Whereas the use of a cosmetic would be ruled out by carcinogenicity in animals, the same would not necessarily be true of a drug that offered effective treatment for a serious disease. In such circumstances, a quantitative estimate of the risk to patients receiving a given dose is needed, and this cannot be provided by current experimental methods.

Observations on humans

For several reasons, clinical and epidemiological observations on humans are also vitally important. They offer the only means for detecting the carcinogenic risks of the multitude of drugs that have not been tested adequately in the laboratory. Even when a drug has been reliably shown not to be carcinogenic in one or a few animal species, it may still cause malignancies in patients – because of variation in the susceptibility of different species, or because it causes cancer only when taken with other medicines (or foods) or when used in the presence of a human disease. Finally, only epidemiological studies can provide quantitative estimates of the risk to patients for comparison with the benefits of the drug.

Many of the unwanted effects of drugs are discovered in the clinical trials that are carried out before and after marketing. Unfortunately, the standard trials in Man cannot be expected to detect carcinogenicity, because they involve only a few hundred or (at most) a few thousand patients, and because these patients are usually observed for only a few weeks or months. We must, therefore, rely on surveillance of drugs after marketing.

In the past, most carcinogenic risks have been detected by *clinical observation*. Doctors who suspect that a drug has caused a cancer may publish a case report in a medical journal, or report their observation to a monitoring centre such as the Committee on Safety of Medicines in Britain. Despite the successes of this approach, it has serious limitations. A drug may be suspected as the cause of a cancer if the latter is of a peculiar type (e.g. the haemangioendothelioma of liver caused by 'Thorotrast'), or if it occurs in association with other drug toxicity (e.g. renal pelvic carcinoma in patients with analgesic nephropathy), or if the risk is exceedingly high (e.g. the bladder cancer caused by chlornaphazine), or if the induction period is very short (e.g. lymphomas in renal transplant recipients). But drugs that cause common cancers in a small fraction of patients after a long delay are likely to escape detection. For example, if a drug trebled the risk of breast cancer after a delay of 20 years, could we expect clinicians to recognize the link?

Apart from the fact that some drug hazards will not even be suspected, clinical observations cannot normally provide proof of an association nor the additional information that is required. Clinical case reports are usually very difficult to assess, because the association of a drug and a cancer in one or a few patients could have occurred by chance. Moreover, we need additional data in order to compare the risks and benefits of prescribing a drug for particular patients. It is important to know not only that the drug is capable of causing a certain malignancy, but also how often it does so, and in what kinds of patients. Hence, although the observations of astute clinicians will continue to be important, epidemiological studies are also essential.

The two main types of epidemiological enquiry used in *ad hoc* studies of drug-induced cancer are *cohort studies* and *case-control studies* (MacMahon and Pugh 1970). Both provide quantitative information about the association between a drug and a disease; they may also identify other factors that modify any risk for an individual. While standard case-control and cohort studies can be used to investigate hazards that have already been suspected, there is also a need for methods of detecting *unsuspected* carcinogenicity. Given the number of drugs on the market (and the continual introduction of new compounds), this is a formidable task. The lack of adequate methods for such routine surveillance is the most glaring gap in our armamentarium against drug-induced cancer.

The case-control and cohort approaches can be adapted for routine drug surveillance. The Drug Epidemiology Unit at Boston University have used a technique of 'case-control surveillance', in which patients admitted to hospital with a variety of diagnoses are interviewed about the drugs that they have used in the past (Slone *et al.* 1977). This method has yielded useful information, but it has several drawbacks. First, the interview method requires many staff and is, therefore, expensive. More importantly, patients will recall only a fraction of the drugs they have taken – especially of drugs used in the remote past. This will reduce the power of the study to detect associations between drugs and diseases, and it will introduce bias if the degree of recall varies among different diseases that are being compared.

The cohort approach has also been used for post-marketing surveillance of new drugs – examples include a study of cimetidine already mentioned (Colin-Jones *et al.* 1982, 1983) and the 'prescription-event monitoring' being conducted by Inman (1981, 1983). Such surveys, however, are usually continued for only a few months or a year or two, while most cancers take many years to develop. Surveillance for 10–50 years would generally be feasible only if the cohort of drug users were followed automatically by means of a cancer registry or national death index. This would be an application of the technique of record linkage – the bringing together of different records about a single person.

Record linkage appears to offer the best opportunity for detecting carcinogenic risks of drugs (Skegg 1980). Rather than studying a cohort of patients taking a single drug, it should be possible to link all the prescriptions dispensed for individuals in a large population with records of their subsequent morbidity and mortality. This would enable detection of associations between drugs and diseases such as cancer, even after a delay of many years. In addition to revealing unexpected hazards of some drugs, a record linkage scheme would provide positive evidence for the safety of many others.

A study of this type was begun in 1969 at the Kaiser-Permanente Medical Center in San Francisco (Friedman *et al*. 1971). Unfortunately the funding for the project was soon withdrawn but, several years later, Friedman and Ury (1980) demonstrated the value of the approach by studying the incidence of cancer among patients whose prescriptions for various drugs had been recorded between 1969 and 1973. Jick and his colleagues (1980) are making similar use of computerized data from a group health scheme in Seattle. In both of these projects, the population included is rather small (about a quarter of a million or less) and the period of follow-up is still short.

The opportunities for large-scale linkage are better in Britain, where prescriptions are collected centrally for pricing and records of hospital admissions and deaths are collected routinely in a form suitable for linkage. A feasibility study in the Oxford region suggested that record linkage would be practicable and useful both for generating and for testing hypotheses about adverse effects of drugs (Skegg and Doll 1981). Calculations showed that, in order to detect carcinogenic effects, a full-scale scheme should include a population of at least half a million, and preferably as many as five million.

The need for action

Better drug surveillance

In 1975, in an article on drugs and cancer, Hoover and Fraumeni commented that record linkage seemed to be an ideal mechanism for drug evaluation, but that 'the reasons for the failure of such record-linking efforts in the past need to be explored to determine if this is a feasible mechanism for drug screening'. In fact, only one significant record linkage study involving drugs had been attempted by that time: the Kaiser-Permanente project in San Francisco. The reasons for its termination appear to have been reliance on expensive computer-based systems for medical records and on special recording of data by doctors (Anello 1977). Despite the passage of another decade and demonstration of the feasibility of using record linkage in Britain, a full-scale scheme has still not been established.

Why has there been no action? The explanation could be fear of the cost although, since the records that would be used in a British scheme are already being collected for other purposes, this would not be as great as might be expected (Skegg and Doll 1981). Another concern relates to the confidentiality of medical records held on computers. As has been mentioned, a drug-monitoring project would make use of data that are already being collected; moreover, with careful design of the system, they could be protected more securely than in conventional records. Nevertheless, there is general concern in the medical profession and in the community about the storage of private information on computers. In summing up a meeting on post-marketing surveillance of drugs in London, Sir Richard Doll (1977) commented:

> . . . if long-term effects, such as cancer, are to be recognised, it can be done only by some form of record linking. It has been hoped by many of us that we would have a system in the U.K. which would link together information about all hospital discharges with the birth and death of the same individual, in operation before now. Such a system was very nearly approved by Ministers, but when it came to the point they were in a delicate state of health for other reasons and they didn't pursue the matter – and they have been in a delicate state of health ever since.

Recently there have been great advances in the development of short-term tests capable of predicting carcinogenicity, and further progress in laboratory methods can be expected. Unfortunately, our capacity to monitor carcinogenic risks in human populations has not made similar progress. It is, of course, for the public to decide whether it is willing to accept an extremely small risk of loss of confidentiality in order to achieve a better standard of drug safety. Researchers have a responsibility to point out the need for action.

Application of existing knowledge

The point has already been made that, although only a small proportion of all cancers are caused by drugs, these should be more readily preventable than most other cancers. Some iatrogenic malignancies could be avoided if existing knowledge were more generally applied.

Certain drugs that cause cancer should no longer be prescribed. The continued use of inorganic arsenic compounds in some countries cannot be justified. It also seems remarkable that, as recently as 1975, 'Thorotrast' was being advocated for localization of brain stem abscesses. As *The Lancet* (1977) rejoined, there are adequate alternatives to this 'potent carcinogen and leukaemogen'.

In the case of other drugs, such as cytotoxic agents, treatment will still be indicated in some circumstances. For each patient, the physician needs to compare the risks and benefits of using a drug. Unfortunately, there is often a lack of reliable quantitative information about either the risks or the benefits. But the information accruing about the incidence of leukaemia in patients receiving alkylating agents shows that these drugs should never be used lightly.

A 5 or 10 per cent risk of leukaemia in ten years would be acceptable for a beneficial treatment of an otherwise fatal disease, but it will not always be acceptable in other circumstances. Schmähl and Habs (1980) stressed the need for caution in 'adjuvant' chemotherapy of malignancies such as breast cancer, since patients who have already been cured by surgery might be subjected to an unnecessary risk. There is also a need for great caution in the use of cytotoxic drugs for treating non-malignant conditions such as rheumatoid arthritis and renal disease. In one study, 3 of 40 children treated with cholorambucil for severe juvenile arthritis and followed for up to 15 years developed acute non-lymphocytic leukaemia (Buriot *et al.* 1979).

It is likely that some of the physicians prescribing alkylating agents and other cytotoxic drugs for non-malignant conditions are not fully aware of the long-term risks, including possible carcinogenic effects. Whitehouse (1983) pointed out that 'while the infrequent user is being discouraged from prescribing anticancer drugs for the treatment of cancer, he is using these drugs more and more for other conditions'. The use of cytotoxic drugs is certainly justified in the treatment of some patients with non-malignant diseases, but one can understand Whitehouse's concern if a 'hit or miss use of drugs' prevails.

Priorities for further research

This review has highlighted the considerable doubt that exists about the possible carcinogenicity of some medicines. Our first priority for research should be to improve methods for predicting and detecting cancer risks – both before and after drugs are marketed. Emphasis should be given to studies of the predictive value of short-term tests and to more effective epidemiological surveillance.

Apart from the drugs mentioned in this chapter, there are others (e.g. phenoxybenzamine) that have been shown to be carcinogenic in animals but have not been studied adequately in humans (IARC 1982, Appendix 2). The effects of such drugs in humans should be evaluated as soon as possible.

Two promising avenues of research relate to the development of structural analogues that might be less hazardous than existing drugs, and the possible use of 'antidotes' to block a carcinogenic effect. For example, Dubertret *et al.* (1979) considered the use in PUVA therapy of 3-carbethoxypsoralen, which was not carcinogenic in the mouse with ultraviolet radiation under conditions in which methoxsalen was extremely carcinogenic. Animal experiments have also suggested that administration of another drug, mesna, might reduce the carcinogenic effect of cyclophosphamide on the bladder (Schmähl and Habs 1982).

Even where such ingenious approaches are not feasible, the recognition that a drug can cause cancer does not necessarily mean that its use should be abandoned. Epidemiologists must provide clinicians with quantitative estimates of the risks, so that these can be compared with the benefits of treatment.

References

Anello, C. (1977). *Identification of adverse reactions to marketed drugs in the United States and the United Kingdom*. Food and Drug Administration, Rockville.

Angervall, L., Bengtsson, U., Zetterlund, C.G., and Zsigmond, M. (1969). Renal pelvic carcinoma in a Swedish district with abuse of a phenacetin-containing drug. *Brit. J. Urol.* **41**, 401–5.

Baxter, P.J., Langlands, A.O., Anthony, P.P., MacSween, R.N.M., and Scheuer, P.J. (1980). Angiosarcoma of the liver: a marker tumour for the late effects of Thorotrast in Great Britain. *Brit. J. Cancer* **41**, 446–53.

Beard, C.M., Noller, K.L., O'Fallon, W.M., Kurland, L.T., and Dockerty, M.B. (1979). Lack of evidence for cancer due to use of metronidazole. *New Engl. J. Med.* **301**, 519–22.

Bengtsson, U., Angervall, L., Ekman, H., and Lehmann, L. (1968). Transitional cell tumors of the renal pelvis in analgesic abusers. *Scand. J. Urol. Nephrol.* **2**, 145–50.

Bengtsson, U., Johansson, S., and Angervall, L. (1978). Malignancies of the urinary tract and their relation to analgesic abuse. *Kidney Int.* **13**, 107–13.

Bridges, B.A., Greaves, M., Polani, P.E., and Wald, N. (1981). Do treatments available for psoriasis patients carry a genetic or carcinogenic risk? *Mut. Res.* **86**, 279–304.

Buriot, D., Prieur, A-M., Lebranchu, Y., Messerschmitt, J., and Griscelli, C. (1979). Leucémie aiguë chez trois enfants atteints d'arthrite chronique juvénile traités par le chlorambucil. *Archs Franç. Pédiat.* **36**, 592–8.

Clemmesen, J. and Hjalgrim-Jensen, S. (1981). Does phenobarbital cause intracranial tumors? A follow-up through 35 years. *Ecotoxicol. env. Safety* **5**, 255–60.

Coleman, C.N., Kaplan, H.S., Cox, R., Varghese, A., Butterfield, P., and Rosenburg, S.A. (1982). Leukaemias, non-Hodgkin's lymphomas and solid tumours in patients treated for Hodgkin's disease. *Cancer Surv.* **1**, 733–44.

Colin-Jones, D.G., Langman, M.J.S., Lawson, D.H., and Vessey, M.P. (1982). Cimetidine and gastric cancer: preliminary report from post-marketing surveillance study. *Brit. med. J.* **285**, 1311–13.

Colin-Jones, D.G., Langman, M.J.S., Lawson, D.H., and Vessey, M.P. (1983). Postmarketing surveillance of the safety of cimetidine: 12 month mortality report. *Brit. med. J.* **286**, 1713–16.

Coustou, F. (1979). Carcinogenic risk of products used in the pharmaceutical and related industries. In *Carcinogenic risks – strategies for intervention* (ed. W. Davis and C. Rosenfeld), pp. 129–49. International Agency for Research on Cancer, Lyon.

Danielson, D.A., Jick, H., Hunter, J.R., Stergachis, A., and Madsen, S. (1982). Nonestrogenic drugs and breast cancer. *Amer. J. Epidemiol.* **115**, 329–32.

da Silva Horta, J., Abbatt, J.D., da Motta, L.C., and Roriz, M.L. (1965). Malignancy and other late effects following administration of Thorotrast. *Lancet* **ii**, 201–5.

Doll, R. (1977). Chairman's summing up. In *Post-marketing surveillance of adverse reactions to new medicines*, pp. 72–3. Medico-Pharmaceutical Forum, London.

Doll, R. and Peto, R. (1981). The causes of cancer. *J. nat. Cancer Inst.* **66**, 1191–308; also published by Oxford University Press.

Drug and Therapeutics Bulletin (1983). Cimetidine and gastric cancer: a reappraisal. *Drug Therap. Bull.* **21**, 65–7.

Dubertret, L., Averbeck, D., Zajdela, F., Bisagni, E., Moustacchi, E., Touraine, R., and Latarjet, R. (1979). Photochemotherapy (PUVA) of psoriasis using 3-carbethoxypsoralen, a non-carcinogenic compound in mice. *Brit. J. Dermatol.* **101**, 379–89.

Fraumeni, J.F. (1967). Bone marrow depression induced by chloramphenicol or phenylbutazone. *J. Amer. med. Ass.* **201**, 150–6.

Friedman, G.D., Collen, M.F., Harris, L.E., van Brunt, E.E., and Davis, L.S. (1971). Experience in monitoring drug reactions in outpatients. *J. Amer. med. Ass.* **217**, 567–72.

Friedman, G.D. and Ury, H.K. (1980). Initial screening for carcinogenicity of commonly used drugs. *J. nat. Cancer Inst.* **65**, 723–33.

Griffin, J.P. (1979). Drug-induced neoplasia. In *Iatrogenic diseases* (ed. P.F. D'Arcy and J.P. Griffin), 2nd edition, pp. 349–59. Oxford University Press.

Grimlund, K. (1963). Phenacetin and renal damage at a Swedish factory. *Acta med. Scand.* **174**, Suppl. 405, 1–26.

Harris, C.C. (1976). The carcinogenicity of anticancer drugs: a hazard in man. *Cancer* **37**, 1014–23.

Hoover, R. and Fraumeni, J.F. (1975). Drugs. In *Persons at high risk of cancer* (ed. J.F. Fraumeni), pp. 185–98. Academic Press, New York.

Horrobin, D.F., Ghayur, T., and Karmali, R.A. (1979). Mind and cancer. *Lancet* **i**, 978.

Horrobin, D.F. and Trosko, J.E. (1981). The possible effect of diazepam on cancer development and growth. *Med. Hypoth.* **7**, 115–25.

Hultengren, N., Lagergren, C., and Ljungqvist, A. (1965). Carcinoma of the renal pelvis in renal papillary necrosis. *Acta chir. Scand.* **130**, 314–20.

Hutchinson, J. (1887). Arsenic cancer. *Brit. med. J.* **ii**, 1280–1.

IARC (1976). *Some naturally occurring substances.* IARC Monographs on the Evaluation of the Carcinogenic Risk of Chemicals to Man. Vol. 10. International Agency for Research on Cancer, Lyon.

IARC (1977). *Some miscellaneous pharmaceutical substances.* IARC Monographs on the Evaluation of the Carcinogenic Risk of Chemicals to Man. Vol. 13. International Agency for Research on Cancer, Lyon.

IARC (1980a). *Some metals and metallic compounds.* IARC Monographs on the Evaluation of the Carcinogenic Risk of Chemicals to Humans. Vol. 23. International Agency for Research on Cancer, Lyon.

IARC (1980b). *Some pharmaceutical drugs.* IARC Monographs on the Evaluation of the Carcinogenic Risk of Chemicals to Humans. Vol. 24. International Agency for Research on Cancer, Lyon.

IARC (1980c). *Long-term and short-term screening assays for carcinogens: a critical appraisal.* IARC Monographs, Supplement 2. International Agency for Research on Cancer, Lyon.

IARC (1981). *Some antineoplastic and immunosuppressive agents.* IARC Monographs on the Evaluation of the Carcinogenic Risk of Chemicals to Humans. Vol. 26. International Agency for Research on Cancer, Lyon.

IARC (1982). *Chemicals, industrial processes and industries associated with cancer in humans.* IARC Monographs, Vol. 1–29, Suppl. 4. International Agency for Research on Cancer, Lyon.

Inman, W.H.W. (1981). Postmarketing surveillance of adverse drug reactions in general practice. II. Prescription-event monitoring at the University of Southampton. *Brit. med. J.* **282**, 1216–17.

Inman, W.H.W. (1983). *PEM News*, No. 1. Drug Surveillance Research Unit, University of Southampton, Southampton.

Jick, H., Walker, A.M., Watkins, R.N., D'Ewart, D.C., Hunter, J.R., Danford, A., Madsen, S., Dinan, B.J., Rothman, K.J. (1980). Oral contraceptives and breast cancer. *Amer. J. Epidemiol.* **112**, 577–85.

Kaufman, D.W., Shapiro, S., Slone, D., Rosenberg, L., Helmrich, S.P., Miettinen, O.S., Stolley, P.D., Levy, M., and Schottenfeld, D. (1982). Diazepam and the risk of breast cancer. *Lancet* **i**, 537–9.

Kincaid-Smith, P. (1978). Analgesic nephropathy. *Kidney Int.* **13**, 1–4.

Kinlen, L.J. (1982). Immunosuppressive therapy and cancer. *Cancer Surv.* **1**, 565–83.

Kleinerman, R.A., Brinton, L.A., Hoover, R., and Fraumeni, J.F. (1981). Diazepam and breast cancer. *Lancet* **i**, 1153.

The Lancet (1975). The 36,000. (Leading article.) *Lancet* **i**, 315–16.

The Lancet (1977). The hazards of Thorotrast. (Leading article.) *Lancet* **i**, 1297.

MacMahon, B. and Pugh, T.F. (1970). *Epidemiology: principles and methods.* Little Brown, Boston.

Neubauer, O. (1947). Arsenical cancer: a review. *Brit. J. Cancer* **1**, 192–251.

Parrish, J.A., Fitzpatrick, T.B., Tanenbaum, L., and Pathak, M.A. (1974). Photochemotherapy of psoriasis with oral methoxsalen and longwave ultraviolet light. *New Engl. J. Med.* **291**, 1207–11.

Reimer, R.R., Hoover, R., Fraumeni, J.F., and Young, R.C. (1977). Acute leukaemia after alkylating-agent therapy of ovarian cancer. *New Engl. J. Med.* **297**, 177–81.

Reinicke, C. (1982). Metals. In *Side effects of drugs annual*, Vol. 6 (ed. M.N.G. Dukes), pp. 216–28. Excerpta Medica, Amsterdam.

Roe, F.J.C. (1983). Toxicologic evaluation of metronidazole with particular reference to carcinogenic, mutagenic, and teratogenic potential. *Surgery* **93**, 158–64.

Rosner, F., Grünwald, H.W., and Zarrabi, H.M. (1982). Cancer after the use of alkylating and non-alkylating cytotoxic agents in man. *Cancer Surv.* **1**, 599–612.

Schmähl, D. and Habs, M. (1980). Drug-induced cancer. In *Drug-induced pathology* (ed. E. Grundmann), pp. 333–69. Current Topics in Pathology, Vol. 69. Springer-Verlag, Berlin.

Schmähl, D. and Habs, M. (1982). Cancer after the use of alkylating and non-alkylating cytotoxic agents in animals. *Cancer Surv.* **1**, 585–97.

Schmähl, D., Thomas, C., and Auer, R. (1977). *Iatrogenic carcinogenesis.* Springer-Verlag, Berlin.

Skegg, D.C.G. (1980). Medical record linkage. In *Monitoring for Drug Safety* (ed. W.H.W. Inman), pp. 337–48. MTP Press, Lancaster.

Skegg, D.C.G. and Doll, R. (1981). Record linkage for drug monitoring. *J. Epidemiol. comm. Hlth.* **35**, 25–31.

Skegg, D.C.G., Doll, R., and Perry, J. (1977). Use of medicines in general practice. *Brit. med. J.* **i**, 1561–3.

Slone, D., Shapiro, S., and Miettinen, O.S. (1977). Case-control surveillance of serious illnesses attributable to ambulatory drug use. In *Epidemiological evaluation of drugs* (ed. F. Colombo, S. Shapiro, D. Slone, and G. Tognoni), pp. 59–70. Elsevier/North-Holland, Amsterdam.

Smith, P.G. and Jick, H. (1977). Regular drug use and cancer. *J. nat. Cancer Inst.* **59**, 1387–91.

Stern, R.S., Thibodeau, L.A., Kleinerman, R.A., Parrish, J.A., and Fitzpatrick, T.B. (1979). Risk of cutaneous carcinoma in patients treated with oral methoxsalen photochemotherapy for psoriasis. *New Engl. J. Med.* **300**, 809–13.

Thiede, T., Chievitz, E., and Christensen, B.C. (1964). Chlornaphazine as a bladder carcinogen. *Acta med. Scand.* **175**, 721–5.

Thiede, T. and Christensen, B.C. (1969). Bladder tumours induced by chlornaphazine. *Acta. med. Scand.* **185**, 133–7.

Tomatis, L., Breslow, N.E., and Bartsch, H. (1982). Experimental studies in the assessment of human risk. In *Cancer epidemiology and prevention* (ed. D. Schottenfeld and J.F. Fraumeni), pp. 44–73. Saunders, Philadelphia.

White, S.J., McLean, A.E.M., and Howland, C. (1979). Anticonvulsant drugs and cancer. A cohort study in patients with severe epilepsy. *Lancet* **ii**, 458–61.

Whitehouse, J.M.A. (1983). Cytotoxic drugs for non-neoplastic disease. *Brit. med. J.* **287**, 79–80.

World Health Organization (1975). *Guidelines for evaluation of drugs for use in man*. WHO Technical Report Series, No. 563. World Health Organization, Geneva.

11 Prevention through legislation

Muir Gray and Charles Fletcher

The use of the State's power to make and enforce rules has played an important part in the prevention of disease for many years. In most developed countries the major reason for improvement in the state of the public health has been the prevention of the common infectious diseases, resulting from the passing of laws to ensure that clean water is provided, that sewage is disposed of safely, and that a healthy environment is provided for people to live in.

Such legislation requires little ethical justification. In some cases the State had to act because the measures required to prevent disease were too great for an individual to implement by himself: it is, for example, very difficult for an individual living in the middle of a large city to provide himself with pure water and clean food. An even stronger justification for the State to prevent disease was the traditional function of law as a means of protecting the individual from harm by third parties. Few people questioned the right of the State to control the factory-owner whose chimney was producing noxious products as he sought to process his material in the cheapest possible way. Few people questioned the complex set of laws and regulations that were set up to regulate the activities of food and drink producers, factory owners, and industrialists. Some debated the amount of legislation; others the cost of its implementation, but few questioned the right of the State to attempt to control the behaviour of those who would harm other citizens (Gray 1979). Such legislation has a major part to play in the prevention of cancer by preventing radioactive and chemical pollution of the environment, by controlling the production and use of food additives, and by protecting the worker from carcinogens in the workplace.

In recent years, however, another type of legislation has been the focus of the debate on preventive medicine: paternalistic legislation, which is designed to prevent disease by making the individual act in a way that reduces the risk of disease. Here the State is not seeking to protect the individual from harm by third parties, but to protect the individual from himself. This type of legislation is the focus of a great deal of ethical debate which is of central importance to cancer prevention because it is the legislation that is principally employed in the attempts to control the commonest known carcinogen – cigarette smoking.

There are many different types of paternalistic legislation. The least controversial concerns the legislation designed to prevent young people from starting smoking, which is long established in many countries. In Norway, for example, the sale of tobacco to children under 15 years was banned in 1899; in Canada the sale of cigarettes to persons under 16 was banned by law in 1908; and in the U.K. the Children and Young Persons Act of 1933 consolidated similar legislation first included in the Children's Act of 1908. The age of majority varies, with most countries proscribing the sale of cigarettes to young people under the age of 16. Although there is some debate about the most appropriate age of majority, because of the differences in regulations governing the sale of cigarettes, the sale of alcohol, and voting, the use of paternalistic legislation to protect children is widely accepted. Measures directed at adults, on the other hand, are criticised strongly.

Before discussing the part that paternalistic legislation has to play in the prevention of cancer it is important to distinguish between 'laws' and 'the Law'.

'Laws' and 'the Law'

Each law is a rule, but should not be viewed simply as a tool designed for specific purpose, because each law is also an expression of certain values prevailing in society. The latter is a very important function and justifies the introduction of laws which are difficult to enforce, such as the law which prohibits the sale of cigarettes to young people. Most police forces do not have the resources to try to enforce it because there are so many places when young people can be sold cigarettes. It is, nevertheless, important that such law exists and that prosecutions are made, albeit only occasionally, because such prosecutions symbolize society's view that the sale of cigarettes to children is wrong and remind the retail trade and individual tobacconists of this view.

There is, of course, the danger that the introduction of a law that cannot be enforced will bring that law, and the Law as a whole, into disrepute (the consequences of the prohibition of alcohol in the U.S. provide striking evidence of this danger), so governments must take care that they do not introduce laws that are impossible to implement.

'The Law' is greater than the sum of all the individual laws. Just as a law is not simply a rule, the Law is not only a rulebook. It is also an expression of the values that prevail, or have prevailed, in a society. A change in the Law reflects a change in the attitudes of the society whose representatives drafted and passed it. Such a change not only follows changes in society, it may also accelerate the rate of change. A legal ban on the advertising of cigarettes would not only reflect attitudes that such a ban was right and that advertising was wrong, but would also change attitudes. Some people believe that cigarettes cannot be very harmful because, they argue, the Government would not allow them to be advertised if they were as harmful as the experts claim. To this group of people the continued existence of advertising and sports' sponsorship supports such beliefs. The introduction of legislation banning sports' sponsorship would challenge their beliefs and would change the beliefs and attitudes of some of them.

It is difficult to measure the impact of changes in the law because they rarely occur in isolation. Usually they are accompanied by changes in beliefs and attitudes, in the manner described in the previous paragraphs, and, in the case of cigarette smoking, other changes take place at the same time. In Norway, for example, the introduction of an Act banning advertising was accompanied by an intensification of education aimed at young people and by the development of services to help smokers who wished to stop. Furthermore, changes in the law can affect more than one of the variables which determine the prevalence of cigarette smoking, for example a ban on advertising might be accompanied by stronger health warnings on cigarette packets.

It is important, therefore, that laws should not be considered or evaluated in isolation. We shall now consider the types of law most commonly used to reduce the prevalence of cigarette smoking.

Types of paternalistic legislation

The various types of legislation governing smoking have been analysed and summarized by the World Health Organization in two important publications: their Expert Committee's *Report on smoking control*, published in 1979 (World Health Organization 1979) and the worldwide survey of anti-smoking legislation published in 1982 (Roemer 1982).

Control of harmful substances in tobacco

Most developed countries now have regulatory measures designed to reduce the tar, nicotine, and carbon monoxide content of cigarettes. In some countries, such as the Federal Republic of Germany, the legal powers which allow the State to lay down standards which must be met by the industry are included in a general law drafted to protect the interests of the consumer. In other countries such regulations are accompanied by measures designed to control toxic substances. A government can issue regulations laying down specific standards which the tobacco industry must meet with respect to the amount of tar, nicotine, and carbone monoxide in cigarettes. If the State sets upper limits for harmful constituents it can then apply pressure on the industry to phase out the brands with concentrations nearest the upper limits. In developing countries, in which there are no such laws, cigarettes high in tar and nicotine are promoted and sold. The use of the law in this way is an effective and important means of reducing the intake of noxious substances but not of reducing the incidence or prevalence of smoking.

Restriction of sales to adults

Some governments have introduced legislation to control the sale of cigarettes to adults in certain circumstances. In Bulgaria, legislation passed in 1980 prohibited the sale of tobacco in educational or health establishments, or in shops within 200 metres of them. Cyprus has totally prohibited the use of cigarette-vending machines in an attempt to restrict the number of outlets for cigarettes; although this legislation is, of course, designed not only to restrict the sale to adults but to restrict the sale of cigarettes to young people.

It is easy to argue that such restrictions are ineffective, because smokers will find other places to buy cigarettes if some points of sale are removed, but the impact of the symbolic implication of such legislation should not be underestimated.

Mandatory provision of information

Many countries now require the printing of a health warning on the cigarette package. In some countries the statement is no more than a vague generalization, such as 'Tobacco is harmful to health', but in some countries the warning is explicit and clear, for example: 'Smokers die younger', or 'Cigarette smoking can cause lung cancer and heart disease'. Furthermore, a small number of countries now require one of a number of alternative warnings to be printed to prevent the smoker becoming so accustomed to a single warning that he eventually fails to notice it. Some countries require a clear statement of the tar and nicotine content of the cigarettes in the packet to complement the verbal health warning.

There has been little evaluation of the effectiveness of this type of measure and considered in isolation it is probably relatively ineffective. If, however, it is employed as part of a comprehensive strategy it probably has a significant impact and as it is relatively cheap to impose it is a measure which is relatively cost-effective.

Restrictions on smoking in public places

This type of legislation can be considered to be both paternalistic and 'traditional'. One of the reasons for its introduction is to provide an environment in which smokers find it easier to stop but the evidence about the harmful effects of passive smoking means that this can also be considered to be a traditional piece of public-health legislation, introduced to protect an individual from harm by third parties. The first law of this type was enacted by the State of Vermont in 1892 but it is only recently that there has been widespread adoption of this approach. This type of measure does not have to depend on state or federal action. It is one which can be implemented by a lower tier of government in many countries. In the U.K., for example, local authorities, county councils, and district councils can pass regulatory measures to prohibit smoking in the buildings for which they are responsible and in the U.S. each state can pass this type of legislation.

A relatively recent approach, pioneered in Finland, has been to reframe the issue by changing the basic assumption from one which accepted that public places were places for cigarette smoking, unless the contrary was stated, to an assumption that public places should be free from cigarette smoking unless cigarette smoking is specifically permitted.

This type of law is difficult to evaluate because its introduction both reflects and contributes to a change in public attitudes. It is, however, reasonable to assume that the introduction of such measures helps to change the image of cigarette smoking by emphasizing its social unacceptability, and such laws definitely benefit non-smokers by protecting them from the smell and noxious effects of the smoke from other people's cigarettes.

Restrictions in the workplace

Few countries have attempted to prohibit smoking in the workplace because of the problems of enforcing the legislation. Workplaces are extremely diverse both in their physical layout and in the social composition of the workforce and it is difficult to draft legislation suitable for all circumstances. However, most developed countries now have laws designed to prevent disease and promote health at work and even in such laws, such as the Health and Safety at Work Act of 1974, in the U.K., do not specifically mention cigarette smoking they offer a framework in which groups of workers locally can request a smoke-free environment.

This type of measure, like that described in the previous paragraph, is partly traditional and partly paternalistic.

Mandatory health education

In a small number of countries and American States health education is required by legislation. The intention of this type of legislation is to ensure that all members of the public are kept informed about the risks of smoking. In Iceland 2 per cent of the value of gross sales of cigarettes must be used to finance health education and in Finland 0.5 per cent of tobacco tax revenue must be used in a similar way.

This is a relatively uncommon type of legislation and its effectiveness is, of course, a function of the effectiveness of health education. It does at least ensure that education includes the subject of cigarette smoking.

Constraints and bans on advertising

A proportion of cigarette smokers argue that if cigarette smoking were really as dangerous as the medical profession stated the government would not permit the industry to advertise and promote their products. The industry, on the other hand, argues that cigarette advertising is simply a matter of encouraging the smoker to switch from one brand to another, citing the example of the U.S.S.R. where there is little advertising but a high prevalence of cigarette smoking. The main arguments of those who wish to see the prevalence of smoking reduced are that advertising implies government and social approval; that it creates an image of smoking as a normal human activity; and that when the advertising is through promotion of a sport, it leads to an association between sport and cigarette smoking that gives a healthy, glamorous image to smoking especially harmful to the young.

A number of countries have enacted a total ban on outdoor advertising and publicity. Iceland, Norway, Finland, and Bulgaria have all done this, the latter being particularly noteworthy as it is a major tobacco-producing country. Other countries seek to restrict both the nature and content of advertising through a voluntary agreement with the industry. The introduction of a total ban on advertising does of course present many problems, not only for the companies that make money from it. If, for example, only one country were to ban magazine advertisements then magazines from other countries which would still continue to insert advertisements would breach the ban. Nevertheless, although there are major practical problems there is strong support for the belief that the advertising and promotion of cigarettes remains one of the most important factors in maintaining the prevalence of cigarette smoking and that restriction of advertising, coupled with other regulatory and educational efforts of the type described in the previous sections, is an important means of reducing the prevalence of smoking and smoking-related diseases.

Alone such legislation will have only a limited impact, as the high prevalence of smoking in the U.S.S.R. demonstrates, but it has an important part to play in any package of legal and educational measures designed to lower the prevalence of cigarette smoking.

Taxation of cigarettes

Fiscal policy can be used in three main ways. The first is to reduce the prevalence of cigarette smoking by using taxes to ensure that cigarettes do not become cheaper either in relation to the price of other goods or in relation to the amount of work that has to be done to purchase them. In some countries steps have been taken to ensure that cigarettes become progressively more expensive relative to the cost of other goods but in many countries taxation is used simply to ensure that they do not become relatively cheaper.

The second use of fiscal policy is to introduce differential taxes so that brands with a low delivery of tar, nicotine, and carbon monoxide are relatively cheaper. The Chancellor of the Exchequer introduced such a measure in the U.K. in September 1978.

A third objective of fiscal policy in countries which grow tobacco is to reduce the subsidy for tobacco growing and promote the substitution of other crops for tobacco. This is much more difficult to achieve because agricultural policy is, as yet, little influenced by health considerations in most countries and the agricultural lobby, pressing governments to promote the interests of farmers, usually seeks to maximize the income of farmers with little concern for any harmful health consequences.

This type of legislation is probably the most effective of all the types of legislation discussed in this section, but it is important to emphasize again that there is no single measure that can prevent the cancers caused by cigarette smoking. A change in the law is only one component of a preventive strategy. Furthermore, it is often one that is more difficult to achieve because of the opposition to paternalistic legislation.

Opposition to paternalism

Opposition to paternalistic measures is common, particularly where the measures are designed to control behaviour that many people regard as pleasurable. The objections that members of the public and politicans have may be philosophical, economic, or both.

Philosophical objection

The argument against paternalistic intervention which is most widely known, and still most widely referred to, is that advanced by J.S. Mill (1859), who wrote:

> . . . the sole end for which mankind is warranted, individually or collectively, in interfering with the liberty of action of any of their number, is self-protection. That is, the only purpose for which power can be rightfully exercised over any member of a civilised community, against his will, is to prevent harm to others. His own good, either physical or moral, is not sufficient warrant. He cannot rightfully be compelled to do or forbear because it will be better for him to do so, because it will make him happier, because in the opinions of others, to do so would be wise, or even right . . . The only part of the conduct of anyone, for which he is amenable to society, is that which concerns others. In the part which merely concerns himself, his independence is, of right, absolute. Over himself, over his own body and mind, the individual is sovereign.

This argument forms the basis for most of the philosophical objections that politicians hold against paternalistic legislation. The State, such politicans argue, should only protect individuals against harm from third parties and should only attempt to promote the well-being of citizens by taking such measures that will ensure that the State remains strong, stable, and secure, for example by extracting taxes from them to pay for an army or a road system.

Such a line of argument has its weaknesses, as even Mill himself recognized (Vallance 1975). Even though Mill wrote before the Welfare State had developed he recognized that individuals who neglected their health could cause harm to others by making demands on the State, giving as an example a man who 'in temperence or extravagance becomes unable to pay his debts, or having undertaken the moral responsibility of a family, becomes from the same cause incapable of supporting or educating them'. When there is a State-financed health service it is difficult to define what is harm to self and what is harm to others, for a person who uses a proportion, no matter how small, of finite health resources inevitably affects other people, and it can be argued that this provides the ethical justification for legal measures to reduce the prevalence of smoking even though they interfere with the liberty of the individual.

To rebut this argument cigarette smokers claim that they make a financial contribution to the health service through the taxes they pay, while people who indulge in other high-risk activities do not. Mountain climbers, for example, do not pay higher taxes than those who do not climb mountains, although they make heavier use of health services. A second criticism of such a justification for measures that affect the liberty of people to buy and smoke cigarettes is that action against cigarette smoking is 'the thin end of the wedge', and that if such measures are introduced to control cigarette smoking the public-health movement will turn its attention to some other aspect of modern life.

John Stuart Mill's passionate defence of liberty still forms the philosophical basis of most attacks on attempts to prevent cancer by legislative means, but those who portray Mill as a champion of the individual also have to take into account the arguments expressed in his essay on Utilitarianism, for these emphasize the interdependence of individuals in society. No-one has absolute liberty. One man's liberty impinges on the liberty of others and the person who uses one part of a finite resource reduces the amount of resources available to meet other needs.

Much of the weakness in Mill's argument stems from a failure precisely to define 'liberty'. The word 'liberty' has such an intoxicating ring to it that it is all too easy for it to be bandied about in debate without any attempt to define it. Liberty, or freedom, appears to be a concept that is so self-evident that it requires no definition but, as is so often the case, a failure to define precisely what is meant by the words being used in an argument results in an argument that is incapable of resolution. Isiah Berlin recognized that this was a fundamental weakness in many of the papers that were written in nineteenth and twentieth century Europe and, in a classic essay entitled *Two concepts of liberty*, he distinguished negative liberty from positive liberty (Berlin 1969).

The former corresponds to the commonsense definition of freedom, such as liberty to smoke cannabis, or to drive without a seat belt, or to purchase cigarettes or alcohol at a market price without an imposed health tax, and it is loss, or the possibility of loss, of one of these freedoms that usually arouses the opposition of the liberty lobby, namely those who accept Mill's views on liberty. Positive liberty, Berlin argues, is much more important, being the liberty to decide how much negative liberty each individual should have. Obviously such decisions are made collectively but the individual should participate in collective decisions through his political representatives. However, many people are deeply disturbed by what they feel to be the loss of positive liberty that has taken place during the last three decades as the influence of the individual, either the individual voter or individual politician, has diminished as the influence of organized lobbies, big business, and the experts has increased. This concept is, however, too complicated for many people who express their distrust of politicians and governments by their opposition to measures that interfere with their negative liberty.

The importance of this distinction for preventive medicine is obvious. There is a danger that the public may oppose the use of legislation to prevent cancer neither because they are opposed to cancer prevention, nor even because they are opposed to the use of paternalistic legislation but because they feel that they have lost the positive liberty of influencing decisions about their negative liberty, and that these decisions are being made by politicans, civil servants, and experts rather than by their political representatives.

To summarize, many politicians have reservations about paternalistic legislation, with a considerable range in the strength of feeling with which they oppose new measures. Members of the public also have reservations about political paternalism, again showing a wide range in strength of feeling. For some members of the public paternalistic legislation symbolizes State control over the individual and is opposed not so much because such individuals oppose the objectives of prevention but because they find the type of legislative measure introduced to prevent disease offers an easily understood issue on which to challenge government.

It is, however, important to recognize that philosophical objections to paternalistic legislation are often a cover for economic objections.

Economic objections: the tobacco lobby

The tobacco industry, like any major industry, has its political supporters. These are people who may oppose paternalistic legislation on philosophical grounds but whose principal interest is to support the tobacco industry, an industry which is not only large and powerful, but also complex and diverse (Calnan 1981). The production of a cigarette involves a long chain from the farmer who grows the crop to the retailer who sells it, and each link in the chain has its own interest in cigarette smoking and its own lobby.

The metaphor of a chain is powerful enough but an even more powerful, and apposite, metaphor was coined by Peter Taylor (1984) when he published a book called *The smoke ring* which emphasizes that all the elements are interconnected.

Taylor's book is a masterpiece that deserves to take its place with the most important books and articles on preventive medicine because he describes in detail, and with precise references, the ways in which politicians and the tobacco industry are mutually interdependent. One of the many dramatic examples he gives is of the relationship between President Reagan and the tobacco farmers. As Taylor points out, tobacco is grown in 51, about one-tenth, of all congressional districts, and the representatives of these districts form a very powerful lobby, a lobby which Reagan required to win to become President. He obtained the support of this lobby by promising that 'I can guarantee my own cabinet members will be far too busy with substantive matters to waste their time proselytising against the dangers of smoking.' This did not, however, prevent President Reagan's Surgeon General Everett Koop from taking a forthright public position (Koop 1983), as his predecessors had before him (Burney 1983; Luther 1983), but it did prevent the introduction of federal curbs on the tobacco industry.

In a country which does not grow tobacco there are also constituency interests because tobacco factories are major employers, whose factories are not infrequently sited in areas of high unemployment. Obviously every constituency has constituents whose livelihood is dependent, principally or partly, on cigarettes: tobacconists, newsagents, and publicans for example, but it is really only where sufficient numbers of people are employed in the manufacture of cigarettes that the Member of Parliament will be pressing to lobby. There are, however, other constituencies than those represented on a map and certain Members of Parliament have links with national organizations, such as those representing tobacconists or workers in cigarette factories, and will thus oppose the introduction of laws drafted to reduce the prevalence of smoking even though they have no direct pressure from their local constituency. Other politicians join the tobacco lobby because they are consultants or advisers, usually receiving payment, to the tobacco companies themselves, or to other companies, such as advertising companies, which obtain income from the tobacco companies.

The tobacco lobby has a clear objective on which the energies of its members can be focused. The health lobby in Parliament, in contrast, is more diverse in its range of interests and less well united. Many politicians are interested in health and health services, but only some members of the health lobby have cigarette smoking as their principal interest. Furthermore, those who are interested in reducing the prevalence of cigarette smoking have less money than the tobacco industry and are not able to provide the same degree of support that the industry provides for the tobacco lobby.

The tobacco lobby's argument has a number of different threads. One is their philosophical opposition, a second that the case against cigarettes is still not completely proven, a third that the economic benefits of the tobacco industry are so great that the contribution it makes to the health of the economy should be taken into account when measures to reduce the public-health hazards of cigarette smoking are under discussion. Their lobby argues that the tobacco industry provides jobs, exports, and revenue for both local and central government and it is true that it does. What the lobby is not prepared to concede, however, is that the costs are so great that these financial benefits cannot be considered in isolation. The lobby uses a wide range of techniques to impress its point upon the Government and upon those politicians who occupy the middle ground, being neither members of the tobacco lobby nor members of the health lobby.

Members of the tobacco lobby act in various ways to protect the industry. They form part of the industry's intelligence system, as antennae in Parliament identifying possible sources of danger. They lobby Government Ministers directly and personally, as Peter Taylor describes in his book, with Members of Parliament from both parties combining to 'ambush' the Chancellor in the Division Lobby (Taylor 1984, p. 70). The lobby, however, has its most serious work to do when new legislation is suggested or introduced. In the U.S. their power was marshalled when Dr Edward Brandt, the Assistant Secretary for Health, was proposing new measures to reduce the prevalence of cigarette smoking (Taylor 1984, p. 9). In the U.K. the most blatant exercise of power was the filibustering of a Private Member's Bill to 'provide for the control and regulation of advertising of tobacco products and of other means of advertising such products.'

Laurie Pavitt is a backbench Labour MP representing the constituency in which stands the Central Middlesex Hospital where Richard Doll did his early work. It was as a result of his contacts with Richard Doll and other physicians who worked at the Central Middlesex that Laurie Pavitt's interest in health was stimulated and he has tried to introduce Private Member's Bills to control advertising on numerous occasions. This occasion appeared to be auspicious because health ministers informally supported the bill, although the bill was presented by Mrs Gwyneth Dunwoody, an opposite Member. The Bill was due to be debated on a Friday, 12 June 1979, following the debate on the Zoo Licensing (No. 2) Bill which appeared to be uncontroversial. However, on 11 June 164 amendments to the Zoo Licensing Bill were tabled by a small number of Members, some of whom were members of the tobacco lobby; for example one was Parliamentary Adviser to a tobacco company while two others represented constituencies with strong tobacco interests. The debate on these amendments, which consisted mostly of minor drafting amendments such as 'leave out "the" and insert "any" ', lasted so long that the Bill presented by Mrs Dunwoody and supported by Laurie Pavitt was effectively filibustered.

One can criticize these tactics but they are conventional political tactics carried out in public and reported verbatim. Of greater concern is the influence that the lobby has behind the scenes. The contribution of the lobby's influence to the decision to move Joseph Califano, President Carter's Secretary of State for Health, and Sir George Young, a Minister in the Department of Health in the U.K., has never been elucidated, but both were moved after displaying a determination to take effective action to curb the industry.

The scope for professional action

What can the medical profession, or any other groups of people interested in the prevention of cancer, do to influence the power politic? At first sight the answer appears to be that very little can be done but there is in fact much that doctors and epidemiologists, both as individuals and collectively, can do to influence the political process.

Collective action

In many countries the medical profession now campaigns for political action. For example, in the U.S. the American Medical Association, and a number of specialist medical groups, have campaigned to support the Surgeon General and to put pressure on Congress; the Medical Association of South Africa is publicly committed to a total ban on all tobacco advertising on all media and a variety of other legislative measures; and the Royal Colleges in the U.K. also play an active role, with their Presidents lobbying the Chancellor of the Exchequer as each budget is being formulated.

The Royal College of Physicians (U.K.) has played a significant part in this work, initially by producing the first College report on smoking and health, which started when Robert Platt, the President, responded with alacrity to the suggestion that the College should produce a report on smoking (Royal College of Physicians 1962). Richard Doll produced data from the British doctors' survey expressed in terms more commonly encountered in betting, an approach which convinced not only members of the public but a number of members of the medical profession who had previously taken little notice of the scientific evidence.

The College Committee took two-and-a-half years to complete its work and a page proof was sent to all Fellows of the College, being approved by them at a meeting of the College in July 1961 with only one dissentient vote. The publishers suggested it would be unwise to print more than 5000 copies but the College treasurer, Dr Dick Bomford, formerly a radio doctor, agreed that the College carry the financial risk of printing 10 000 copies. A copy was sent to Mr. Geoffrey Todd, Secretary of the Tobacco Advisory Committee, who made a number of valuable comments and who asked the Committee to circulate 20 copies of the report to the tobacco industry before publication, which they did.

The report was published on Ash Wednesday in 1962 with the President, Robert Platt, asking the reporters at the press conference if they would fly an airline if one in eight of their planes crashed every decade. The impact was enormous, with banner headlines in all the evening papers on the day of publication and on the daily papers the next morning. All the copies were sold within a few days and 20 000 further copies were printed for the U.S. Cancer Society, the report being one of the factors which led President Kennedy to ask the Surgeon General to prepare the first of the valuable U.S. Public Health Reports on the health consequences of smoking.

The College was pleased with the immediate effect of its first report but was disappointed by the response of the Government. Enoch Powell, then Minister of Health, said that he accepted the conclusions of the report and although he took little direct action he did set up a Departmental Advisory Committee on Smoking which met monthly and was responsible for persuading the Ministry to finance important surveys of public attitudes towards smoking (McKennell and Thomas 1967), smoking among schoolboys (Bynner 1969), and smoking among medical students (Bynner 1967). The Committee was supported by Sir George Godber, the Chief Medical Officer, who made forthright reports each year in his Annual Report on 'The state of the public health'. Other small gains were made, for example the Labour Government, on coming to power in 1964, prohibited cigarette advertising on television and the manufacturers accepted the voluntary code of advertising control.

The College Committee published a report on air pollution in 1970 (Royal College of Physicians 1970), demonstrating that the effects of air pollution were much less severe than the effects of cigarette smoking, and during the time that had elapsed since the first report, the evidence demonstrating the dangers of smoking had become very much stronger, particularly that derived from the second report of Doll and Hill (1952) on their study of doctors, but despite the increasing evidence cigarette consumption had not continued the decline that had started following the publication of the 1962 report.

The College Committee, with Sir Max Rosenheim in the Chair, published a second report in 1971 (Royal College of Physicians 1971), expressing their views in strong language. The Secretary of State, Sir Keith Joseph, Conservative, was impressed by the report, describing it as 'a lobby which could not be resisted', but his actions, though more vigorous than those of Enoch Powell nine years previously, fell far short of the actions the report had demanded. For example, warnings were put on cigarette packets but they were much weaker and less prominent than had been recommended, and the grant for health education was increased but was still negligible in comparison with resources spent by the tobacco industry.

The College Committee was of the opinion that more forceful action was required than could be expected of either the Department of Health or of the College Committee, and at a press conference launching the second report on smoking and health the College President announced the formation of what he called 'Action on Smoking and Health' (ASH), modelled in part on the 'Interagency Council' on smoking and health which acted as a co-ordinating body in the U.S. The first director was a doctor, a former Parliamentary Under-Secretary at the Ministry of Health in the Labour Government who had lost his seat in the election of 1970, and the work of ASH was supported both by the College and by the Department of Health, which made a grant that was intended to be a single launching grant.

However, the major British charities concerned with cancer and vascular disease did not wish to support ASH and it was not until the arrival of its second director that the decision was made to transform ASH from a co-ordinating body which acted as a source of advice and information to a political pressure group providing a 24-hour information service for press and broadcasters, information for Members of Parliament, and evidence to the Advertising Standards Authority of breaches in the voluntary code of advertising restriction. An all-party Parliamentary Working Group on Smoking and Health was set up, drawing together sympathetic Members of Parliament from all political parties, and with the aid of sympathetic civil servants, the case to the Department of Health for continuing funding was made and accepted.

In the 1970s the other Royal Colleges also became involved in direct lobbying of Ministers of State but the main source of political pressure centrally remains Action on Smoking and Health, a political pressure group set up by, and supported by, the medical profession.

The medical profession is involved in campaigning in many other countries, notably in Australia where doctors have been involved in a range of activities from direct lobbying of State Parliaments to the staging of newsworthy events designed to embarrass the tobacco industry and maintain public interest. For example, 150 doctors held a public meeting on the steps of the Parliament House in Western Australia when the Smoking and Tobacco Products Advertisements Bill was being introduced. This resulted in its approval by the Lower House, though the Upper House, influenced by a massive campaign funded by the industry, rejected it. The Australian BUGA-UP (Billboard Utilizing Graffitists Against Unhealthy Promotions) campaign is now well known because the techniques used by the campaigners to amend the messages of the cigarette hoardings are often witty and arresting.

Finally, it is encouraging to note that a growing number of medical journals are giving prominence not only to the adverse health effects of cigarette smoking but also to the need for political action. The *British Medical Journal*, *The Lancet*, *The Journal of the American Medical Association*, and the *Americal Journal of Public Health* are all strongly committed to cancer prevention through legislation.

There seems little likelihood that the medical profession and the tobacco industry will ever abandon their adversarial relationship for the industry still tries to cast doubts on the evidence: the Chairman of Rothmans International has stated in the European Parliament, of which he is a member, that 'I would emphasise that there is no medical evidence that a few cigarettes, say ten or fifteen a day, are bad for you' (Nicholson, 1980).

Individual action

If the medical profession sometimes seems daunted when faced with the power and complexity of the political process, it is not surprising that many individuals feel that there is little that they can do to try to prevent the harmful effects of cigarette smoking by influencing the political process.

Some physicians of course are uniquely placed to take action. Successive Surgeons General have committed the United States Public Health Service to the need for legislative controls, often in the face of political opposition and, in the early days, in the face of criticism from their colleagues; the first statement on smoking and health by the Surgeon General, in 1957, was greeted with a critical editorial by the Editor of the *Journal of the American Medical Association*. In the U.K. the Chief Medical Officer is in an analogous position and Sir George Godber made a major contribution to the public health by the prominence he gave to cigarette smoking as a health hazard.

Most physicians are, however, not in a position of central influence but it is important for the individual not to underestimate the contribution that he can make. As political lobbying becomes increasingly well organized, both the lobbying of the tobacco industry and the lobbying of major medical associations and voluntary bodies, it might seem that the scope for individual action decreases. Paradoxically this is not the case because politicians are becoming increasingly sceptical of centralized lobbying and are increasingly resistant to its effects. In any Parliament the majority of politicians do not lobby either for or against the tobacco industry. There will always be only a small number on each side who are passionately committed and for political change to occur the majority who are mildly interested must be motivated to take action. Although centralized lobbying does influence the uncommitted politician, such a person is often more influenced by the supplication of a small number of his constituents.

In the United Kingdom most Members of Parliament would be very interested in the opinions of doctors working and living in their constituencies, but unfortunately individual physicians make very little contact with politicians. For example, one Member of Parliament who was widely known nationally for his commitment to preventive medicine had never once been approached by any of the doctors in his constituency about cigarette smoking and the only contact he had was when he initiated it. If an uncommitted politician were to receive four or five letters or visits from physicians or epidemiologists, and were to see that these were not part of a centrally organized lobby but a genuine expression of concern that politicans might well move from being neutral to being interested in, and committed to, action to control the smoking epidemic. It is therefore very important for physicians not simply to act by supporting their national organizations, but to take individual action (Daube and Gray 1983).

One individual physician who has of course made a major impact has been Richard Doll and it has been one of his principal characteristics that he has not entered directly into political lobbying for the changes that his epidemiological work have indicated as being essential if we are to improve the public health. He has certainly supported the work of groups such as ASH but his main strength has been that he has been seen as a neutral observer describing a relationship and leaving the public and physicians to draw the inevitable conclusions. He was the first, and is perhaps still the only British epidemiologist whose name alone will convince journalists that a topic is newsworthy, who is cited in the House of Commons and House of Lords, and in many hearings in the U.S. Sir Keith Joseph, when Secretary of State for Social Services, said in Parliament in 1971, 'It was the Doll and Hill experiment . . . which totally convinced me that cigarette smoking inflicts very grave and avoidable suffering on large numbers of our fellow countrymen.' (Hansard 1971). The impact of the work of Richard Doll, firstly with Bradford Hill and then with other research workers, has been far-reaching, not only epidemiologically but politically, demonstrating that cancer prevention requires not only individual action but also political action.

Acknowledgement

We are grateful to Michael Daube and David Simpson, the former and present Directors of ASH (Action on Smoking and Health) for the help they gave us in preparing this chapter and for the contribution they have made, and are making, towards improving public health by persuading governments to recognize the impact of cigarette smoking and their responsibility to reduce that impact.

References

Berlin, I. (1969). Two concepts of liberty. In *Four essays on liberty*. Oxford University Press.

Burney, L.E. (1983). Policy over politics: The first statement on smoking and health by the Surgeon General of the United States Public Health Service. *N.Y. State J. Med.* **83**, 1252–3.

Bynner, J.M. (1969). *The young smoker*. A study of smoking among schoolboys carried out for the Ministry of Health. SS 383. HMSO, London.

Bynner, J.M. (1967). *Medical students' attitudes towards smoking*. A report on a survey carried out for the Ministry of Health. SS 382. HMSO, London.

Calnan, M. (1981). A review of government policies aimed at primary prevention. In *The prevention of cancer* (ed. M. Alderson), pp. 101–35. Edward Arnold, London.

Daube, M. and Gray, J.A.M. (1983). The politics of prevention – the scope for individual action. *Preventive medicine in general practice*, (ed. J.A.M. Gray and G.H. Fowler), p. 86–93. Oxford University Press.

Doll, R. and Hill, A.B. (1952). Mortality in relation to smoking: ten years' observations of British doctors. *Brit. med. J.* **i**, 1399–405; 1460–5.

Gray, J.A.M. (1979). *Man against disease*, pp. 115–23. Oxford University Press.

Hansard. (1971). House of Commons, 23 April.

Koop (1983). A dialogue with Surgeon General Koop: confronting America's most costly health problem. *N.Y. State J. Med.* **83**, 1260–3.

Luther, L.T. (1983). The Surgeon' General's first report on smoking and health: A challenge to the medical profession. *N.Y. State J. Med.* **83**, 1254–5.

McKennell, A.C. and Thomas, R.K. (1967). *Adults' and adolescents' smoking habits and attitudes*. A report on a survey carried out for the Ministry of Health. SS 353/B, HMSO, London.

Mill, J.S. (1859). *On liberty*, p. 135. Fontana.

Nicholson, D. (1980). *Proc. Euro. Parl.*, 12–13. Feb.

Roemer, R. (1982). *Legislative action to combat the world smoking epidemic*. WHO, Geneva.

Royal College of Physicians (1962). *Smoking and health*. Pitman Medical, London.

Royal College of Physicians (1970). *Air pollution and health*. Pitman Medical, London.

Royal College of Physicians (1971). *Smoking and health now*. A new report and summary on smoking and its effects on health. Pitman Medical, London.

Vallance, E. (1975). Introduction. In *The state, society and self-destruction*. Allen and Unwin, London.

Taylor, P. (1984). *The smoke ring*. The Bodley Head, London.

World Health Organization (1979). *Controlling the smoking epidemic*. Report of the WHO Expert Committee on Smoking Control. Technical Report series No. 636. WHO, Geneva.

12 Prevention of cancer by education: the case of smoking

Muir Gray and Konrad Jamrozik

To a very large extent 'prevention of cancer by education' means prevention of smoking. At least 90 per cent of cancer of the trachea and bronchus (lung cancer) is attributable to tobacco smoking (Royal College of Physicians 1971) and this disease, virtually always fatal, is already the most common cancer of men in Western countries and is poised to overtake cancer of the breast as the commonest cancer of women. On a world scale, for none of the other major cancers – those of the liver, breast, colon, stomach, or uterine cervix – are the risk factors so well understood or as simple to avoid. Tobacco smoking has been estimated to be responsible for 30 per cent of *all* fatal cases of cancer in the U.S. (Doll and Peto 1981). Faced with this evidence prevention of smoking must be the first concern of any education campaign aiming to reduce the incidence of cancer in the community.

Widespread use of tobacco began in Europe at most only four generations ago. It took two generations for the harmful effects of cigarettes first to become apparent, and much research over the next 20 years was devoted to confirming the harmful effects and to investigating the mechanisms by which tobacco smoke caused disease. Although all of the questions have not been answered, there is no doubt that smoking is the leading avoidable cause of ill-health and premature death in developed countries, if not the whole world (World Health Organization 1975), and this has lead several countries to adopt policies designed to ensure that the next generation is 'smoke-free'. Sweden and Norway, in particular, appear to be making great strides in pursuit of this aim, and it is notable that each has adopted the tripartite anti-smoking strategy advocated by the International Union Against Cancer (Gray and Daube 1980). The three components of this strategy are:

(1) legislation and regulation to curb smoking and pro-smoking influences;
(2) public information and education campaigns;
(3) smoking-cessation activities.

Although each of these components has some impact of its own, in combination the strategies are mutually reinforcing and, in reflecting the commitment of the government and of the community, will accelerate the re-establishment of non-smoking as the norm.

The role, scope, and impact of legislation in controlling tobacco-related cancer in developing countries have been reviewed in the previous chapter, and we will focus on the contribution of health education to (a) preventing people from starting to smoke and (b) helping people to stop.

Preventing people from starting to smoke

The natural history of cigarette smoking

In recent years theories about the reasons why young people smoke have undergone a transformation. The earliest theory was simply that young people start to smoke as part of the process of 'growing up', of becoming an adult. This theory, which was derived largely from the sociological study of adolescence, was then elaborated and a number of different reasons for smoking were hypothesized, in all of which smoking was depicted as playing an instrumental part in the transition from childhood to adulthood. The common theories that evolved from the belief that smoking was primarily a *rite de passage* are that adolescents smoke for the following reasons:

(1) to act like a grown-up: the image of smoking is tough and sexy, cool and sophisticated, and it was claimed that children smoke to mimic their heroes;
(2) to feel like a grown-up: behaving like an adult was said to help the adolescent who was nervous and insecure;
(3) to rebel: it was argued that if parents and teachers simply said 'don't smoke' the rebellious adolescent would do the reverse.

Recent research, more influenced by psychological than sociological theory, has suggested that smoking should be regarded less as a means of achieving adult status and more as a means of being a teenager, that is to say as a means of interacting with other teenagers and doing the things that teenagers regard as normal (Evans 1981).

The first cigarette

Many young people take their first cigarette as a means of solving what has been called a 'momentary dilemma' (Covington 1981; Thier 1981). The research in the Ray-S project in California suggests that young people do not start smoking because they have made a conscious decision 'to smoke' or 'to become a smoker' but because they are offered cigarettes in situations in which they find acceptance easier than refusal, typically when the casual offer of a cigarette is made by one young person to another young person who admires, respects, or fears him. Cigarettes, therefore, are tools that young people use to facilitate their relationship with one another rather than 'rites of passage' to adult life. In the Ray-S project young smokers reported 14 different types of reason for smoking, ranging from the use of cigarettes to preclude rejection, to the use of cigarettes as a means of ingratiating oneself with another. Only 5 per cent of young people stated that they smoked to find enjoyment and only one-fifth of those young people who smoke regularly enjoyed their first cigarette (Table 1).

Developing dependence

After the first cigarette most young people smoke sporadically, and often with difficulty. Few people find smoking physically pleasant during the early phase and the probability that the young person will become a regular smoker is a function of a number of different variables, notably:

(1) his appreciation of the hazards of smoking: some young people refuse to believe that it is harmful or argue that it 'won't happen to me';
(2) his ability to identify himself with the long-term consequences of smoking: to some teenagers the age of 21 is old and the prospect of a heart attack at 51 is not alarming, as the young person may simply be unable to conceive of himself being that age;
(3) the attitudes and behaviour of his parents, siblings, and friends: smoking is like an infectious disease, the more contact you have with it the more likely you are to acquire it;
(4) the prevailing ethos in his school and his attitude towards the school ethos;
(5) the success with which he copes with the social demands of adolescence; children who are self-confident and have good self-esteem are less likely to smoke than the child with low self-esteem who feels he is insignficiant.

In the early stage of the young person's flirtation with cigarettes the offer of each cigarette poses a momentary dilemma for the young person and the same factors that influence his decision to accept or refuse the first cigarette are influential. The social and psychological factors listed above determine whether the young person will become dependent on cigarettes or become a non-smoker.

Table 1. The first cigarette: pupils' reactions, by smoking behaviour (per cent)

Pupils' reactions	Tried smoking once			Used to smoke			Smokes occassionally			Smokes regularly			Total		
	Boys	Girls	All	Boys	Girls	All	Boys	Girls	All	Boys	Girls	All	Boys	Girls	All
England and Wales															
Felt sick/ill	46	47	47	23	27	25	22	22	22	35	30	32	36	35	35
Felt sorry	8	18	13	3	10	6	4	6	5	2	2	2	5	11	8
Felt disappointed	9	7	8	8	1	4	4	2	3	4	4	4	7	4	6
Felt grown up	5	6	5	20	16	18	16	19	18	17	15	16	12	12	12
Enjoyed it	2	2	2	10	7	9	23	16	19	18	20	19	10	10	10
Felt nothing	28	22	25	32	28	30	27	26	27	18	15	17	26	22	24
Can't remember	8	9	9	11	18	14	14	13	13	20	23	22	12	15	13
Number of pupils (= 100%)†	*330*	*286*	*616*	*148*	*142*	*290*	*100*	*125*	*225*	*163*	*159*	*322*	*742*	*712*	*1454*
Scotland															
Felt sick/ill	46	49	47	26	34	30	35	26	30	28	39	34	36	39	37
Felt sorry	8	9	9	3	5	4	3	7	5	1	3	2	5	6	6
Felt disappointed	7	5	6	4	5	5	–	4	2	2	3	2	4	5	4
Felt grown up	5	4	5	15	5	10	6	15	11	12	11	11	9	8	9
Enjoyed it	2	1	2	6	5	5	16	16	16	19	9	14	9	7	8
Felt nothing	26	27	26	27	29	28	24	25	24	16	16	16	23	24	24
Can't remember	13	10	12	23	22	23	18	12	15	30	25	28	20	17	19
Number of pupils (= 100%)†	*291*	*203*	*494*	*143*	*137*	*280*	*88*	*105*	*193*	*172*	*152*	*324*	*695*	*599*	*1294*

† Percentages add up to more than 100 because some pupils gave more than one reaction
From Dobbs and Marsh (1983)

An educational strategy

In the past health education intended to prevent young people from starting to smoke was aimed principally at children. However, such an approach is ineffective, for what is required is an integrated strategy designed to influence not only the child but the world in which he lives – the world which influences his beliefs, attitudes, and behaviour – namely his family, friends, school, and the society of which all three are parts.

Educating the child Education, like medicine, is prone to fashions and, as in medicine, fashions survive longer in some places than in others. It is usually possible in education to identify two extreme points of view and to place educators, schools, and teachers at some point in the spectrum between these extremes. The development of health education about cigarette smoking has been influenced by two of the main debates that have prevailed in the educational world in the last decade.

Education for exams or for life? If children are to be influenced by health education they have to be exposed to it, and the last 10 years have seen a significant increase in the number of schools including health education in the curriculum, first as a separate subject in the curriculum, then as a theme running through many subjects. For some topics, notably 'sex education', the inclusion of health education has led to debate about the respective contributions of family and school in shaping attitudes and values. A vociferous pressure group has argued that it is the responsibility of the family, not the school, to inculcate attitudes and values and thus to influence the young person's behaviour. Many parents, however, welcome the help of the school in educating their children for life and appreciate that teachers and health educators are not trying to supplant the family as a source of beliefs, attitudes, and values but to supplement it. Parents, including those who smoke, particularly welcome the efforts made by the school to help their children remain non-smokers.

Is the aim to inform or to influence behaviour? The assumption that children and adults are ignorant and simply require information about health and disease is now known to be inaccurate. It is now appreciated that people are not ignorant about health but that they have beliefs about virtually every health problem, beliefs which have been developed on the basis of information received from parents, friends, and the media, that is from many sources other than doctors or health educators. Health education has to start therefore from the assumption that the beliefs that the individual holds are useful and valuable to him, even if they are not in line with the beliefs held by epidemiologists, doctors, and health educators. For example, the belief that 'it won't happen to me' may arise simply from the mistaken belief that people whose relatives did not develop smoking-related diseases are in some way immune from the effects of cigarette smoke – 'my grandfather's 82 and healthy and he has smoked for 50 years'. More commonly, however, this belief is not based on ignorance but is the means that the individual uses to cope with the anxiety that derives from the fact that he accepts that all smokers are at risk, but cannot stop smoking and has to adopt denial or fatalism – 'there's a bullet with your number on it' – to cope with his anxiety (Gray 1979; Gray and Fowler 1983).

The assumption is now that people have beliefs about smoking that are useful and satisfactory, and that health education has to take these beliefs into account if it has any hope of influencing them. This, however, raises a second question: should the aim of health education be to do no more than influence beliefs and attitudes? This has been the prevailing view until recently but there is now a number of people who would argue that the aim of education should be to influence behaviour as well as beliefs. If the objective is to influence behaviour a different approach is required from that if the aim is simply to influence beliefs, for a change in beliefs and attitudes does not necessarily lead to a change in behaviour.

Young people need accurate information about topics such as the immediate physiological effects of cigarette smoking, the long-term hazards, and the magnitude of the risk of smoking relative to other risks. The provision of this type of information can influence smoking behaviour. This has been shown in Australia (Homel *et al.* 1981) and in the U.K., where the 'HEC [Health Education Council] my body' project has been successful in influencing not only beliefs but also behaviour. The 'HEC my body' project, which is based on the principles used to develop the school health curriculum in the U.S. – the Berkeley Project – is principally concerned with the respiratory and cardiovascular systems and focuses on both the short- and long-term effects of smoking. It has now been shown that children who participated in the 'HEC my body' project had a significantly lower incidence of experimentation with smoking up to two years after participation than children from a control group of schools (Wilcox *et al.* 1981; Wilcox and Gillies 1983).

However, it is now accepted that this approach alone, though effective for some children, is not effective for all and others need to be helped to acquire the specific skills to help them resist the social pressures to smoke, particularly those exerted by their peers.

Educating the family Adolescence is a phase in which the young person puts distance between himself and his parents to resolve his existential uncertainty. Only rarely does he reject his family entirely, and many young people are influenced by their parents even though they may appear to be disaffected. Parents have a very important part to play in the prevention of smoking but it is important that they are involved long before adolescence. Parents need:

(1) help and support to stop smoking in the antenatal period if they are smokers;
(2) encouragement to continue as non-smokers throughout the child's life if they manage to stop smoking during pregnancy, or education about the dangers of smoking in front of their children if they continue to smoke. Most parents who smoke welcome advice about the steps they can take to reduce the probability that their children will adopt the same habit;
(3) specific information about the most effective way to speak to their children about cigarette smoking when they reach the age at which experimentation begins. Smoking and non-smoking parents need different types of advice;
(4) specific information about the most effective way to help their children if they discover that they have started to smoke; again different advice is needed for smoking and non-smoking parents.

A failure to co-operate with parents has been one of the weak points in health education but steps are now being taken to harness the influence that parents have, and wish to use, to stop their children smoking cigarettes. The main work in this field has been done in Norway (Aaro 1982), a country which has tackled smoking prevention with notable imagination, enthusiasm, and success, and the U.K.'s Health Education Council is developing is own 'HEC school-parent smoking project'.

Educating the school One fact to emerge from recent research is that the school has an influence on smoking prevalence that is independent of the social characteristics of its pupils. Different schools drawing pupils from the same catchment areas have different smoking prevalence rates, and the move from primary to secondary school has been shown to be associated with a significant change in the attitudes of the young people towards cigarette smoking. The school ethos is influential but the term 'ethos', meaning the 'genius of an institution or system', though appropriate, is too vague to be useful in planning an educational strategy. Some of the factors contributing to the ethos have now been identified though much more work, using an anthropological approach, requires to be done.

Some of these factors obviously relate to the school's attitude towards cigarette smoking, for example whether or not the school has a specific policy about cigarette smoking and whether the school has a consistent set of sanctions for smokers or whether punishment is meted out arbitrarily and inconsistently. The behaviour of the teachers is also important, for example whether they smoke anywhere in the school or only in the staff room. However, other aspects of the school's ethos which are not directly related to cigarette smoking are also probably influential. A low level of academic ability has been shown to be associated with cigarette smoking but it now seems that it is not so much the lack of academic success as the school's attitude towards it which is important. In an interesting study in Scotland it was demonstrated that twice as many teenage smokers described themselves as 'fed up with school' compared with non-smokers (Ledwith 1982). It seems to be the low level of self-esteem of those pupils who do not succeed academically, which in turn reflects the attitude of the school towards academic success, that is the important factor, rather than the lack of academic success *per se*.

The ethos of the school is a compound of many factors. The beliefs and attitudes of the headmaster are obviously important but even within a school there may be considerable variation from year to year and from form to form. No effective means of influencing the school ethos has yet been identified but this is a focus of current research. For example, the Health Education Council has supported the development of a Health Development Questionnaire which schools can use to measure smoking prevalence rates and assess the impact of teaching. The use of such simple tools for audit undoubtedly has an influence not only on the teaching but the school ethos.

Educating the peer group The growing appreciation of the fact that most young people start to smoke because they do not wish to refuse a cigarette proffered by a peer, rather than as a result of a deep-seated motivation to appear adult or attain adult status has resulted in increasing interest in the influence of the peer group and the scope for influencing the young person's response to peer group pressure. Group discussion of cigarette smoking is popular but an unstructured discussion is ineffective. More recent approaches have been the introduction of peer-led teaching and the teaching of techniques to help young people resist social pressure. The former technique encourages youngsters to select group leaders from among their peers to lead discussion on smoking and the place of the cigarette in the life of the teenager, relying on the fact that the most popular and influential pupils will, in general, be the ones chosen by their peers. In the latter technique the young person is given not only information about the hazards of smoking and the opportunity to discuss the pressure to smoke exercised by peers and advertisements but also the opportunity to practise saying 'no' in the types of situation in which cigarettes are proffered. This approach is used at a later age than the factual information about smoking and health and there are encouraging early results.

Educating society Measures affecting society as a whole can help to create an environment in which the young person is less likely to accept the proffered cigarette, to experiment with smoking, and to proceed from the experimental phase to become an established smoker. The price of cigarettes is at least as important for children as for adults. In addition the advertising of cigarettes and their association with sport through sports sponsorship perpetuates the image of smoking as an acceptable social custom, particularly when the promotion of cigarettes is contrasted with society's proscription of cannabis.

As has been shown in Norway (Aaro *et al.* 1982) a programme of political action is as important in the prevention of smoking in childhood as it is in helping adults to stop smoking.

One piece of legislation of particular importance is that which prohibits the sale of cigarettes to children, but even where such a law exists it is commonly disregarded by tobacconists. It would of course be impossible to enforce such a law by the imposition of external controls, and it is inappropriate to regard such a law simply as an instrument which can be used by policemen and courts to control the behaviour of tobacconists. A law is not only an instrument or tool, it is also a symbol, codifying the actions that society considers to be unacceptable. Rather than trying to modify the behaviour of tobacconists by an increase in police surveillance, in an attempt to use the tool more often, it is probably more effective to try to change the beliefs and attitudes of tobacconists so that they appreciate the symbolic meaning of such a law and thus take action as individuals to refuse to sell cigarettes to children. There are too many outlets for effective policing; the only effective form of control is self-control which will be reinforced by the presence of a legal proscription even though it is rarely invoked. The survey of smoking among secondary schoolchildren in the U.K. found that children who were too young to buy cigarettes legally were sold £60 million worth of cigarettes in 1982 (Dobbs and Marsh 1983): a problem that demands urgent action.

Resources and research

More research is needed, particularly on the evaluation of the effectiveness of different types of intervention. This type of research is expensive both because of the number of schools and children that have to be included and because of the time that such studies take. For example, the first phase of a Health Education Council project to modify the techniques developed in Minnesota and Houston to help young people resist social pressure – the SET (Smoking Education for Teenagers) project – will take three years and evaluation will require additional time. This type of research therefore requires central funding.

The implementation of these programmes also requires the investment of resources. No single programme can hope to be effective. Schools need a number of different programmes for pupils of different ages and the education of the young person at risk requires integration with interventions to influence family, friends, schoolteachers, and society. To develop and implement this type of strategy requires individuals whose main occupation is health education and they require, both centrally and locally, adequate resources to help young people resist the pressure to smoke.

The need for strategy

It is of paramount importance that the types of measure described in this chapter be introduced not as disparate elements, related to one another solely by the common theme, but as elements of an educational strategy. As the International Union Against Cancer has emphasized so effectively, the prevention of smoking in childhood will be relatively ineffective if the campaign consists solely of an unconnected series of tactical moves, even if each of those tactics is of proven effectiveness (Wake *et al*. 1982). What is needed to cope with strategy of the tobacco industry is an educational strategy in which these components focus on a single objective and complement one another. Each country, each education authority, and each school needs such a strategy to help children cope with one of the main health hazards.

Helping people to give up smoking

Surveys have repeatedly found that a majority of smokers say that they would like to give up the habit. While the 'widespread harassment of smokers' makes uncertain the extent to which these sentiments are a reflection only of changes in the prevailing attitudes to smoking (Kozlowski *et al*. 1980), it seems likely that giving up the habit appears somewhere on the 'personal agenda' of most smokers. As well as 'benefits' such as pleasure, smoking brings cost – financial costs, minor physical symptoms, and, increasingly, the social and personal costs of choosing to remain with a minority or being seen as being unable to give up an unhealthy habit. These are immediate consequences of smoking, largely unrelated to any possible long-term consequences to health developing in the remote future, and the natural response of any organism is to minimize such aversive factors while maximizing positive gains. The task facing health education is to bring individual smokers to the point where the perceived costs outweigh the apparent advantages of continuing to smoke. Once this point is passed in the individual's own reckoning smoking will be abandoned as there is 'nothing' to be gained from it.

Educating the individual smoker

By the early 1980s millions of smokers had already passed the point of no return mentioned above, and most of them did so completely independently of formal health education activities. This is not to say that the latter are not effective, as there is good evidence that programmes based in the community (Puska *et al.* 1979), the workplace (Rose *et al.* 1982), or in medical clinics (Hjermann *et al.* 1981; MRFIT Research Group 1982) can all help individual smokers to give up smoking sooner than they might otherwise have done so (see Fig. 1). However, the scope of such programmes is limited, and the 'cost per convert' is high. Moreover, the unrealistic expectation that they would yield a demonstrable saving of lives has, in the main, not been fulfilled, because it has not been appreciated that the benefits for a community of stopping smoking are likely to take almost as long to become apparent as did the adverse effects of starting to smoke.

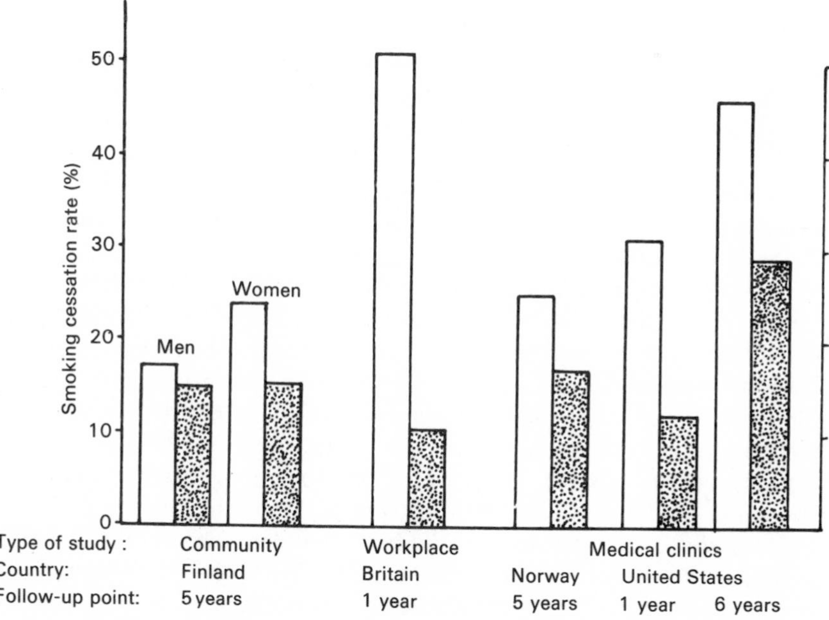

Fig. 1. Smoking cessation rates achieved in intensive anti-smoking programmes Although these four trials took place in different countries and used different entrance criteria (three trials included men only), different intervention regimens, and different follow-up periods, in each of them more subjects in the special intervention group (blank bars) than in the normal care group (stippled bars) gave up smoking.

At the same time, the potentially most economical way of influencing a large proportion of smokers, that of using every contact with the health professions as an opportunity for health education, has received much lip service but relatively little serious study. Admittedly the relatively small acceleration of the smoking-cessation snowball that can be achieved by routine anti-smoking advice, at most a double of the 'spontaneous' rate (Russell *et al.* 1979) may seem hardly worthwhile to the individual practitioner, but, as Rose (1981) has convincingly argued, a small effect spread over a wide proportion of those at risk stands to bring greater overall benefit than intensive efforts directed at the minority at high risk.

Research into routine anti-smoking advice is in its infancy compared with the efforts made to understand how smoking causes disease or even why people smoke at all. It is obviously much more difficult to collect data 'in the field' than it is to submit groups of volunteers in psychological laboratories or special anti-smoking clinics to batteries of questionnaires designed to validate a specific theory in the mind of the investigator. Yet, in the final analysis, it is 'in the field' where most of the suicide-by-smoking is taking place and where the challenge really lies.

At present all that we know is that routine verbal advice from doctors is effective, and that the effect is augmented if the doctor also gives each patient a simple anti-smoking booklet (Russell *et al.* 1979). Showing the patient personal evidence of an immediate and potentially harmful effect of smoking, such as a raised carboxyhaemoglobin level, is a further improvement (Jamrozik *et al.* 1984) (see Fig. 2) and may be effective with smokers from lower socio-economic groups, those who have been least responsive to other anti-smoking measures in the past. Nevertheless, simple questions concerning the relative effectiveness of advice from doctors, nurses, and even non-professional health staff, or of advice given on one occasion versus repeated advice have hardly been touched. More complex issues, such as how best to meet patients' protestations of 'weight gain' or 'addiction', and support for the new ex-smoker during the first few days or weeks without cigarettes (the important problem of staying stopped) remain almost virgin soil. Perhaps most difficult of all is assessment of the motivated patient who is unable to give up smoking unaided, so as to offer the second-line treatment having the greatest likelihood of success for that individual, be it nicotine chewing-gum, a smoking-cessation clinic, acupuncture, or hypnotherapy. It may well be that many health professionals are reluctant to give anti-smoking advice routinely because they have no clear idea of how to proceed should advice alone prove inadequate.

Finally, it is very important not to underestimate the need of smokers for information, because there is clear evidence that all smokers do not know the dangers of cigarette smoking, as the survey of smoking attitudes and

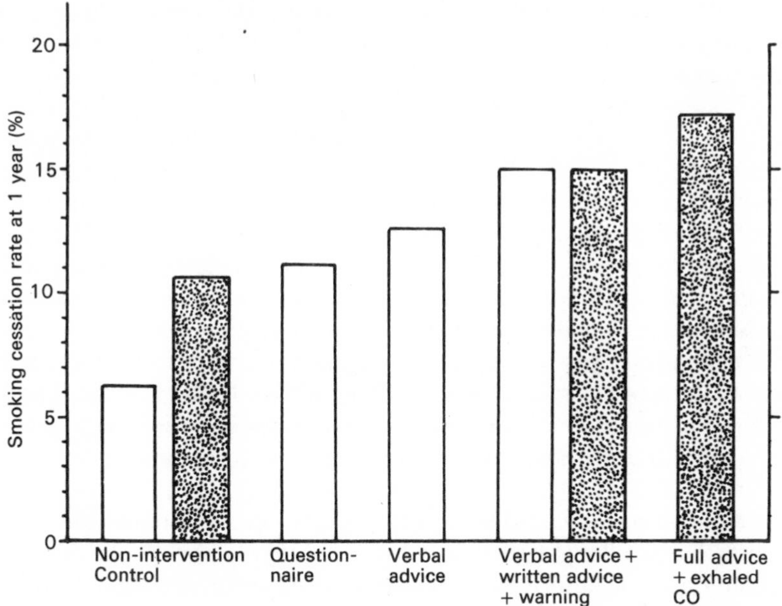

Fig. 2. Results in two trials of routine anti-smoking advice in general practice. The full advice 'package' including an anti-smoking booklet and a warning about follow-up is clearly associated with an increase in smoking cessation compared with the non-intervention control group. The two studies were conducted in London (blank bars) and Oxford (stippled bars) in 1974 and 1979, respectively; the accelerating trend away from smoking is reflected in the higher 'spontaneous' cessation rate observed in Oxford.

behaviour demonstrated (Marsh and Matheson 1983). For example, 40 per cent of smokers did not accept that there was a risk of heart disease associated with cigarette smoking and of those smokers who did accept such an association some smokers thought that only very heavy smokers were at risk: only 14 per cent of smokers believed that heart disease was more likely among smokers than non-smokers, that smokers consuming less than 20 a day were at risk, and that abstinence of less than six years would significantly reduce that risk. Even more surprising was the fact that only 11 per cent of smokers believed the same proposition with respect to lung cancer.

Educating the community

As well as bringing individual smokers to a decision to give up the habit, health education has a role to play in keeping the issue alive in the whole community. Since, in many developed countries, the smoker is confronted by a printed reminder that smoking damages health each time he or she takes a cigarette from the packet few could deny the existence of at least some evidence that smoking is harmful. It is no small triumph that, within the space of a generation, a contention that rests fundamentally upon a series of statistical associations has been turned into common knowledge. How much credit the health educators can claim for the accelerating trend away from smoking that has appeared over the same period (Office of Population Censuses and Surveys 1981) is impossible to quantify and is probably not particularly important. What does matter is how best to use the funds made available for general health education now, paltry as they are in comparison with the advertising budgets of the tobacco companies. Given that the basic association of smoking with ill-health is widely known, health education should now pursue two courses in parallel, those of combating disinformation and of correcting misinformation.

Combating disinformation The tobacco industry and its satellite advertising interests have a long history of disseminating to the public incorrect information or 'disinformation' concerning cigarette smoking. The most harmful of these false truths is that smoking 'in moderation' is 'safe', when in fact all of the epidemiological evidence points to the absence of any threshold of risk below which the individual is unlikely to develop smoking-related disease. The safety in moderation argument has been heard in Parliament from Members representing constituencies with cigarette factories. It is also used to justify the continuation of tobacco advertising so that the consumer can be made aware of the latest 'milder' brands to reach the market. Patients occasionally report being told by a doctor that 'five or six cigarettes a day won't do you any harm.' Thus there is a need for the public, Parliament, and the health professions to be made aware of the strong medical evidence that even moderate smoking is dangerous to health (see Fig. 3).

A second favourite theme of the industry is that curtailment of tobacco advertising will have immediate and catastrophic consequences for the economy, the Exchequer, for employment, and for the advertising-dependent institutions such as the media and, increasingly, sport and the arts. The industry is also wont to quote the Norwegian experience as showing that an advertising ban does not affect consumption: this statement itself provides a refutation of the economy-employment argument! The truth is that since the decision to introduce a Tobacco Act was taken in 1970 there has been a slow downturn in sales in Norway averaging 0.3 per cent per annum, and therefore no precipitous loss of jobs or of government revenue. (Meanwhile of course the health lobby is hailing a halt in the long-continued rise in annual per caput consumption as a major

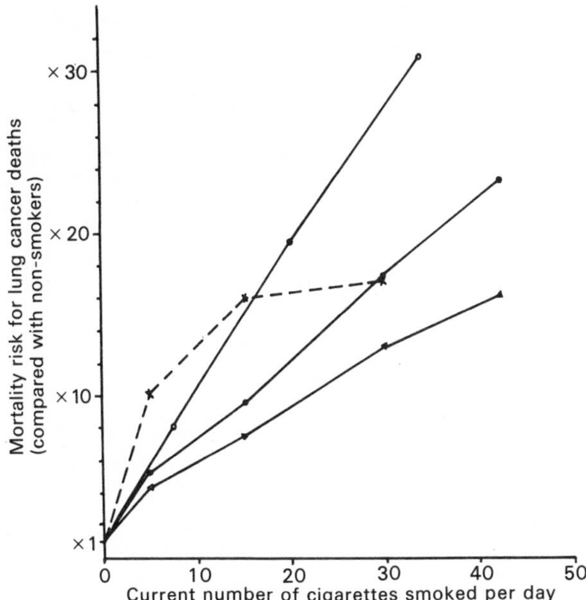

Fig. 3. Morality ratios for deaths from lung cancer in men from four large prospective studies. Three of the studies show a clear increase in risk of lung cancer associated with smoking five cigarettes a day. (Source: WHO Technical Report No. 636.)

victory, see Fig. 4.) Again, the details of this argument need to be spelt out carefully to the public, the parliamentarians, and to the employees in the tobacco industry. Although obvious when one stops to think, it also has to be pointed out that there is no shortage of advertisements on independent television in Britain, even though cigarette advertising was abolished in 1965; other advertisers have filled the gap.

The tobacco lobby also uses a series of more philosophical arguments concerning the 'right to smoke' and the 'right to advertise a product that it is legal to sell' (Waterson and Henry 1981). These are, quite deliberately, more difficult to debate since the counter-arguments are also to some extent philosophical and therefore liable to differing interpretations by smokers and non-smokers. The fallacies in the industry's arguments are perhaps better exposed by direct confrontation before a critical press than by more formal health education (Chapman 1983).

Correcting misinformation Although the general public has probably received the message that 'smoking damages health' and even that 'smoking causes cancer', there are numerous instances where only half of

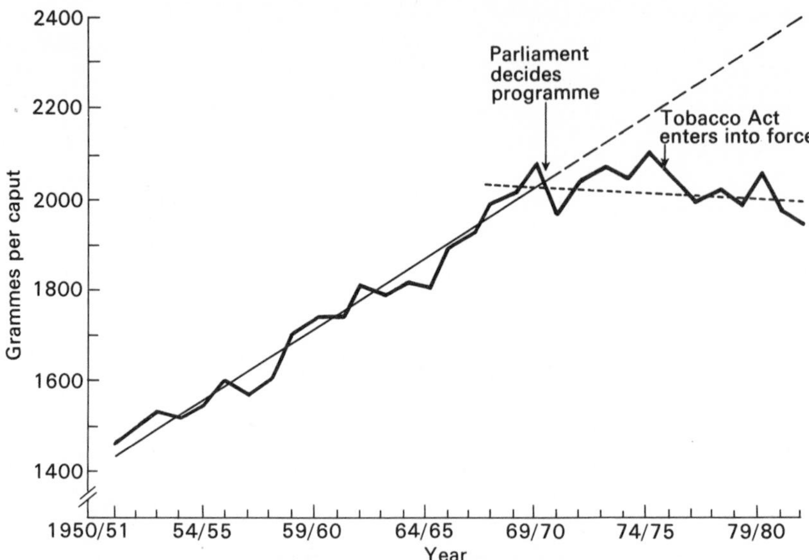

Fig. 4. Sales of smoking tobacco + manufactured cigarettes per caput, age 15 years+, Norway, 1950–51 to 1981–82. The regression line for the period 1950–51 to 1969–70 shows a clear annual increase in consumption. After the 1970 decision to implement a legislative programme, the increase ceased, and was replaced by a slow decrease averaging 0.3 per cent per annum. (Source: Norwegian National Council on Smoking and Health.)

the message is understood, and the resulting misconceptions are used by individuals to rationalize their continued smoking.

Richard Peto (1980) has written on the subject of conveying the quantitative enormity of the risk, and the fact that three in four smokers do not die of smoking-related disease does not mean that the habit is not dangerous. There is confusion in some people's minds between lung cancer, caused by smoking, and non-smokers dying from pulmonary metastases from primary sites in other organs. Few people know someone with lung cancer, but even fewer appreciate that the prevalence of the disease is so low because it is rapidly fatal, not because it is among the cancers that doctors are now able to cure. There are risks associated with smoking at any time during pregnancy; avoiding the 'drug' during the first trimester is not enough. Moreover, a resumption of smoking after the child is born carries a significant risk of respiratory disease during its infancy (Colley *et al.* 1974) and of the child becoming a smoker in its turn. Both of these points have been neglected by intensive anti-smoking campaigns focusing on the antenatal period alone.

The Fourth Report of the Royal College of Physicians (1983) has deliberately emphasized the cardiovascular diseases associated with smoking because of concern that the public at large has not appreciated that these are numerically more important than lung cancer.

Smokers have got the message that cigarettes might kill them, and are tired of that drum being beaten. Just as health warnings on cigarette packets should be changed regularly to retain some freshness, so health educators should vary the quantum of information that they are trying to convey, in the hope of keeping 'active' the smoking file on each smoker's personal agenda.

Limits to health education

If the content of health education messages has been limited in the past, then so has their scope. Although financial constraints have always been present, many of these limits would seem, on closer scrutiny, to have been self-imposed almost on 'moral' grounds. While Black and Strong (1982) have expressed concern that preventive medicine is an example of professional empire-building, the decision of the individual smoker whether or not to quit ultimately remains a personal one. When it comes to specific contexts, the enlarging body of evidence on the consequences of passive smoking (Royal College of Physicians 1983) is finally giving individual non-smokers the confidence to 'educate' smokers about the rights of others to breathe unpolluted air. But in the wider arena, formal health education is guilty of neglecting several quite legitimate target areas.

Until relatively recently the whole anti-acquisition campaign has been directed at the mid-to-late teenager group, that is, the age identified by the current generation of established adult smokers as the one at which they became regular smokers, a generation or more ago. It was only once evidence emerged that children begin experimentation with cigarettes long before this that the emphasis slowly changed to early secondary, and then to the later primary school age groups. We have yet to face up to the implications of findings such as those of Baric (1979) that pre-school children are already aware of cigarettes and what to do with them.

Most of our activities have been concerned with smoking and smokers. Doctors might ask their patients about smoking (Jamrozik and Fowler 1982) but they probably rarely record a history of non-smoking (Fleming and Lawrence 1981) nor systematically take time to reinforce this behaviour. We are aware that it may well be futile to warn children that smoking is strongly associated with the leading causes of death in middle age. While we could probably teach them a lot more about society and life in general by exposing the ways advertisers try to seduce children into becoming smokers, this approach has apparently been dismissed as being too 'un-medical' to be used legitimately by those concerned with the promotion of health and with establishing their credentials in the medical world (Chapman 1983).

Lastly, through concentrating on adults with moderate to heavy cigarette consumption and neglecting the 'social smokers' and the 'geriatric smokers', we are perpetuating a fundamental weakness in the overall campaign. There are good medical reasons why both of the latter groups should be encouraged to give up – 'social smokers' because there is no safe limit to smoking, and 'geriatric smokers' because it is never too late to give up and because duration of smoking is more strongly related to lung cancer than is consumption (Peto *et al.* 1975). But if our ultimate aim is to make the cigarette an aberration limited to the twentieth century, then a major reason for encouraging each of these groups of smokers to stop is to remove adult models from the younger generation's view and thus to accelerate the re-establishment of non-smoking as the norm.

Conclusion

Up to three in ten fatal cases of cancer occurring in developed countries today are due to a single avoidable cause – tobacco smoking. Since outright prohibition of tobacco is impractical, the major thrust of the public health response to this modern epidemic falls to health education. Reducing the numbers of people starting to smoke and convincing established smokers to give up the habit are two separate but complementary ways of reducing the prevalence of smoking and hence the burden of smoking-related disease borne by the community. Although the two target groups involved present quite different challenges, experience so far provides some lessons in common for future health education campaigns. Most important of these is that our previous working models of what governs an individual's behaviour – that the teenager smokes to become an adult and that the adult continues to smoke because of ignorance of the possible consequences – have been far too simplistic. This became apparent only when we began to evaluate systematically the results of campaigns based on such theories. Although the ball has started rolling and smoking is on the wane, it is conceivable that this change represents only the 'easy pickings'. Although simple approaches of proven worth and wide applicability should not be neglected, to guarantee a steady erosion of the harder core in the future these techniques may have to be modified to take into account the individual's beliefs about smoking, and attention may have to be paid to other sources of influence in the general social environment. Tobacco-related cancer remains an unncessary cause of suffering and it is as desirable to eradicate it completely as it was to eradicate smallpox.

References

Aaro, L.E., Brulard, E., Haukness, A., and Løchsen, P.M. (1982). Smoking among Norwegian schoolchildren 1975–1980: the effect of anti-smoking campaigns. *Scand. J. Psychol.* **23**.

Baric, L. (1979). *Primary socialisation and smoking*. Health Education Council Monograph Series No. 1. Health Education Council, London.

Black, N. and Strong, P.M. (1982). Prevention: who needs it? *Brit. Med. J.* **285**, 1543–4.

Chapman, S. (1983). *The lung goodbye: a manual of tactics for counter-acting the tobacco industry in the 1980's*. Consumer Interpol, Sydney.

Colley, J.R.T., Holland, W.W., and Corkhill, R.T. (1974). Influence of passive smoking and parental phlegm on pneumonia and bronchitis in early childhood. *Lancet* **ii**, 1031–4.

Covington, M.V. (1981). Youth and decision-making dilemmas: new approaches to smoking uptake and prevention. Paper presented at the International Seminar on School Health Education, Southampton.

Dobbs, J. and Marsh, A. (1983). *Smoking among secondary school children*. OPCS Social Survey Division. HMSO.

Doll, R. and Peto, R. (1981). *The causes of cancer*. Oxford University Press.

Fleming, D.M. and Lawrence, M.S. (1981). An evaluation of recorded information about preventive measures in 38 practices. *J. royal Coll. gen. Pract.* **31**, 615–20.

Gray, J.A.M. (1979). *Man against disease*. pp. 141–51. Oxford University Press.

Gray, J.A.M. and Fowler, G.F. (1983). *Preventive medicine in general practice*. Oxford University Press.

Gray, N. and Daube, M. (1980). *Guidelines for smoking control*. UICC Technical Report Series, Vol. 52. International Union Against Cancer, Geneva.

Hjermann, I., Holme, I., Byre, K.V., and Leren, P. (1981). Effect of diet and smoking intervention on the incidence of coronary heart disease. *Lancet* **ii**, 1303–10.

Homel, P.J., Daniels, P., Reid, T.R., and Lawson, J.S. (1981). Results of an experimental school based health development programme in health education. *Int. J. Hlth Educ.* **25**, 263–70.

Jamrozik, K. and Fowler, G. (1982). Anti-smoking education in Oxfordshire general practices. *J. roy. Coll gen. Pract.* **32**, 179–83.

Jamrozik, K., Vessey, M., Fowler, G., Wald, N., Parker, G., and Van Vunakis, H. (1984). Controlled trial of three different anti-smoking interventions in general practice. *Brit. med. J.* **288**, 1499–1503.

Kozlowski, L.T., Herman, C.P., and Frecker, R.C. (1980). What researchers make of what cigarette smokers say: filtering smokers' hot air. *Lancet* **i**, 699–700.

Ledwith, F. (1982). *A study of smoking in primary and secondary schools in the Lothian Region*. Department of Community Medicine, University of Edinburgh.

Marsh, A. and Matheson, J. (1983). *Smoking attitudes and behaviour*. OPCS Social Survey Division. HMSO.

Multiple Risk Factor Intervention Trial Research Group (1982). Multiple risk factor intervention trial: risk factor changes and mortality results. *J. Amer. med. Assoc.* **248**, 1465–77.

Office of Population Censuses and Surveys (1981). *General household survey* – 1981/2, pp. 13–15.

Peto, R. (1980). Possible ways of explaining to ordinary people the quantitative dangers of smoking. *Hlth Educ. J.* **39**, 1.

Peto, R., Roe, F.J.C., Lee, P.N., Levy, L., and Clack, J. (1975). Cancer and ageing in mice and men. *Brit. J. Cancer* **32**, 411–25.

Puska, P., Tuomilehto, J., and Salonen, J. (1979). Changes in coronary risk factors during comprehensive five-year community programme to control cardiovascular diseases (North Karelia Project). *Brit. med. J.* **ii**, 1173–8.

Rose, G. (1981). Strategy of prevention: lessons from cardiovascular disease. *Brit. med. J.* **282**, 1847–51.

Rose, G., Hamilton, P.J.S., Colwell, L., and Shipley, M.J. (1982). A randomised controlled trial of anti-smoking advice: 10 year results. *J. Epidemiol. commun Hlth* **36**, 102–8.

Royal College of Physicians (1971). *Smoking and health*. Pitman Medical, London.

Royal College of Physicians (1983). *Health or smoking*. Pitman Medical, London.

Russell, M.A.H., Wilson, C., Taylor, C., and Baker, C.D., (1979). Effect of general practitioners' advice against smoking. *Brit. med. J.* **ii**, 321–5.

Thier, H.D. (1981). Teenagers and beginning smoking. Paper presented at the International Seminar on School Health Education, Southampton.

Wake, R., McAlister, A., and Nostbakken, D. (eds) (1982). *A manual on smoking and children*. International Union Against Cancer, Geneva.

Waterson, M.J. and Henry, H.W. (1981). The case for advertising alcohol and tobacco products. In *Health education and the media* (ed. D.S. Leathar, G.B. Hastings, and J.K. Davies). Pergamon Press, Oxford.

Wilcox, B., Gilles, P., and Reid, D. (1981). *The effect of the 'My Body' school health education project upon children's smoking behaviour*. Tobacco and Youth Conference report, Fandzione Giorgio, Cini-Isola, di S. Giorgia Maggiore, Venezia.

Wilcox, B. and Gillies, P. (1983). A longitudinal study of the effect of 'My Body' on children's behaviour and knowledge of smoking. *Fifth International Conference on Smoking and Health*.

World Health Organization (1975). *Smoking and its effects on health: report of a WHO Expert Committee*. WHO Technical Report Series No. 568. WHO, Geneva.

World Health Organization (1979). *Controlling the smoking epidemic: report of the WHO Expert Committee on smoking control.* WHO Technical Report Series No. 636. WHO, Geneva.

13 Cancer risks and cancer prevention in the Third World

Nigel Gray

What constitutes the Third World?

By and large the Third World consists of countries (Bannock 1972) that are characterized by lack of industrial development and lack of national income sufficient to finance investment. They are mainly agricultural primary producers using subsistence farming methods although some have substantial natural resources. Chronic overpopulation is usual and contributes in many cases to deteriorating trade balances and real incomes. The Food and Agriculture Organisation (FAO 1980) has classified 174 'developing market economies'. This group includes a wide variety of nations with diverse ethnic backgrounds. Some have a long colonial history and hence a considerable degree of Western social organization, even though they may be poor in terms of production and money. Many populations are included which are characterized by highly developed and formalized religious beliefs and practices.

Although it may seem somewhat quaint to list Bermuda, Saudi Arabia, Nauru, and Singapore as developing countries, by and large the Food and Agriculture Organization classification provides a reasonable basis. The list of developing countries also includes: Algeria, Nigeria, Ghana, Senegal, Uganda, Tanzania, Ethiopia, Mexico, Venezuela, Afghanistan, Jordan, India, Pakistan, Bangladesh, Thailand, Indonesia, and Papua New Guinea among others. The omission of China, Kampuchea, Korea, Mongolia, and Vietnam by FAO is due to their classification elsewhere as 'centrally planned economies'. Clearly these countries ought to be considered as developing in a public health sense.

The developing countries are, in many ways, victims of the affluent world, which exploits their primary produce and dumps upon them its surplus tobacco. The full spectrum of their impending increase in cancer risk is yet to be revealed, although the possibilities for preventing this are becoming clear. The state of relevant research in the West offers exciting opportunities for cancer prevention in the Third World. However, the sheer size of the problems of social organization and politics which stand in the way of preventive strategies must dampen the enthusiasm of any optimist and it is impossible, in 1985, to predict which way the cancer trends will run.

Cancer patterns

Information on the occurrence of cancer in developing countries is limited in quality and quantity. It is nevertheless unlikely that any important cancer would not declare itself in a review of available mortality, incidence, and hospital admission statistics. Precise assessment of risk is possible only in the better organized developing countries, but it is not essential for consideration of preventive strategies. Nor should it be assumed that preventive strategies will not be applied unless substantial and excess risk is demonstrated. The history of the affluent countries demonstrates that cancer prevention has great popular and political appeal and that it may attract great resources, particularly when unopposed by vested interests. For example, the Papanicolau smear was widely used in affluent countries long before its cost effectiveness and ability to accelerate an already declining mortality was established. Developing countries such as Colombia (Correa and Zavala 1982) have also established this secondary prevention programme.

Cancer patterns are probably changing in most parts of the world at rates which cannot yet be determined. The decline of stomach cancer seen in the U.S. and Japan may also be occurring in China but lung cancer is almost certainly increasing in China and every other country where the manufactured cigarette has invaded a consumer market previously occupied by the various forms of indigenous tobacco usage. These are substantial assumptions but they are well based on probability – information on trends is virtually non-existent.

It is, perhaps, generally appreciated that cancer is rapidly climbing the ladder of comparative mortality in developing countries. It is certainly less well known that it is the leading cause of death among males in such a city as Shanghai (Bing *et al.* 1982) a city in which it does not have to compete with the heart disease death-rate of the affluent overfed, nor the infection of the undernourished and overcrowded.

Future trends may be influenced by preventive action but will be affected also (in some cases quite soon) by the progressive appearance of the cumulative effect of established cultural habits (tobacco-chewing, smoking) as populations achieve longer lifespans due to control of infection and undernutrition.

Cancer prevention

The term 'prevention' requires definition. Obviously avoidance of smoking results in prevention (primary prevention) of tobacco-induced cancer. Cervical cancer may be avoided by use of the Papanicolau smear (National Institute of Health 1980), i.e. detection and removal of precancerous tissue or 'secondary' prevention. Similarly, secondary prevention may be achieved by screening (regular examination) of betel/tobacco chewers in a programme which would detect both precancerous changes and clinical cancers. Whereas primary prevention of oral cancer (by avoidance of chewing) is to be preferred, any public-health programme aimed at oral cancer will extend of necessity from primary prevention to secondary prevention and to treatment of both early and late clinical disease, for pragmatic and logistic reasons. Treatment of clinical disease is cancer 'control', not 'prevention'.

Although control is not the topic of this chapter, we must discuss the broader issues simply because preventive and control programmes in developing countries will frequently be based on existing treatment facilities, and public education programmes aimed at prevention will stimulate the presentation of clinical disease. No health worker can be enthusiastic about delivering public education messages about oral or cervical cancer unless the medical treatment system is both supporting the preventive programme and supplying proper treatment for established disease. If treatment of established disease produces a reasonable success rate then both primary and secondary prevention is likely to be more popular, due to the lesser threat involved at the time of induction into the programme. For example, an uninformed patient offered a cervical smear or oral examination for the first time will be encouraged if it is known that the disease, if present, can be effectively treated and that a positive diagnosis is not a death warrant. An initial successful and normal test is reassuring to both patient and friends and means that the next screening experience provides a lesser psychological hurdle.

The theoretical possibilities for cancer prevention are considered in the following paragraphs for three reasons. First, to clarify the possibilities for the application of existing knowledge; secondly, to set the directions for future research; and thirdly, to focus attention on the severe practical problems associated with both research and application of existing knowledge in developing countries.

It should be emphasized here that certain experiments in prevention may reasonably be based on relatively poor theoretical evidence, and justified on the grounds that they are harmless, that the potential benefit is great and that the potential carcinogen has other bad effects. For example, it can do no harm to attempt to remove aflatoxin from the diet, nor to remedy suspected nutritional deficiency of vitamin A, nor to control hepatitis B infection.

Removal of a known cause

There is little need to review in depth the evidence that tobacco is a carcinogen. This evidence is extensive, consistent, and unshaken by the dissonance of the tobacco industry. It has been regularly reviewed by the U.S. Surgeon General (1967–82) who has published over 4000 pages on the topic.

Several types of study give us guidance as to the place of tobacco as an international carcinogen in humans:

(1) studies relating tobacco dose to cancer response (Doll and Peto 1978);
(2) studies demonstrating reversal of risk in ex-smokers (Doll and Peto 1976; Kahn 1966);
(3) case-control studies in many countries demonstrating the same preponderance of disease among smokers/chewers and its relative absence in non-users (Simarak *et al.* 1977; Gupta *et al.* 1980).

Analysis of the constituents of tobacco smoke provides no reason to believe that tobacco can be smoked in any part of the world without substantial risk. Tobacco smoke contains initiators, promotors, and complete carcinogens (Wynder and Hoffman 1967). The evidence relating chewing habits to cancer is less conclusive but perfectly acceptable. In part this is because it is difficult to apply a relative weighting to the roles played by the tobacco leaf, betel nut, various herbs, and slaked lime in the incidence of oral cancer among those who chew. Tobacco/betel chewers experience a relative risk of developing oral cancer of about five compared with a three times greater risk for those chewing betel mixtures without tobacco. Bidi smoking alone produces a 14-fold increase in risk for oropharyngeal cancer compared with the risk in non-smokers (Jussawalla 1982). However, the attraction of research aimed at producing a less carcinogenic chewing mixture is limited by the fact that such mixtures vary almost infinitely, and that the addition of a corrosive such as lime to tobacco/betel mixtures releases alkaloids in the free base form, thus producing a more satisfying blood level of the uplifting alkaloids desired by chewers (*Merck Index* 1976).

The cancers that would be reduced if smoking and chewing declined include mouth, pharynx, oesophagus, larynx, lung, and bladder (Maclure and McMahon 1980). In theory, over one million cases of human cancer can be prevented annually (Parkin *et al.* 1984) if populations can be persuaded not to smoke or to chew tobacco-containing mixtures. There is no doubt that tobacco is causally involved in more avoidable cancer than any other known carcinogen.

Removal of a link in the chain of causation

Transmissable agents Epidemiological and basic cancer research have revealed some fascinating possibilities. Hutt (1982) has pointed out that six of the seven common cancers in Africa are candidates for a viral origin. He quotes cancers of the liver, cervix and penis, Burkitt's lymphoma, nasopharyngeal carcinoma, and Kaposi's sarcoma, and Kinlen discusses this topic in detail in Chapter 7. To the potentially causal transmissable agents that may be related to these cancers, we must add the parasite responsible for schistosomiasis.

Human experience does not yet show examples of cancer prevention by intervention aimed at removal of an apparently important contributary factor in any of these cancers and in most cases proof will come only from some large, long-term experiments. Fortunately there are other, very good, public health reasons for researchers in infectious disease to work on vaccines against hepatitis B, Epstein–Barr virus, the virus of genital herpes, cytomegalovirus and the schistosomiasis parasite. All of these agents cause unpleasant clinical disease regardless of their role in cancer. Elimination of these agents from experimental populations may be needed to provide the ultimate proof that they are involved in causing cancer.

Hepatitis B virus and hepatocellular cancer The mechanism of causation of hepatocellular carcinoma is not yet clear. The relative parts played by aflatoxin, alcohol, and cirrhosis may remain obscure for some time yet. However, the details of the association between hepatocellular cancer, cirrhosis, and hepatitis B virus are well established (Alter 1982) and the likelihood that hepatitis B infection is a necessary component of the causal chain is high, as is the probability that appropriate vaccination against hepatitis B will reduce the risk of developing hepatocellular cancer in susceptible populations. The evidence may be summarized as follows:

(1) the worldwide distribution of hepatitis B surface antigen (HBsAg) carriers matches that of hepatocellular cancer well;
(2) the prevalence of HBsAg among hepatocellular cancer patients is much higher than among matched controls. Beasley *et al.* (1981) found the risk for development of hepatocellular cancer to be 233 times greater among Taiwanese HBsAg carriers than controls in a prospective study;
(3) in carriers of HBsAg who develop hepatocellular cancer, hepatitis B infection precedes liver damage;
(4) hepatitis B DNA has been shown to be integrated into the DNA of tumour cells in patients with hepatocellular cancer.

Although the strength of the association between hepatocellular cancer and HBsAg carriers implies that elimination of the HBsAg carrier state may reduce or eliminate hepatocellular cancer, the epidemiology of hepatitis B is complex and the mechanism of establishment of the carrier state is such that any vaccination campaign aimed at attacking the carrier state faces some difficult logistic problems. There is clear evidence (Szmuness 1980) that vaccination will prevent infection with hepatitis B. Further, trials have shown (Barin 1982; Beasley and Stevens 1978) that neonates respond well to vaccination and that the presence of passively administered antibody does not prevent a primary immune response to vaccination either in older infants or in neonates whose reponse is not so marked, and this reduces the frequency of the carrier state.

The fact that some 40–50 per cent of chronic carriers in some Far Eastern populations appear to contract infection at birth may be related to genetic factors as well as to exposure to infection during or soon after birth. It is likely that a combination of active and passive immunization commencing at birth will soon be developed which will prevent the establishment of the carrier state. Such a programme is very likely to inhibit the development of hepatocellular cancer in the long term, although we can only speculate to what extent. The prospective human studies required to confirm absolutely that hepatitis B vaccination reduces hepatocellular cancer incidence may take four to five decades and will require a simply administered, affordable, vaccination programme.

Currently, hepatitis B subunit vaccines are available in modest quantity and high cost in a number of countries. Research on new vaccine-production techniques is promising (Alter 1982), particularly the development by Smith *et al.* (1983) of a vaccine in which HBsAg is expressed in infectious vaccinia virus recombinants. It is important that a vaccine made for use against a potential tumour virus does not contain replicating virus. Fortunately, purified HBsAg alone protects against hepatitis B and no viral nucleic acid is necessary for this purpose.

The relationship between hepatitis B and hepatocellular cancer lends itself readily to laboratory work and field trials. The work relating aflatoxin ingestion to hepatocellular cancer is less easy to do. Munoz and Linsell (1982) reviewed the correlation between hepatocellular cancer incidence and aflatoxin ingestion, hepatitis B, alcohol, and other potential carcinogens. The association between alfatoxin ingestion and hepatocellular cancer is uniformly quite strong although some elements of the cancer registration data are unsatifactory. In theory there is a good chance that dietary aflatoxin plays a part in the cause of hepatocellular cancer but it is unlikely that satisfactory data will appear to confirm or deny this conclusion in the near future. Intervention to improve storage techniques and reduce aflatoxin ingestion is worthwhile simply to reduce exposure to a toxin which produces unpleasant and sometimes fatal illness. Neat experiments to assess the effects on hepatocellular cancer incidence will be difficult as aflatoxin contamination of foodstuffs varies because of seasonal, economic, and other factors.

Epstein–Barr virus (EBV), Burkitt's lymphoma, and nasopharyngeal carcinoma This remarkable virus manifests itself in varied ways. It is clearly the cause of infectious mononucleosis in developed countries and is likely to be causally involved in the production of nasopharyngeal carcinoma in Chinese people (Simons and Shanmugaratnam 1982), and Burkitt's lymphoma in African children (Epstein 1976).

Although the clinical effects of Epstein–Barr virus vary greatly in different countries, the epidemiology is typically that of a virus of modest infectivity transmitted via the saliva. Primary infection occurs in childhood in developing countries but is often delayed until late adolescence or early adulthood in developed countries. Infection produces seroconversion, permanent immunity, and incorporation of the viral genome into some of the circulating B lymphocytes, plus intermittent virus excretion. Virus excretion is more frequent in developing countries and among immunosuppressed patients. It has been postulated that the immunosuppressive effects of malaria and parasite infection account for the higher frequency of virus excretion in developing countries (Simons and Shanmugaratnam 1982).

It is not clear why the Epstein–Barr virus behaves as an apparent tumour virus in Chinese and Africans but causes a relatively benign if unpleasant infectious disease in the affluent world. The difference may be related to the age at which infection occurs (DeThé 1977), to genetic factors, or to the activity of co-factors, such as malaria or diet, in the developing countries.

As with the association of hepatocellular cancer and hepatitis B, that between Epstein–Barr virus and cancer seems likely to be causal. In both cases the evidence is strong but circumstantial. The best way to determine whether Epstein–Barr virus actually causes cancer would be to find out whether a vaccine which interferes with Epstein–Barr virus infection also interferes with the development of cancer. As Epstein (1976) has pointed out, the West Nile district of Uganda contains a dense population with a sufficiently high incidence of Burkitt's lymphoma to allow detection of a fall in incidence to be recognizable. Since Burkitt's lymphoma occurs in young children, answers to the questions of vaccine efficacy and causality should be clear five or six years after introduction of a vaccine. Obviously ultimate proof that Epstein–Barr virus has a causal role in nasopharyngeal cancer will take much longer, as high incidence rates in Chinese are not seen until adult life. Epstein (1976) has summarized the reasons why Epstein–Barr virus is thought to be oncogenic. They are:

(1) properly authenticated cases of Burkitt's lymphoma and nasopharyngeal cancer only occur in individuals infected by the virus;
(2) viral DNA is present in tumour cells and determines the expression in them of virus coded neo-antigens;
(3) virus production can be activated in some tumour cells by various laboratory procedures;
(4) the virus is a powerful stimulator of lymphoproliferation *in vitro*;
(5) the virus confers the property of continuous growth on normal human B lymphocytes together with many changes analogous to malignant transformation;
(6) Epstein–Barr virus is carcinogenic experimentally in South American subhuman primates and fulfils Koch's postulates.

The fact that vaccines free of viral nucleic acid have been shown to work against both hepatitis B and Marek's disease of chickens (Lesnick, Ross 1975), which is due to a herpes virus closely related to Epstein–Barr virus, suggests that a suitable vaccine can be made. It is possible (Epstein 1980) that a vaccine against Epstein–Barr virus membrane antigen will be suitable. Once a vaccine has been developed and made available it will be possible to perform the important experiment in prevention of Burkitt's lymphoma quite quickly.

Burkitt's lymphoma and malaria: Burkitt (1983) reviewed the association between Epstein–Barr virus, Burkitt's lymphoma, and holo- or hyperendemic malaria. Burkitt's lymphoma is nowhere common without malaria. It remains to be seen whether attempts by WHO to eradicate malaria in some parts of Africa will affect the incidence of the tumour. In theory malaria ought to be controllable although, so far, it has proved recalcitrant.

Nasopharyngeal carinoma and salted fish: The environmental determinants of nasopharyngeal cancer have received considerable attention (Simons and Shanmugaratnam 1982). Household smoke, occupational factors, tobacco, Chinese tea, alcohol, and soy sauce have been considered among many other candidate co-factors. Salted fish has been extensively studied (Ho, Huang, and Fong 1978) and many of the studies show a strong association between childhood consumption and nasopharyngeal cancer. Salted fish consumed in Hong Kong has been shown to contain various volatile nitrosamines.

Nasopharyngeal carcinoma and HLA antigens: The evidence that certain populations almost certainly have an inherited predisposition rests mainly on three observations (Simons and Shanmugaratnam 1982):

(1) there is a consistently high risk among southern Chinese living under varying environmental conditions;

(2) there is an elevated risk among peoples believed to have genetic admixture with Chinese;
(3) the low risk in other populations persists when living in high-risk countries (e.g. Indians in Singapore).

Within populations of southern Chinese extraction several strong associations with specific HLA genes have been established and it appears clear that a proportion of the excess risk for nasopharyngeal cancer in this population can be attributed to HLA-linked genes. The importance of these findings in demonstrating potentially high-risk subpopulations on which to focus primary and secondary preventive programmes is substantial.

Cervical cancer and viruses The epidemiology of cervical cancer is extensively documented (The Walton Report 1982). Increased incidence is associated with early intercourse, multiple sexual partners, early pregnancy, large families, low socioeconomic status, and poor personal hygiene. It is rare in nuns and Jewish women. Cervical cancer is four to six times more common in prostitutes than in low-risk populations (Keighly 1968; Pereyra 1961). It is widely regarded as a venereal disease (Kessler 1976). The evidence that a transmissable agent is involved is impressive (Buckley *et al.* 1981).

It is difficult to select the real carcinogenic factors from the candidate group of viruses, sperm protein, and paracoital debris (Reid *et al.* 1978). Three types of virus are commonly associated with cervical cancer: herpes simplex type 2 (HSV2), cytomegalovirus, and papilloma viruses. HSV2 is still regarded by many as the prime candidate (Rapp and Jenkins 1981) and has certainly been the most extensively studied. Evidence suggesting a role for HSV2 includes:

(1) the high frequency of association between the virus and the cancer;
(2) the fact that HSV2 infection frequently precedes cervical dysplasia and carcinoma *in situ* (Nahmias *et al.* 1970);
(3) the detection of virus specific antigens and antibodies, and virus-specific nucleic acid in cervical cancer biopsies (Elgin 1982);
(4) the fact that HSV2 will transform cells in culture and that these cells produce tumours after innoculation into experimental animals (Duff and Rapp 1971).

Cytomegalovirus has some similar characteristics. It is considered to be transmitted sexually (Willmott 1975); is associated serologically with cervical cancer though less strongly than HSV2 (Pacsa *et al.* 1975); and has been shown to transform cells *in vitro* which will produce tumours when innoculated into animals (Geder 1976).

Papilloma viruses are frequently associated with venereal disease; they produce several forms of warts including condylomata acuminata (genital warts). Genital warts may become malignant after long latent periods and may be associated with carcinoma *in situ* (Rapp and Jenkins 1981) (see p. 150).

HSV2 is a strong suspect and is also a good prospect for development of a vaccine and a widespread vaccination programme on general public-health grounds. Its role in cervical cancer could possibly be clarified within a decade of a vaccine becoming available. Thus primary prevention in developing countries must await further research.

Fortunately the cervix is accessible to examination and is examined from time to time by primary care personnel in many high-risk patients in many developing countries for routine obstetric and sometimes gynaecological reasons. Secondary prevention is therefore possible and is part of routine care in many Western countries. It is also practised in Mexico, Columbia, Peru, Argentina, and Chile (Correa and Zavala 1982), and in a limited way in other developing countries.

Kaposi's sarcoma and cytomegalovirus Reports from the U.S. suggested that cytomegalovirus might be involvedd in Kaposi's sarcoma (Cooper 1983). Recent work has established that the Auto Immune Deficiency Syndrome which frequently precedes Kaposi's sarcoma is due to a retrovirus (Gallo 1983).

Bladder cancer and schistosomiasis Cheever (1978) and Ibrahim (1982) have reviewed the evidence relating this infection to cancer of the bladder in Egypt and elsewhere. Both reviews are striking in their references to the number of obvious studies which have *not* been done despite knowledge of a strong association described at the turn of the century (Goebel 1905). Nevertheless the link has impressed Doll (1982) and a causal role for the humble snail and its worm seems biologically probable if epidemiologically unproven.

Schistosomiasis is another of the infections which the developing countries could well do without on grounds other than cancer. It ought to be a controllable disease and controlling it may well affect cancer incidence.

Conclusion The theoretical concept that the incidence of some cancers can be reduced by controlling infectious diseases is attractive and intriguing but does more to point up new areas for research than to contribute to cancer prevention in the 1980s. There is little hope that infectious causes of cancers occurring in developing countries will attract the research budgets needed for resolution of their aetiological role. It is perhaps, in some ways, a good thing that most of these agents appear to cause unwanted clinical disease in affluent countries also. We owe a great debt to a small number of

Western scientists, whose curiosity has crossed the international borders of biology, for the application of modern research techniques to the problems of the developing world. They have given us grounds for an optimism quite unforeseeable a decade ago.

Non-transmissible environmental agents The historical search for removable environmental carcinogens has produced an astonishingly short list of real culprits (Doll and Peto 1981), and a remarkable volume of speculation involving relatively simple everyday substances such as fluoride and saccharin. Less work may be required to prove a substance is carcinogenic than to prove it is harmless and the ultimate social decisions as to usage may be made by courts, parliaments and newspapers rather than laboratories. Most of the identified carcinogens are products of the industrial society, as is most of the debate. The hunt for carcinogens in food is hindered by the complexity of diet, and of the metabolic breakdown products of diet, which is such that laboratory research is severely hampered by uncertainty as to which substances to study. Epidemiologists have provided some useful general clues which may apply to developing and developed countries, but cannot be expected to do more than establish generalities in the absence of facilities and opportunities to do controlled trials.

The application of laboratory knowledge on carcinogens is difficult because laboratory carcinogens (nitrosamines for example) have not been proved to have precise cause and effect relationships with cancer in humans, despite their presence in frequently taken forms of food in populations with relevant cancer risk.

The reverse is also true. Epidemiological field studies in Africa, Iran, and China have identified populations showing precancerous changes in the oesophagus associated with a high incidence of oesophageal cancer (Linsell and Peters 1982). However, careful and logical laboratory studies have not yet clearly identified the carcinogen or specific nutritional deficiencies involved.

So what should we be trying to remove from the environment? Candidates would seem to include nitrosamines, aflatoxin, salted fish, excess calories and fat, over-refined cereals. Attempts to reduce all these dietary components will do no harm, but in the case of the first three, reduction still needs to be justified by field trials which demonstrate their causal role in human cancer.

Additions to the diet

Although generalized undernutrition clearly leads to lower death rates from heart disease, there is little evidence that cancer in developing countries is greatly decreased or increased by nutritional deficiency. However, the important work relating intake of yellow-green vegetables to both cancer incidence and survival (Hirayama 1979) offers a very important opportunity for relevant research and early application of knowledge.

The situation has been thoughtfully reviewed by Peto *et al.* (1981). A dietary increase in ß-carotene or retinol produces a geneal increase in blood retinol levels, but we will discover whether this reduces cancer incidence only by doing suitable controlled trials. They point out that such trials offer one of the few hopes of reducing cancer incidence available to us at present, other than that presented by reducing tobacco use.

Since there is an obvious theoretical possibility of preventing cancer by increasing blood retinol in developed and developing countries, this area of research is one of our highest priorities. The clinical trial currently under way in American doctors may answer the relevant questions in a few years' time (Vain 1983).

Clinical trials At first sight it may seem unrealistic to suggest that preventive interventions can be tested by clinical trial procedures in developing countries, especially in view of Western failures in this field over recent decades, of which two notable examples will suffice: the failure thus far to confirm and extend the studies of Shapiro and Strax (1971) on the efficacy of population screening for early detection of breast cancer, and the failure to submit the cervical screening programme to controlled trials in its early stages of development. Both of these omissions have led to years of unnecessary speculation, argument, and public health uncertainty.

With this experience, can we expect to do better in developing countries? The answer may be a cautious affirmative for two reasons. First, there are many well-identified test populations with serious and unresolved cancer problems in developing countries. Secondly, there are many developing countries in which public-health decisions may be made rationally and backed by the power of a paternalistic government.

Epidemiological data on cancer in developing countries

Although there are gross limitations to the conveniently available data on cancer in developing countries it is quite possible to form a realistic picture of the evolving cancer pattern. Such a picture is adequate for discussion and the development of preventive strategies. When the time comes to apply such strategies it will be highly desirable and in some cases essential to establish data sources that monitor change and demonstrate the effects. Monitoring will be of crucial importance in demonstrating the effects of expensive interventions, e.g. hepatitis B vaccine, chemopreventive techniques but, it will be less important where intervention is cost-free and of obvious efficacy, e.g. banning cigarette advertising in India or Papua New Guinea.

Measurements available include cancer incidence (Waterhouse *et al.* 1982; Hirayama *et al.* 1980); mortality analysis (Segi *et al.* 1981; WHO 1982); population estimates (UN 1979); and estimates of relative frequency from hospital-based cancer registries or surveys of hospital admissions. There are serious omissions and biases in many of the data sources, some of which are obvious and some not. International borders do not always reflect racial distribution or lifestyle characteristics, although these are reasonably well known and allow some extrapolation of cancer patterns from good sources into poorly measured areas in which only spot checks may be available, e.g. from Singapore to surrounding Chinese and Malay populations.

From the above information it is possible to work out which cancers represent major problems in developing countries. A valuable attempt to quantify this cancer burden has been made by Parkin (1983). Clearly, some fairly broad assumptions are necessary for these estimations. They include:

(1) that incidence and mortality are identical for various highly fatal tumours, e.g. oesophagus, stomach, liver, lung;
(2) that a known incidence–mortality ratio in a population-based registry allows deduction of incidence for similar areas which collect only mortality;
(3) when only relative frequency is available, that incidence can be derived from a crude 'all sites' rate which is guessed from rates available in population-based registries in demographically similar areas.

Table 1 is abstracted from Parkin *et al.* (1984). It compares the population age distribution of some developed and developing countries.
Thus there are roughly 47 000 000 Chinese, 33 500 000 East Africans, 24 000 000 Americans, 21 000 000 Western Europeans, and one and a half

Table 1. Population structure in the Third World

Area	Population (millions)	Age distribution	
		% under 15	% over 16
East Africa	115	45	2.9
West Africa	121	46	2.5
China	895	37	5.2
North America	236	25	10.3
Western Europe	152	23	13.6
Australasia	17	28	8.7

Table 2. Importance of selected cancer rates in selected areas of the world

Rank	West Africa		North America		China		South East Asia	
	Male	Female	Male	Female	Male	Female	Male	Female
1	Liver	Cervix	Lung	Breast	Stomach	Cervix	Mouth/ Pharynx	Cervix
2	Lymphatic	Breast	Prostate	Colorectal	Oesophagus	Stomach	Lung	Breast
3	Prostate	Lymphatic	Colorectal	Lung	Liver	Oesophagus	Oesophagus	Mouth/ Pharynx
4	Stomach	Liver	Bladder	Lymphatic	Lung	Breast	Stomach	Oesophagus
5	Mouth/ Pharynx	Stomach	Lymphatic	Cervix	Colorectal	Colorectal	Lymphatic	Stomach

million Australasians available to develop cancer in the high-risk age group over 65 years.

Trends in cancer incidence in developing countries will be quite sharply influenced by the controls of infection and undernutrition which will result in the progressive ageing of the world's larger populations, in which current lifestyles may have already established substantial cancer risks which are not apparent because of premature mortality due to causes other than cancer. This situation should be a strong stimulus to governments of developing countries to introduce preventive strategies to avoid unnecessary development of expensive therapeutic facilities to treat avoidable cancers.

Table 2 shows the rank order by sex of selected cancer sites in selected areas of the world (Parkin *et al.* 1983). Table 3 is from the same source and provides an estimate of rank order of the commonest high-volume cancers worldwide.

Table 3. Rank order by sex of major causes worldwide

Rank	Male	Female	Total
1	Bronchus	Breast	Stomach
2	Stomach	Cervix	Bronchus
3	Colorectal	Stomach	Breast
4	Mouth and pharynx	Colorectal	Colorectal
5	Prostate	Bronchus	Cervix
6	Oesophagus	Mouth and pharynx	Mouth and pharynx
7	Liver	Oesophagus	Oesophagus
8	Bladder	Lymphatic	Liver
9	Lymphatic	Liver	Lymphatic
10	Leukaemia	Leukaemia	Prostate
11	–	Bladder	Leukaemia
12	–	–	Bladder

As developing countries become more affluent we can expect to see transferred to them some of the costs and benefits, in terms of cancer risk, of Western lifestyles. These should include natural decreases in cancers of stomach and cervix and possibly of mouth and pharynx. They may include increases in cancers of lung, breast, and colon/rectum. It is less clear what will happen to cancer of the oesophagus. Cancer of the liver is likely to decrease eventually, as hepatitis B vaccination takes effect. Other changes are, at this time, speculative as the research which will allow us to prophesy change is yet to be completed. It is necessary to re-emphasize that cancers of the lung, mouth, and pharynx are largely avoidable.

The practicalities of cancer prevention

Cancer of the cervix

Cancer of the cervix is responsible for one-tenth of Chinese female cancer mortality (China Map Press 1982); its incidence is in excess of 80 per 100 000 women per annum in Bulawayo, Colombia, and Bombay (Hirayama *et al.* 1980); it is the commonest female cancer presenting to the Dr. Sutomo Hospital in Surabaya (Sukardja 1982); and it is also common in the Phillippines (Elicano 1982), and South America (Correa and Zavala 1982). This cancer is progressively coming under control in Western populations. It is largely avoidable by use of the Papanicolau smear and may one day be the target for a vaccination programme. Continuing research into its cause is a very high priority. Secondary prevention programmes can be organized in developing countries but have not been attempted in most. A high-risk group can be defined epidemiologically and ought to be susceptible to selective screening in those developing countries with primary care facilities in villages and at birth.

What should developing countries do? An optimal international strategy can be readily devised; it would include:

(1) research into identification of the transmissible cause: this may require the development of gene-free vaccines aimed at the prime candidates, then controlled intervention experiments;
(2) identification of high-risk populations: this is not theoretically difficult. The parameters have been set by the epidemiologists. The practical problems are not great;
(3) delivery of secondary prevention programmes: easy enough in theory and demonstrably possible in Colombia (Correa and Zavala 1982). Patients need to be educated, examined, smears processed, early and late lesions treated. Substantial resources are needed.

What is actually likely to happen? The research will almost certainly be done in the West. Intervention trials will probably be done in both East and West. The experiment that determines whether HSV2 causes cervical cancer may be a byproduct of vaccine programmes established simply to eradicate herpes genitalis as a social disease in the West.

Whether secondary prevention programmes are applied in developing countries is more a question of emotions, politics, and health resources than of science. Colombia is an example if not necessarily a model. China could probably implement a widespread screening programme within a decade, if so minded. Many other developing countries could not. There is no more reason to expect developing countries to base public health decisions on cost-benefit estimates than there is in the West, and decisions to develop interventionist and costly public health programmes may well accompany increasing sophistication and education of populations. As countries become more sophisticated they may improve sanitation, hygiene, birth control, and increase the general use of soap and water. Cervical cancer may decrease naturally as this occurs, although increased sexual freedom may slow such a decrease.

Hepatocellular carcinoma of the liver

Liver cancer occurs in about one quarter of a million people each year. It occurs at an earlier age than most other cancers. Forty per cent of the total occurs in China, where it is the third commonest tumour in men. It is the most frequent tumour seen in many parts of Africa. In the developing countries the incidence is related to hepatitis B antigenaemia and to aflatoxin ingestion. Alcohol probably makes a relatively minor contribution in the Third World.

It is very likely that hepatitis B vaccination will reduce the incidence of hepatocellular cancer in due course. However, this process may take a very long time unless a carefully organized perinatal vaccination program can be applied to prevent development of the HBsAg carrier state. Such a programme is inconceivable in countries lacking adequate primary care and obstetric services. There is a possibility that this cancer can be attacked in the country which suffers most from it, China. The prevention of hepatitis B infection and the prevention of cirrhosis associated with chronic hepatitis or the hepatitis B virus carrier state are in themselves high-priority health objectives. The difficult organizational task is the delivery of suitable vaccination immediately after birth. It seems that we are on the brink of knowing what to do about liver cancer, but that we are not very likely to be able to do it because of problems of social organization rather than medical knowledge.

Much the same may be said about aflatoxin and the possibility of removing it from the diet. Again the problem requires organization, better grain-storage facilities, and educated agricultural planning. These are not easy to achieve even in highly developed countries with temperate climates. It seems unlikely that the aflatoxin problem will attract sufficient priority unless or until its place as a hepatic carcinogen is absolutely established. Research, including some controlled intervention experiments, appears to be a first essential.

Epstein–Barr virus-associated cancers

Nasopharyngeal carcinoma We already have some clear research results. The population at risk is known: southern Chinese. High-risk groups can be identified by HLA typing. Epstein–Barr virus is implicated and may be a key causal factor. Salted fish may also contribute. Early detection is difficult but may be assisted by serological surveys (Zeng *et al.* 1982).

Research priorities have been spelt out in detail (Simons and Shamangarutnam 1982) and the prime requirement is clear – a vaccine free of genetic material for use against Epstein–Barr virus. Such a vaccine would certainly be tested against glandular fever in the West and probably against Burkitt's lymphoma in African children. These intervention studies are feasible as suitable populations are available and they can be done within a reasonable time. Whether such an intervention trial against nasopharyngeal cancer would claim a priority in China is uncertain as it would take several decades to do. It might, however, be done in Singapore where population monitoring is highly developed and will continue to improve, and where interest in cancer control and international co-operation is considerable.

Other environmental determinants, particularly salted fish, require further epidemiological study, as does HLA-associated risk. Experiments in early detection using serological screening offer the most immediate hope of practical results. It is nevertheless unlikely that non-experimental public health programmes aimed at reducing nasopharyngeal carcinoma cancer will be introduced within the next decade.

Burkitt's lymphoma The situation here is more encouraging, for the reasons stated above: the high-risk population is known, and the efficacy of vaccination against Epstein–Barr virus would be evident in six to eight years. Infection takes place after birth so the organizational problems noted in the discussion of hepatitis B virus vaccination are less severe. The effect of malaria eradication experiments may also be clear in 5–10 years.

Despite these optimistic elements, a vaccine still has to be developed, and the intervention trials have to be funded and structured. There is a real possibility that these things actually will be done, as Burkitt's lymphoma has attracted world attention and offers our best and most immediate opportunity of discovering whether vaccination against a virus will actually abort a human cancer.

Bladder cancer

This cancer is one of the world's most common tumours and appears to have several causes. The contribution made by smoking is important but not quantifiable for the Third World. Schistosomiasis is a probable contributory factor. Reduction of infection by orthodox hygiene improvement has proved possible but difficult (Ibrahim 1982). It is likely that schistosomiasis will remain a problem for some decades unless molluscicides improve or the human immune response to parasitic infection can be better manipulated. Short-term optimism seems unjustified but there is every reason to encourage immunological research.

Other cancers

Mention should be made of some less common cancers which may differentially affect the Third World. These include cancer of the penis, which is common in East Africa (Hutt 1982), and in Bali and may be related to poor hygiene and lack of circumcision. Improved hygiene can be recommended but increased rates of circumcision may not be desirable as the practice invites operative infection and septicaemia which may be a more frequent cause of death than cancer of the penis.

Cancer of the biliary tract and gall-bladder is reported to be surprisingly common in some parts of South America, such as Bolivia–New Mexico (Hirayama 1982). Lymphoma is reported to be unusually common in Saudi Arabia (Shoboski 1982), as is skin cancer related to skin ulceration in Papua New Guinea (Henderson 1982); and breast, lung, and stomach cancer in Polynesians (Henderson 1982). All of this information is somewhat preliminary and requires confirmation. Existing data have been well summarized by Hirayama (1980); there is nothing yet to suggest that any large pockets of substantially different cancer patterns exist. However, as cancer registration spreads it is likely that many subpopulations will be found to carry a disproportionally high risk of certain cancers which may be related to changeable factors already known from Western experience, e.g. breast cancer in Polynesians may be related to obesity. It is important that the general programme of documentation of cancer patterns which owes so much to the International Agency for Research on Cancer continues to attract funds and expand.

Of the eight most common cancers listed in Table 3, all but colorectal cancer and breast cancer show a disproportionate incidence in the Third World. Application of existing knowledge could reduce those of bronchus, mouth, pharynx, cervix, and probably liver. Nothing can be done to influence stomach cancer on the basis of present knowledge except to persist with the development of better food preservation which is speculatively responsible for the decline of this cancer in the West.

Tobacco-associated cancers

Tobacco is by far the most widely used of the world's known carcinogens. It is avoided by many people for health reasons and by some for religious or moral reasons. World production of tobacco amounts to 1.47 million tons (*Tobacco Reporter* 1983), but no estimate has been made for the proportion of the world population that uses tobacco.

Nowhere is our international dilemma in cancer prevention more obvious than in this field. Continuing tobacco usage appears to be mediated by a combination of habit and drug dependence. All forms of tobacco use seem to have the capacity for inducing dependence on nicotine and its allied alkaloids. Consequently a large proportion of users experience great difficulty in giving up their habit. This is the central reason why primary cancer prevention is best achieved by exerting social pressures which will prevent the initiation of tobacco use.

In attempting to reduce tobacco consumption we are trying to combat two quite different influences. First, the established cultural norms which predate our knowledge of tobacco-induced disease, and secondly, the cultural and political pressures deliberately applied by the international tobacco industry. In some developing countries the tobacco industry is owned by the government, which also has a duty to protect the public health.

Doctors and all those who work in public health are invariably and inevitably in direct conflict with promotion of tobacco usage of any sort. In developing countries it is possible that inertia and ignorance are partly responsible for the lack of application of policies aimed at reduction of use. Sadly, and too often, governmental failure is more related to the corruption of policy by the international tobacco industry, which steadfastly rejects the evidence relating smoking to disease. The fact that many British Members of Parliament declare tobacco-related financial interests (Daube 1981) is a demonstration of the problems associated with controlling the world's largest cause of avoidable cancer, even in developed countries. Britain is not the only country to have politicians who reflect the economic interests of the tobacco industry, but it does have a parliamentary system which encourages the disclosure of such interests.

In the Western world clear and agreed policies exist which, if applied, can be expected to reduce smoking rates by, perhaps, several per cent per year (Gray and Daube 1980). That these policies are applied in only a few countries represents a political problem which can be expected to lessen as the health lobby gains in experience. Where active and comprehensive programmes are pursued (Bjartveit 1983) we can be optimistic. For example, smoking rates in men have fallen, over 10 years, by 10 per cent in Britain, 11 per cent in Norway, and 8 per cent in Sweden. Smoking is increasingly a habit of less well-educated poorer people.

One serious effect of the success of Western anti-smoking programmes is the focusing of the tobacco industry's attention on the untapped markets of developing countries. The problem for developing countries is more complex and possibly more serious for three reasons:

(1) existing tobacco usage patterns are well established and, as yet, little opposed by public knowledge or government action;

(2) as the populations age as a result of the control of infection and malnutrition, the effects of long-standing use of tobacco may emerge as a substantial increase in cancer rates;
(3) the tobacco industry is deliberately attempting to expand the international market for manufactured cigarettes. It is uncertain whether these efforts will effect a transfer from indigenous smoking and chewing, or whether the cigarette-associated problem of lung cancer will create an addition to the total cancer burden. Certainly a combination of habits is likely to be more dangerous.

What will be the effect of 10 or 20 years of cigarette smoking on an individual who has chewed tobacco/betel/lime for 20 or 30 years? What daily dose of smoke will reach the lungs of a chewer/smoker previously used to less easily inhaled 'bidi' smoke? We can only speculate on these questions. A gentle transfer within, say, the Indian market towards low-tar cigarettes, as a*substitute* for bidi and/or chewing, might conceivably be an overall benefit. However, such a change is only likely in a market well controlled by taxes, the complete eradication of promotion, and employing health warnings and public education programmes. The greater probability is that the easily smoked and inhaled Western cigarette will find an additional place in parts of the marketplace previously occupied by non-smokers or occasional smokers/chewers, and that government policy-makers will be as slow to respond to the problem as their counterparts in the West.

Indigenous smoking and chewing habits There are some hundreds of variations in tobacco use in various developing countries. They include:

(1) *Chewing*: Combinations of tobacco, lime, betel, and various herbs. Chewed, held in the mouth (sometimes overnight). Frequently mixed to personal taste and rarely mass marketed. Chewing is common throughout Asia, Africa, and Melanesia, but apparently much less common in China
(2) *Smoking*: Both manufactured and home-grown products. Varies from the water-filtered hookah to the high-tar densely rolled cigar with many local variations: Examples are
   (a) bidi: a thin cigarette made of locally grown tobacco rolled in a dried tembumi leaf;
   (b) chillum: a clay pipe with a wet cloth which acts as a filter;
   (c) hookah: a smoking device in which tobacco seasoned with molasses and sometimes with narcotics is placed in a bowl topped with burning charcoal; water is used as a filter;
   (d) biri: hand-rolled thin folds of coarse tobacco; used in Bangladesh;

(e) brus: a long cigarette made of partially cured tobacco treated with molasses; used in Papua New Guinea;
(f) cigarettes: hand-rolled or manufactured; mixed with cloves in Indonesia.

It is extremely difficult to estimate the comparative dose of carcinogens delivered by these products. In Papua New Guinea (Anderson 1974) inhalation is reported by 18 per cent of male brus smokers but 56 per cent of manufactured cigarette smokers. The tar and nicotine content of brus is much higher than in the manufactured cigarette (Brott 1981) but the daily dose is only two or three against 10–20 cigarettes.

Clearly the best thing we can do for developing countries is to persuade them to adopt policies aimed at reducing the number of smokers and increasing the ex-smokers. Allowing the tobacco industry to continue to promote smoking on the grounds that the newer products are lower in tar and nicotine and are 'safer' is a very risky policy. The U.S. Surgeon General's (1981) comprehensive review of death rates among users of low-tar and low-nicotine cigarettes presents the view that these products are associated with death rates not much lower than those occurring among continuing smokers of 'high-tar' cigarettes. However, as Table 4 shows, a modern low-tar cigarette is very low in comparison with earlier brands and it should be noted that:

Table 4. Changes in yields of cigarettes in U.S. (Gori and Lynd, 1978)

	Tar (mg)	Nicotine (mg)	Carbon monoxide (mg)
'Typical cigarette' pre-1960	43	3	23
'Benson & Hedges Lights' 1978	10.1	0.81	12.1
'Carlton' 1978	1.5	0.155	2.6

(1) Wald and Doll (1981) consider that some of the decrease in British lung cancer deaths is due to the general fall in tar content occurring in the 1960s and 1970s;
(2) tar content has been little measured in developing countries but is often higher than in the West, in some cases dramatically so. Table 5 shows the range of tar delivered by cigarettes in some countries in which measurements have been made.

There is a strong case for reducing the tar and nicotine content of cigarettes sold in developing countries. This can be done quite easily. A reasonable upper limit for the 1980s is between 15 and 20 mg of tar per cigarette. The

Table 5. Tar content of cigarettes in selected countries

	Range or upper limit (mg)
Australia	1–18
Brazil	2–24
Canada	22
Egypt	20
Finland	18
Japan	6–25
Oman	20
Philippines	28–50
Saudi Arabia	14
U.S.	1–30
Singapore	19–33

sale of manufactured cigarettes yielding 40 or 50 mg is inexcusable. Eradication of such products is one of the highest priorities for the Third World.

Lower yields of tar and nicotine can be readily achieved by simple legislation, as in Egypt (Omar *et al.* 1982) which restricts levels of imported and locally produced cigarettes to 20 mg of tar or less. Many countries import unnecessarily high-tar cigarettes. Singapore (1980) is a good example.

Table 6. Tar content of cigarettes – 1980

Brand	Australia	U.S.	Singapore	Country of origin
Benson & Hedges	14	15	31	Singapore
Camel	18	16	27	U.S.
Kent	13	12	19	U.S.
Lucky Strike	15	24	23	U.S.
Marlboro	14	16	21	U.S.
Peter Stuyvesant	16	–*	33	Singapore
Winston	16	16	23	U.S.

* Peter Stuyvesant not sold in the U.S.

Only when tar is measured more widely will we know what is actually being made in, or dumped upon, developing countries. Simple analysis of tar yields in developing countries is a high priority, as is legislation to reduce it.

Policies for reduction of tobacco use Appropriate policies for Western countries, as agreed upon by the World Health Organization, the International Union Against Cancer, the International Union Against Tuberculosis, and the International Society and Federation of Cardiologists, can be simply summarized:

1. Change the smoker's habits – by education programmes aimed at persuading adults to stop and children not to start; by smoking cessation clinics as needed; and by informing the public as a whole (see page 50)
2. Change the cigarette – by legislation controlling yields of tar, nicotine, and other appropriate constituents.
3. Change the cultural background – by banning promotion of tobacco and sales to minors, by restrictions on smoking in public places, by increasing taxes regularly, by correct packet labelling.

Developing countries can also use these policies to attack the expanding market of the manufactured cigarette. Developing countries also need to resist the inducements offered by the tobacco industry to create local growing and manufacturing industries. There is no virtue in substituting a cash crop of tobacco for a food crop. Nor is there virtue in destroying natural forests to provide fuel for tobacco curing.

Policies to discourage chewing and the smoking of home-made or locally grown indigenous products are much more difficult to develop. Only experience and experiment will provide these. Some important policy areas are nevertheless clear.

1. *Research*. Recognition and definition of the smoking/chewing problem as a problem is a prerequisite for any government approach. The medical establishment is as important a resource here as it was in the U.S. and Britain in the 1960s. It is emphatically not necessary to repeat research inculpating tobacco as a carcinogen, only to define usage patterns, enumerate deaths is likely to be attributed to tobacco, and estimate the extent of disease needing costly treatment.

2. *Taxation*. Experience in the West shows taxation to be effective in reducing consumption. Can tobacco be effectively taxed? – At the point of sale, or at grower level? Will taxation on chewing and local products promote a transfer to manufactured cigarettes? A comprehensive taxation policy ought to address these issues and, in any individual country, to bring about general price increases and usage decreases.

3. *Legislation*. Banning tobacco *promotion* is a first step. Controlling yields of the manufactured and imported products that are sold is a second. Controlling production for personal use is likely to be ineffective and unpopular.

4. *Public information.* Developing countries very often do have adequate, frequently government-controlled, radio and sometimes television facilities. The history of cigarette sales in the West suggests that many people will abandon tobacco habits once informed authoritatively that they are harmful. All the available information channels should be used, including those offered by religious groups.

5. *School and primary care programmes.* Where schools exist they are a potent weapon for informing the younger generation and, indirectly, its parents. Community action programmes can be based on schools and primary care services.

It is not possible to predict what will happen to smoking and chewing habits in developing countries over the next two decades. Many of the governments involved have great centralized power and a paternalistic tradition, while others have the opposite. If the broad spectrum of the problem is recognized and addressed by comprehensive action there is no reason why tobacco use should not decline as it is declining in the West. For the reasons given earlier, those countries which ignore the problem may face a much greater escalation of disease than anyone expects, as increased ageing and newly adopted habits compound the risks already established by decades of indigenous smoking and chewing (see page 289).

Conclusion

The most striking feature of this review is the broad spectrum of prevention strategies which are theoretically possible in the Third World, in contrast to the West. While most of the world has a tobacco problem, the developing countries face the additional, and enormous, burden of infection-related cancers which may conceivably become controllable in the next decade.

Research has brought us to the point where we can see possible ways of preventing cancers of the liver, nasopharynx (in Chinese), oropharynx (in chewers and smokers), lung, cervix and Burkitt's lymphoma. We are now in a position to define the three greatest needs of the Third World: to do some further quite specific research; to do some intervention experiments; and to apply the knowledge we already have. The specific research includes:

(1) the development of a cheap and practical vaccination programme against hepatitis B;

(2) the development of a vaccine against Epstein–Barr virus that is free of viral nucleic acid and is also cheap and deliverable;

(3) the identification of the viral culprit responsible for cervical cancer; then the development of a vaccine against this agent;

(4) further case-control studies to establish the place of aflatoxin and other dietetic sources of nitrosamines (salted fish) in cancer of the liver and nasopharynx.

Intervention experiments depend upon research findings but we obviously need to know:

(1) whether chemoprevention works;
(2) whether vaccination against Epstein–Barr virus reduces the incidence of Burkitt's lymphoma. If it does then it would be reasonable to infer that it could work against nasopharyngeal cancer in the Chinese and to examine ways of establishing such vaccination as a realistic long-term programme;
(3) whether vaccination against HSV2 reduces the incidence of cervical cancer;
(4) whether removal of dietetic nitrosamines reduces the incidence of cancer of the liver in patients already suffering from hepatitis B virus antigenaemia because controlling the diet might work more quickly than controlling hepatitis B virus.

The application of existing knowledge could quite rapidly reduce the vast numbers of cancers attributable to tobacco. This means application of policies already known and tested in parts of the Western World. These need to be adapted and evolved for use in the Third World. Legislative abolition of tobacco promotion, reduction of tar content, and implementation of taxation strategies offer the most immediate benefits. The practitioners of medicine must play their part in opposing the expansionist aims of the tobacco industry and those countries with surpluses to sell.

If we believe that cancer research will provide the weapons for controlling the major cancers of the Third World, then we must ask the next crucial question. Will these weapons be used? Matters of politics and social organization provide reasons for both pessimism and optimism.

The reasons for pessimism are all too obvious in many developing countries. While overcrowding, infection, and subnutrition are rampant, cancer prevention will be low priority unless it is easy, and either inexpensive or profitable. Although tobacco use can be reduced to the profit of government, sensible decisions may be resisted (as they have been in the West) for reasons of simple corruption. The chances that present or future knowledge will be universally applied are trivial, and we must face the fact that eradicating both tobacco and infection-related cancer will be much more difficult than eradicating smallpox.

On the other hand, there are also powerful reasons for optimism. China has somehow managed substantially to control overpopulation and subnutrition over a few decades. Whether this is due to Confucius or communism is less relevant than the fact that public health has triumphed twice and may do so again. Paternalistic government may well decide to discourage tobacco use and provide resources for vaccination against hepatitis B. Nor should we forget that Sikhs do not smoke, that Moslems do not drink alcohol, and that cleanliness and clear sexual mores are characteristic of many Third World populations. Religion may provide a means for communication and behaviour change in populations which are poorly organized and illiterate. Authoritarian or dictatorial governments may sometimes make undemocractic but sensible decisions. Finally, creative man may succeed even in the most turbulent times: we must remember that it was possible to monitor the Epstein–Barr virus exposure of 42 000 Ugandan children despite the incumbency of Idi Amin.

Western cancer research is providing the knowledge needed to prevent cancer in the Third World. This research has been funded with great intellectual and financial generosity. The West has controlled its infectious disease and can be expected to apply future research knowledge with alacrity. It has not controlled its tobacco problem with the same speed. There remains a good chance that many developing countries will contain tobacco-associated cancer more rapidly than we expect. However, control of infection-related cancer will require resources of people and money well beyond the capacity of the Third World. We can only hope that the generosity shown in research will also be shown when the time comes to implement research results.

References

Alter, H.J. (1982). The evolution, implications and applications of the hepatitis B vaccine. *J. Amer. med. Ass.* **247**, 2272–5.

Anderson, H.R. (1974). Smoking habits and their relationship to chronic lung disease in a tropical environment in Papua New Guinea. *Bull. Phys. Path. Resp.* **10**, 619–33.

Bannock, G., Bangore, R.E., and Rees, R. (1972). *The Penguin dictionary of economics*. Penguin Books, England.

Barin, F., Goudeau, A., Denis, F., *et al.* (1982). Immune response in neonates to hepatitis B vaccine. *Lancet* **i**, 251–3.

Beasley, R.P., Hwang, L.W., Lin, C.C., *et al.* (1981). Hepatocellular carcinoma and hepatitis B virus. *Lancet* **ii**, 1129–32.

Beasley, R.P. and Stevens, C.E. (1978). Vertical transmission of HBV and interruption with globulin. In *Proceedings of the 2nd Symposium on Viral Hepatitis* (ed. G.Y. Vias, S.N. Cullin, and R. Schmidt), pp. 333–45. Franklin Institute Press, Philadelphia, Pennsylvania.

Bing, L., Junyao, L., and Hswien-wen, H. (1982). National survey of cancer mortality in China. In *Cancer prevention in developing countries* (ed. K. Aoki, S. Tominago, T. Hirayama, and Y. Hirota), pp. 21–32. The University of Nagoya Press, Nagoya.

Bjartveit, K. (1983). In *Proceedings of the Fifth World Conference on Smoking & Health*. (In press.)

Brott, K. (1981). Tobacco smoking in Papua New Guinea. *Wld Smoking Hlth* **6**, 33–7.

Buckley, J.D., Doll, R., Harris, R.W.C., and Vessey, M.P. (1981). Case control study of the husbands of women with dysplasia or carcinoma of the cervix uteri. *Lancet* **ii**, 1010–15.

Burkitt, D.P. (1983). The discovery of Burkitt's lymphoma. *Cancer* **51**, 1777–86.

Cheever, A.W. (1978). Schistosomiasis and neoplasia. *J. nat. Cancer Inst.* **61**, 13–18.

China Map Press (1981). *Atlas of cancer mortality in the People's Republic of China*. Beijing.

Cooper, D.A. (1983). Epidemic Kaposi's sarcoma and opportunistic infections. *Med. J. Aust.* **1**, 564–6.

Correa P. and Zavala (1982). Patterns of cancer frequency in Latin America. In *Cancer prevention in developing countries* (ed. K. Aoki, S. Tominaga, T. Hirayama, and Y. Hirota), pp. 227–236. The University of Nagoya Press, Nagoya.

Daube, M. (1981). In *Smoking and smoking related diseases*, pp. 36–52. Unit for Continuing Education, Department of Community Medicine, University of Manchester.

De Thé, G. (1977). Is Burkitt's lymphoma related to a perinatal infection by Epstein–Barr virus? *Lancet* **i**, 335–8.

Doll, R. (1982). Underlining concepts of cancer control in the future. In *Cancer prevention in developing countries* (ed. K. Aoki, S. Tominaga, T. Hirayama, and Y. Hirota), pp. 587–94. The University of Nagoya Press, Nagoya.

Doll, R. and Peto, R. (1976). Mortality in relation to smoking: 20 years' observations of male British doctors. *Brit. med. J.* **2**, 1525–36.

Doll, R. and Peto, R. (1978). Cigarette smoking and bronchial carcinoma: dose and time relationships among regular smokers and lifelong non-smokers. *J. Epidemiol. Comm. Hlth* **32**, 303–13.

Doll, R. and Peto, R. (1981). *The causes of cancer*. Oxford University Press.

Duff, R. and Rapp, F. (1971). Oncogenic transformation of hamster cells after exposure to herpes simplex virus type 2. *Nature New Biol.* **233**, 48–50.

Elgin, R.P., Sharp, F., MacLean, A.B., *et al.* (1982). Herpes simplex virus-type 2 coded material in cervical neoplasm. In *Pre-clinical neoplasia of the cervix*, (ed. J.A. Jordan, F. Sharp, and A. Singer). Royal College of Obstetricians and Gynaecologists, London.

Elicano, T. (1982). Chacteristic features of cancer in Philippines. In *Cancer prevention in developing countries* (ed. K. Aoki, S. Tominaga, T. Hirayama, and Y. Hirota), pp. 587–94. The University of Nagoya Press, Nagoya.

Epstein, M.A. (1976). Epstein–Barr virus – is it time to develop a vaccine program? *J. nat. Cancer Inst.* **56**, 697–700.

Epstein, M.A. (1980). In *The human herpesviruses* (ed. A.J. Nahmias, W.R. Dowdie, and R. Schinazi), pp. 432–9. Elsevier, New York.

Food and Agricultural Organization Production Yearbook, 1980 (Vol. 34). FAO, Rome.

Gallo, R.C., Sarin, P.S., Gelmann, E.P., *et al.* (1983). Isolation of human T-cell leukemia virus in acquired immune deficiency syndrome (AIDS). *Science* (N.Y.) **220**, 865–7.

Geder, L., Lausch, R., O'Neill, F., and Rapp, F. (1976). Oncogenic transformation of human embryo lung cells by human cytomegalovirus. *Science*, N.Y. **92**, 1134–7.

Goebel, S.M. and Colley, D.G. (1905). Ueber die bei Bilharziakrankheit Vorkommsoen Blasen Tumoren mit besonderer Beruechsichtigumg des Carcinoms. *Z. Krebsforsch* **3**, 309–13.

Groi, G.B. and Lynch, C.J. (1978). Towards less hazardous cigarettes. *J. Amer. Med. Assoc.* **240**, 1255–9.

Gray, N. and Daube, M. (1980). *Guidelines for smoking control* 2nd edn, International Union Against Cancer Technical Report Series, Vol. 52, Geneva.

Gupta, P.C., Mehta, F.S., and Irani, R.R. (1980). Comparison of mortality rates among bidi smokers and tobacco chewers. *Ind. J. Cancer* **17**, 149–52.

Henderson, B.E. (1983). Cancer in the South Pacific. In *Cancer prevention in developing countries* (ed. K. Aoki, S. Tominaga, T. Hirayama and Y. Hirota), pp. 83–90. The University of Nagoya Press, Nagoya.

Hirayama, T. (1979). Diet and cancer. *Cancer* **1**, 67–81.

Hirayama, T., Waterhouse, J.A.H., and Fraumeni, J.F. (1980). *Cancer risks by site.* International Union Against Cancer Technical Report Series, Vol. 41, Geneva.

Hirayama, T. (1982). Summary of the whole five days' discussions and the underlining concepts of cancer control in the future. *Cancer prevention in developing countries* (ed. K. Aoki, S. Tominaga, T. Hirayama, and Y. Hirota), pp. 581–6. The University of Nagoya Press, Nagoya.

Ho, J.H.C., Huang, D.P., and Fong, Y.Y. (1978). Salted fish and nasopharyngeal carcinoma in southern Chinese. *Lancet* **ii**, 626.

Hutt, M.S.R. (1982). Cancer in East and Central Africa: aspects of incidence and prevention. *Cancer prevention in developing countries* (ed. K. Aoki, S. Tominaga, T. Hirayama, and Y. Hirota), pp. 217–25. The University of Nagoya Press, Nagoya.

Ibrahim, A.S. (1982). Epidemiology of cancer of the urinary bladder in Egypt. pp. 217–25. *Cancer prevention in developing countries*, (ed. K. Aoki, S. Tominaga, T. Hirayama, and Y. Hirota), pp. 499–512. The University of Nagoya Press, Nagoya.

Jussawalla, D.J. (1982). In *The UICC smoking control workshop*, (ed. S. Tominaga and K. Aoki), pp. 40–7. The University of Nagoya Press, Japan.

Kahn, H.A. (1966). In *Epidemiological approaches to the study of cancer and other chronic diseases* (ed. W. Haenszel), pp. 1–125. National Cancer Institute Monograph No. 19. National Cancer Institute, U.S. Department of Health Education and Welfare, Public Health Service.

Keighley, E. (1968). Carcinoma of the cervix among prostitutes in a women's prison. *Brit. J. ven. Dis.* **44**, 254–5.

Kessler, I. (1976). Human cervical cancer as venereal disease. *Cancer Res.* **33**, 783–91.

Lesnick, F. and Ross, L.J. (1975). Immunization against Marek's disease using Marek's disease virus-specific antigens free from infectious virus. *Int. J. Cancer* **12**, 153–63.

Linsell, C.A. and Peers, F.G. (1977). Field studies on liver cell cancer. In *Origins of human cancer*, (ed. H.H. Hiatt, J.D. Watson, and J.A. Winsten), pp. 549–56. Cold Spring Harbor, New York.

Maclure, K.M. and MacMahon, B. (1980). An epidemiologic perspective of environmental carcinogenesis. *Epidemiol. Rev.* **2**, 19–48.

Merck Index (1976). 9th edn, p. 6346. Merck & Co., Railway, New Jersey.

Munoz, N. and Linsell, A. (1982). Epidemiology of cancer of the digestive tract (ed. P. Correa and W. Haenszel), pp. 161–95. Martinus Nijhoff Publishers, The Netherlands.

Nahmias, A.J., Josey, W.E., Naib, Z.M., Luce, C.F., and Guest, B. (1970). Antibodies to herpes virus hominis types 1 & 2. II Women with cervical cancer. *Amer. J. Epidemiol.* **91**, 547–54.

National Institute of Health (U.S.). (1980). Cervical cancer screening: the pap smear, summary of an NIH consensus statement. *Brit. med. J.* **281**, 1264–6.

Omar, S., El Aaser, A.B., Hussein, M., Galal, A., El Merzatani, M., and Sayed, G.M. (1982). *Prevention of the smoking epidemic in a developing country* (Egypt). WHO, Geneva.

Parkin, D.M., Stjernsward, J., and Muir, C.S. (1984). *Estimates of the worldwide frequency of twelve major cancers*. WHO, Geneva. (In Press)

Pasca, A.S., Kummerlander, L., Pejtsik, B., and Pali, K. (1975). Herpesvirus antibodies and antigens in patients with cervical anaplasia and in controls. *J. nat. Cancer Inst.* **55**, 775–81.

Pereyra, A.J. (1961). The relationship of sexual activity to cervical cancer: cancer of the cervix in a prison population. *Obstet. Gynaecol.* **17**, 154–9.

Peto, R., Doll, R., Buckley, J.D., and Sporn, M.B. (1981). Can dietary beta-carotene materially reduce human cancer rates? *Nature* **290**, 201–8.

Rapp, F. and Jenkins, F.J. (1981). Genital cancer and viruses. *Gynecol. Oncol.* **12**, S25–S41.

Reid, B.L., French, P.W., Singer, A., Hagan, B.E., and Coppleson, M. (1978). Sperm basic proteins in cervical carinogenesis correlation with socioeconomic class. *Lancet* **ii**, 60–2.

Segi, M., Tominaga, S., Aoki, K., and Fujimoto, I. (eds) (1982). *Cancer mortality and morbidity statistics: Japan and the world.* GANN Monograph on Cancer Research No. 26. Japan Scientific Societies Press, Tokyo.

Shapiro, S., Strax, P., and Venet, L. (1971). Periodic breast cancer screening in reducing mortality from breast cancer. *J. Amer. med. Ass.* **215**, 1777–85.

Shoboski, O. (1982). Cancer frequency in Saudi Arabia. In *Cancer prevention in developing countries* (ed. K. Aoki, S. Tominaga, T. Hirayama, and Y. Hirota), pp. 135–144. The University of Nagoya Press, Nagoya.

Simarak, S., DeJong, U.W., Brewslaw, N., Dahl, C.J., Ruckphaoput, K., Scheelings, P., and Maclennan, R. (1977). Cancer control of the oral cavity, pharynx/larynx and lung in North Thailand: case-control study and analysis of cigar smoke. *Brit. med. J.* **36**, 130–40.

Simons, M.J., and Shanmugaratnam, K. (eds) (1982). *The biology of naso-pharyngeal carcinoma.* International Union Against Cancer Technical Report Series Vol. 71. Geneva.

Smith, G.L., Mackett, M., and Ross, B. (1983). Infectious vaccinia virus recombinants that express Hepatitis B virus surface antigen. *Nature* **302**, 490–5.

Sukardja, I.D.G. (1982). Cancer statistics at Dr. Sutomo Hospital Surabaya – Indonesia. In *Cancer prevention in developing countries* (ed. K. Aoki, S. Tominaga, T. Hirayama and Y. Hirota), pp. 73–82. The University of Nagoya Press, Nagoya.

Szmuness, W., Stevens, C.E., Harley, E.G., *et al.* (1980). Demonstration of efficacy in a controlled clinical trial in a high-risk population in the United States. *New Engl. J. Med.* **303**, 833–41.

The Walton Report (1982). *Report of the Reconvened Task Force on Cervical Cancer Screening Programs*, Canada.

Tobacco Reporter (1983). 1983 world crop estimate indicates higher production. *Tobacco Rep*. **110**, 8.

U.S. Department of Health, Education and Welfare (1979). *Smoking and health: a Report of the Surgeon General*. U.S. Department of Health, Education and Welfare, Public Health Service, Office on Smoking and Health.

U.S. Department of Health and Human Services (1981). *The changing cigarette, report of the U.S. Surgeon General*. Department of Health, Education and Welfare, Public Health Service.

United Nations, Department of International Economic and Social Affairs (1980). *Concise Report on the World Population Situation in 1979*. Population Studies No. 72.

Wald, N., Doll, R., and Copeland, G. (1981). Trends in tar, nicotine, and carbon monoxide yields of U.K. cigarettes manufactured since 1934. *Brit. med. J*. **282**, 763–5.

Waterhouse, J., Muir, C., Correa, P., and Powell, J. (1976). *Cancer incidence in five countries*, Vol. III. IARC Scientific Publications No. 15. Lyon.

Willmott, F.E. (1975). Cytomegalovirus in female patients attending a venereal disease clinic. *Brit. J. ven. Dis*. **51**, 278–80.

World Health Organization Statistics Annual (1982). Vital statistics and causes of death 1978–82. WHO, Geneva.

Wynder, E.L. and Hoffman, D. (1976). *Tobacco and tobacco smoke: studies in experimental carcinogenesis*, p. 498. Academic Press, New York.

Zeng, Y., Zhang, J.M., Li, L.Y., *et al*. (1982). Serological mass survey for the early detection of nasopharyngeal carcinoma in Sangwu County, China. *China Int. J. Cancer* **29**, 139.

Index